Doctor From Bugtussle

Wendell W. Wilson, M.D.

To Jerry Barnes
Enjoy the book

© Copyright 1995. Wendell W. Wilson. All rights reserved.

ISBN 0-9647202-1-3 (paperback edition)
ISBN 0-9647202-2-1 (hardback edition)

Published by:
Hillbilly Books
P.O. Box 430
Old Hickory, Tennessee 37138

Cover design by Ron Watson
Produced by JM Productions, Brentwood, TN

Printed in the United States of America

Acknowledgments

During the last three years, I have found that while attempting to produce this book that many people are needed to help a would-be author complete the task. For those people who have been so helpful in every respect so that I could finally "see the light at the end of the tunnnel," a great big Thank You! I could never have realized completion of the writing nor publishing the document without your help and support.

❖ ❖ ❖

First, I want to thank my wife, Jessie, for her faithful support and encouragement, as well as for helpful suggestions and some constructive criticisms that helped me stay on track during the time I had a few difficulties in continuing with the project. She has been my anchor at those times that I could have "abandoned ship" and never realized an end to this work.

❖ ❖ ❖

To Perry Biddle, who has encouraged in many ways to write in the way that I felt it was best to tell my story. It was a healing process for both: for me, to recover from a short bout of mild depression and a feeling of uselessness following my retirement after forty years of a busy family practice; and for him, in recovering from physical disabilities following a near-fatal automobile accident. We have both thrived while working together on *Doctor From Bugtussle*. I can never thank him enough for his encouragement, support, and helpful suggestions during this time.

❖ ❖ ❖

A "thank you" to my brothers and sisters who helped me in recalling some incidents to make them more authentic when retold in this writing.

❖ ❖ ❖

To Mrs. Juanita Flatt, an ex-employee and faithful friend: Thank you for those long, long hours you spent in deciphering my jumbled typing and almost unreadable handwritten notes while re-typing the manuscript, as you made them into readable sentences and full storeies. Without your faithful, hard work we could not have "put it all together."

❖ ❖ ❖

To the Editor, Joe Johnson: Thank you for the long hours spent in helping make this a more readable story.

❖ ❖ ❖

And lastly to the publishers, who have helped me tremendously through the maze of all the necessary paperwork of applying for various documents to complete a publication. This has all been a very enlightening and learning process. One that I will never forget!

— W.W.W.

Foreword

Wendell Wilson is a master storyteller like so many other raconteurs from the hills of Tennessee. I have listened to his stories many times over the past years as he has read them to me and we have discussed them, looking forward to getting them published. I am excited about the finished versions of these stories from the life of a busy family physician.

I have known Dr. Wilson, the "Doctor From Bugtussle," since 1974 when I became his pastor and he became our family physician. Dr. Wilson became not only my doctor but my friend.

After the manuscript of *Doctor From Bugtussle* was in draft form, I read it and enjoyed the stories yet another time. Reading them was like eating salted peanuts — I couldn't stop with just a few! The stories are exciting accounts of his early life, his work on the family farm near Bugtussle, Tennessee, his college and medical school education, his stints in the U.S. Navy, and his family practice in Memphis and in Old Hickory, Tennessee.

We are coming to understand that stories are at the heart of what it means to be human beings. We live stories, and stories pull together the meaning of our lives. Dr. Wilson has not only pulled together the stories of his life for his own enjoyment, but now in this published form he shares them with his family, friends, and thousands of former patients and the public at large. These stories are like windows through which we can see into the life and times of the "Doctor From Bugtussle."

The author has given us a fascinating historical account of life in rural Tennessee when life was simpler but harder. His father, a country doctor, practiced without the miracle drugs and sophisticated medical technology which Wendell used in his practice. But his father knew his patients in their family setting and modeled the "caring family physician" for his son.

The author also shows us his special relationship with his mother, who demonstrated great patience and perseverance as she lovingly raised a large family.

There is an old southern saying that if a youngster doesn't acquire a nickname, then he or she "isn't worth their salt." According to this criterion Dr. Wilson is a very worthy person since he has had many monikers over the years. He was named Wendell for the famous Justice Oliver Wendell

Holmes. His middle name, Winfred, came from the name of one of his father's best friends. When he was about fourteen and began playing football at school, he was nicknamed "Scrub" since he was slight of stature. Later while working in a tea room during college days the boss called him "Wennel" since he couldn't pronounce "Wendell." A college friend nicknamed him "Clark Gobble" since he wore a pencil moustache like Clark Gable's. Then in medical school he was given the name "Woodrow" by a German professor who had escaped Nazi Germany and who was familiar with President Woodrow Wilson's life. Finally he became "Dr. Wilson" and was highly respected by patients and collegues alike. As you read *Doctor From Bugtussle* you can trace the stages of Dr. Wilson's life by his nicknames. However, the variety of nicknames did not seem to have an adverse effect on Dr. Wilson's self-identity!

This book is not only a "good read" but it will help young people, especially those who are planning to go into medicine, understand the trials, tribulations, and joys of family medicine. Dr. Wilson tells of the joy of delivering babies which helped offset the stress of dealing with the pain and grief of other patients.

My life is richer for having Dr. Wendell W. Wilson as a friend. I am delighted to recommend this book to you as a way of coming to know Dr. Wilson as your friend too, and sharing his triumphs, love affairs, dreams and failures, disappointments, hurts, and a lifetime of healing.

As Dr. Wilson has shared these stories with me during the past five years I have encouraged him to be as transparent as possible and to tell his story "warts and all." He has done this. I think readers will find their own lives richer for having read and enjoyed *Doctor From Bugtussle*.

— Rev. Dr. Perry H. Biddle, Jr.

Contents

Foreword
by Rev. Dr. Perry H. Biddle, Jr. v

Preface x

1. Where It All Began 1
2. Miss Dee, Our Mother 6
3. Doctor Tom, Our Dad 17
4. The Early Years 27
5. Growing Up 45
6. High School 68
7. College Years 78
8. Medical School 123
9. Internship 177
10. The Navy Medical Corps 191
11. Residency 219
12. Private Practice 230
13. Unusual Cases and Unforgettable Families 255
14. House Calls and Emergencies 281
15. The Doctor As A Patient 303
16. A Forty-Year Career 310

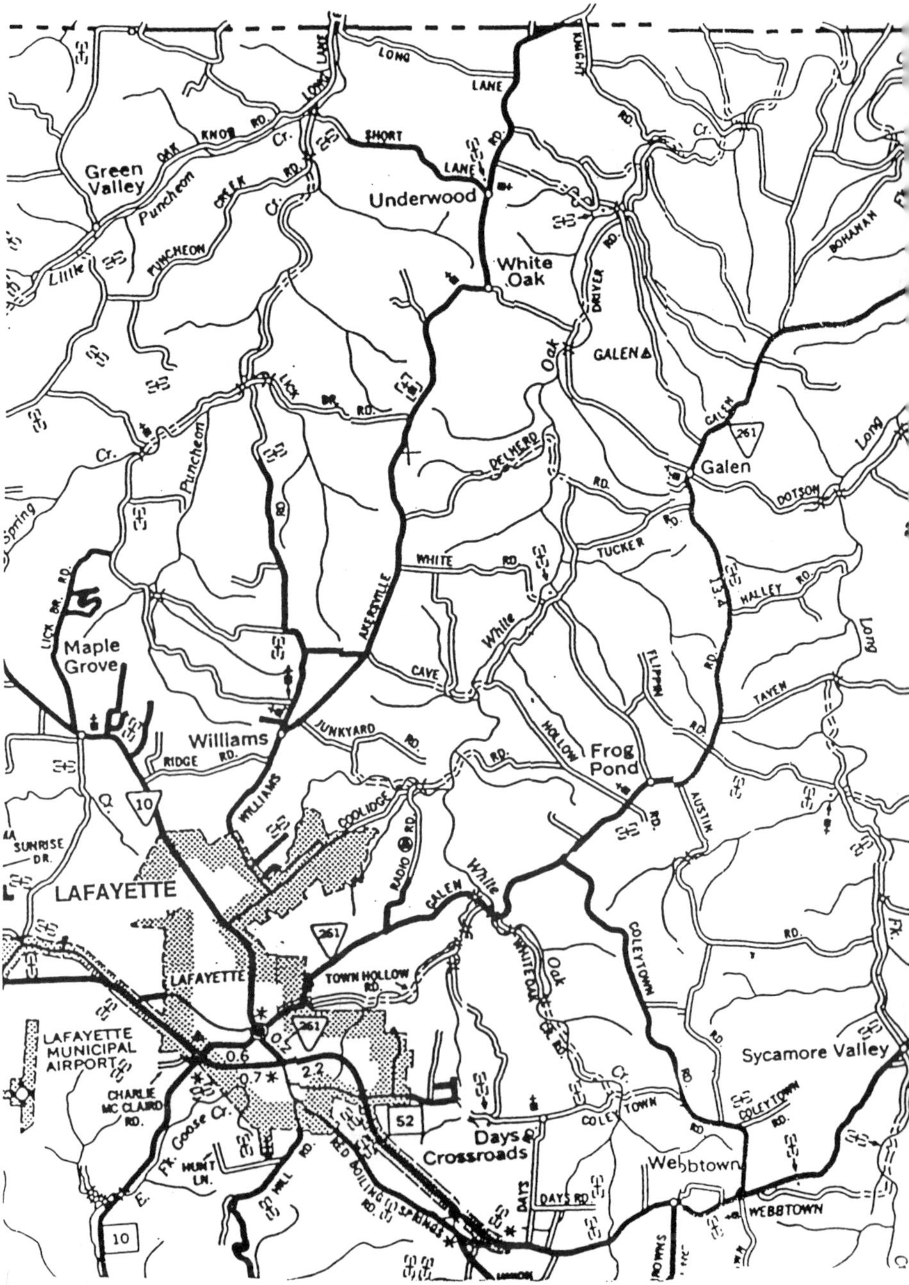
Green Valley
Underwood
White Oak
Galen
Maple Grove
Williams
Frog Pond
LAFAYETTE
LAFAYETTE MUNICIPAL AIRPORT
Sycamore Valley
Days Crossroads
Webbtown
LONG LANE
SHORT LANE
KNOB RD.
PUNCHEON
LICK BR. RD.
DELMERD
WHITE RD.
TUCKER RD.
HALLEY RD.
CAVE
JUNKYARD RD.
RIDGE RD.
AKERSVILLE
WILLIAMS
COOLIDGE
RADIO RD.
TOWN HOLLOW RD.
COLEYTOWN
DOTSON
TAYEN
AUSTIN
FLIPPIN
SUNRISE DR.
CHARLIE MC CLAIRD RD.
HUNT LN.
RED BOILING SPRINGS RD.
DAYS RD.
WEBBTOWN
BOHANAN
DRIVER RD.
KNIGHT RD.
GALEN

ix

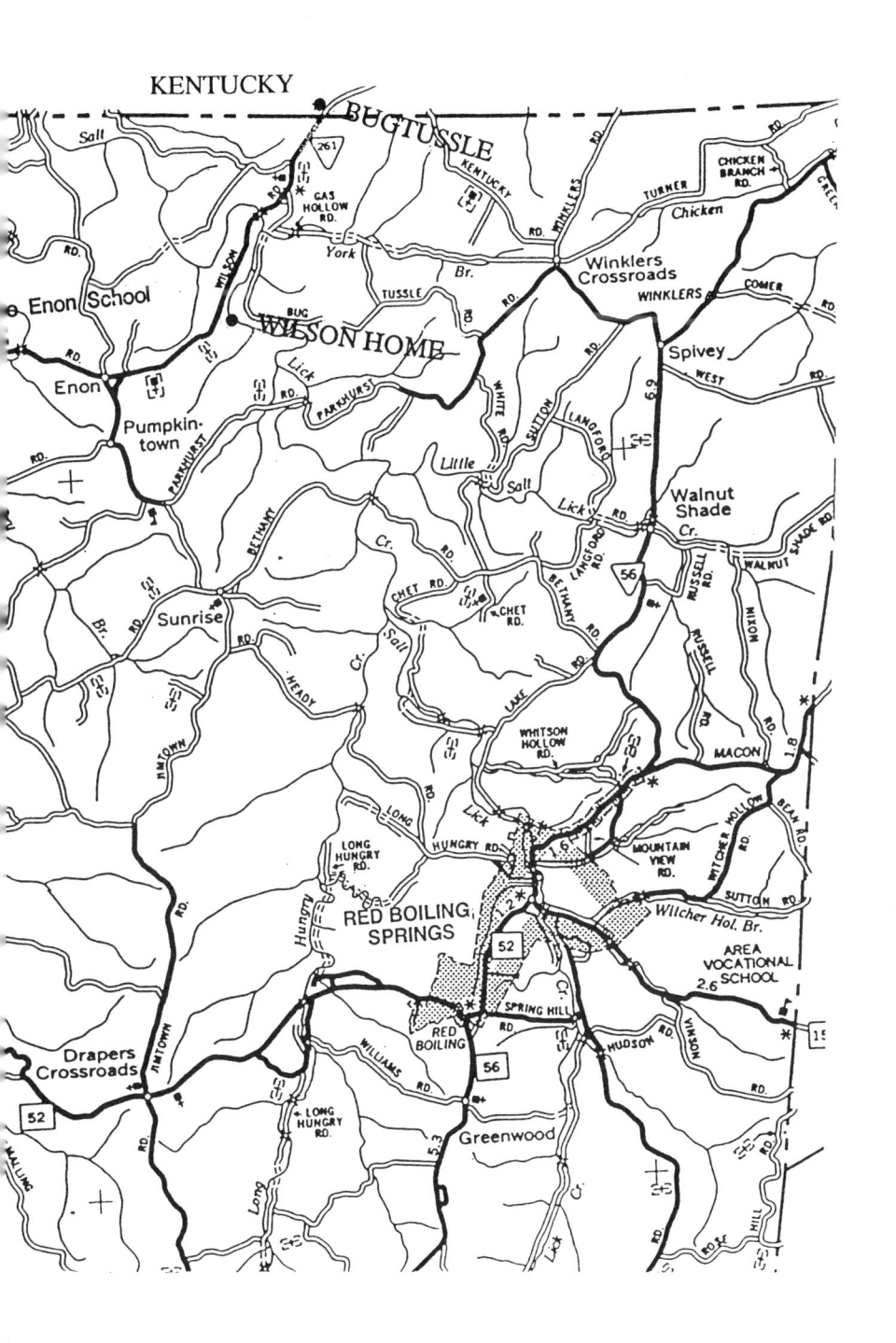

Preface

At the insistence of my daughters and some close friends to whom I had related some of my life's stories, *Doctor From Bugtussle* was conceived in 1992. The period of "gestation" was long, tedious and sometimes painful. While writing each phase of the journey through life, my memory bank would open, then I would recall other incidents which had occurred that I had failed to record. For this reason many of the earlier pages were re-written two or three times. As writing continued through the months the "memory bank" opened more readily. Soon recall became easier, and writing was more enjoyable. When this happened, time literally flew by as I re-lived incident after incident. I was so absorbed in these that the re-living was so realistic that the characters were alive with me. My emotions waxed and waned with each incident as I wrote, and found myself laughing aloud at the hilarious ones and sometimes even felt tears coming to my eyes with sad or heart-rending ones. These emotions raised my desire to continue with the many stories that have been recalled in the pages of this book.

This, my first attempt at writing, has been a wonderful, stimulating, rewarding and enjoyable experience for me. Life has taken on a new meaning as I feel that now I am again useful and doing something for my fellow man. I hope you, the reader, will enjoy reading *Doctor From Bugtussle* as much as I have enjoyed writing it.

— Wendell Wilson

Where It All Began

At 8:00 a.m. on June 22, 1951, my niece, Gloria, and I, left Memphis, Tennessee, headed for Old Hickory, Tennessee, where I was to begin a new practice. I was driving a small car and pulling a four-wheel trailer, loaded to the top with household goods. As we journeyed along, I was having thoughts about the move and not much about the speed at which we were moving. As we would travel down long grades, I soon realized that something was wrong as the small car would sway back and forth, and the braking was not too effective. I realized that I was about to wreck and came back to reality. After that the trip was uneventful. We made it through Nashville without incident and stopped in Madison at my brother's place of business. As we walked in, he greeted me with, "Glad you got here safely. Looks like you'll be busy. Dr. Johnson has called three times. He's anxious for you to call the office as soon as you arrive."

Knowing how he never seemed to be very anxious, I had called immediately, identifying myself and got a quick response.

"Dr. Wilson!! I'm sure glad you're here."

"What can I do for you, Dr. Johnson?"

"I need you to see a patient in the emergency room at Madison Hospital just as soon as you can make it."

"I'll be glad to. What's the problem?"

"She's been injured in a car wreck, but I'm not sure about the extent of her injuries. Can you get there soon"

"Yes. I'll leave in a few minutes and report as soon as we can evaluate her."

As I hung up the phone, I called out to Harold, "Will you take care of my passenger? I'm on my way to the emergency room."

"Sure, don't worry about it."

"Thanks, I'll call you later."

How I backed that loaded car and trailer out onto a busy, main thoroughfare and headed for the hospital, God only knows, I don't. On my way to the hospital, my mind racing and the adrenalin flowing, a million things crossed my mind, mostly what I was getting into with the patient

Doctor From Bugtussle

waiting in the emergency room. But I was also wondering—have I lost my mind? I was leaving a very busy, successful practice in a medical center where I had been fortunate to be associated with a brilliant, highly respected general and thoracic surgeon, whom I assisted in 90 percent of his cases, as well as performing major surgery on my own patients. The senior member of the group was an equally capable and highly respected Internist who was a father figure to me. I left all of this to enter a practice in a small town not too far from a Medical Center (Vanderbilt). In spite of what I was leaving, within my heart I knew this move was the right thing.

My reverie was interrupted as the hospital came into sight. The adrenalin started flowing more freely again at the prospect of what was awaiting in the emergency room.

As I parked the car and trailer, a nurse appeared outside the emergency room door. "Are you Dr. Wilson?," she asked.

"Yes, I am."

"Boy! Are we glad to see you, doctor!! The patient is in here."

As she led the way into the emergency room, I had a feeling the problem was a major one. My feeling was right. As we entered the room, I paused. What I saw was not unfamiliar to me, and not pleasant either. Lying on the table was a white female in her mid-thirties, unconscious, and apparently in shock. Her face, neck, chest, and upper arms were covered with blood. Her face had several superficial lacerations, and blood was still oozing from the wounds. Her nose was distorted; there was a laceration across its bridge also. Blood was oozing from it as well as from the nostrils. The lower half of her left ear was torn away from the face, and was still bleeding. Her face was swollen and discolored, and so was her chest. Oxygen was being administered by a nasal catheter. She was breathing on her own with no apparent airway obstruction. The left thigh was discolored, swollen, and distorted. It was apparent that we had a lot of work to do.

"What is her status at present, Nurse?," I asked.

In a highly professional manner she gave her report: "She is unconscious but breathing on her own. Blood pressure 90/50, pulse 118 and regular, respiration 28 and regular. Lab work has been done and there are four units of blood ready when needed. Lab report shows anemia with red-cell count of 3,250,000 and hemoglobin of 9. Blood sugar is 200. She is a known diabetic and not well-controlled as a rule. She has been x-rayed from head to toe also. These show a displaced fracture of her nose. There is also a markedly displaced fracture of her mid-left femur (thigh) with the head of the femur driven through the acetabulum (pelvis) or socket."

Since there were no fractures of the face, neck, or skull, we elected to repair the lacerations and reduce her nasal fractures under local anesthesia. I talked to the family, explaining everything in detail and called Dr. Johnson with the report. I called an orthopedist of the family's choice. Then we went to work in the operating room.

"How is she doing now, Mr. Bowen?," I heard someone inquire.

"Fair, but stable," was the reply.

"What is she getting in the IV solution now?"

"Dextrose 5 percent in saline."

"Let's give her two units of blood immediately, slow the IV down, and change to lactated ringers when the glucose is finished."

While this conversation was in progress, I was scrubbing, and the nurse had the surgical instruments and sutures ready. The other had "prepped" the face, nose, and ear.

First, we controlled the bleeding, then we repaired the facial lacerations. The ear was evaluated, and I was able to replace it to a normal position and suture it there. We repaired the nasal lacerations, suctioned and cleaned the nasal cavities, reduced the fracture, and packed the involved nasal cavity. The surgery went well, her general condition improved, her blood pressure rose to near normal and she began to react to her pain. Then I felt she would recover and, barring any complications, would lead a normal life. After her post-operative evaluation, I glanced at the clock and only then did I realize how long we had been doing the surgical procedures. It had been five-and-one-half hours from the actual time we began.

The orthopedic surgeon took care of her fractured femur after our surgery was completed. Her diabetes was controlled by diligent care of an internist and she made an uneventful recovery. I visited her twice daily while she was hospitalized and was happy with the results from the surgery of her facial region. Her scarring was hardly noticeable, the nose was straight, and the ear looked normal. Mrs. Allen remained a grateful and careful patient for more than twenty years and expired from an acute myocardial infarction (heart attack).

Upon leaving the hospital the night of Mrs. Allen's surgery, I realized it had been twelve hours since I had eaten. I began to feel tired and hungry. The adrenalin started flowing freely again as I remembered that there was a trailer for me to unload. I had to find help for that.

As I walked out of the emergency room, I looked up to thank my God for watching over us during the last many trying hours. A fine mist of rain sprayed me in the face as I looked up, and I thought, *What have I done wrong, Lord? Surely the rest of this day will be quiet and peaceful.*

I backed the car and trailer out and hurried to Old Hickory. I had previously arranged to pick up a key to the "new" house at a local drug store. By the time I arrived the rain was falling a bit harder. The pharmacist greeted me with open arms.

"Good to see you again, Dr. Wilson," he said. "Here is your house key. Is there anything else we can do for you tonight?"

"Yes, sir," I replied, "tell me where I can find somebody to help me unload a trailer."

"Right here, we have just the man for the job. Come here, Fred," he called to the teenager who was his delivery boy, cleanup man, etc.

"This is Dr. Wilson, Fred, and he needs you to help him unload some furniture from a trailer."

"I'll be glad to help."

"I'd appreciate if you will," I gratefully replied.

We shook hands and left for the house on Clark Street. When we arrived, neither of us knew there was another problem awaiting us. It was still daylight when we started the unloading, so we didn't need electric power.

As darkness began to engulf us, we plugged up a table lamp, but no light came on. We tried a ceiling light with the same result. The power was not on. Back to the drug store we went.

"Did you get unloaded ok, fellows?" the friendly pharmacist asked.

"Yes," I replied, "we got unloaded, but there's no electricity."

"Oh, we can take care of that," he assured us.

"Come here, Tenor. This is Dr. Wilson. He needs some help," he said as he introduced me to Tenor Long.

"Hello, Mr. Long, glad to meet you but not this way."

"Glad to meet you, Doctor. What can I do for you?"

"I just moved into a house on Clark Street and have no electric power."

"I think we can help you with that. Let me make a phone call."

I listened.

"Hello, Red, this is Tenor. I need some help to get the power into the new doctor's house. Can you meet us at 1008 Clark Street?"

We could hear Red on the other end: "Sure, I'll see you in about ten minutes."

Red Cunningham beat us there. We greeted each other than we went to work.

About fifteen minutes later, he had bypassed the meter and power was back on.

"Thank you Mr. Cunningham, and thank you, Mr. Long. You're real friends. I won't forget you," I promised, and I never did. They soon became patients and remained so until Mr. Cunningham died and I became disabled. Mr. Tenor Long is still living at age 89. We have talked about that night many, many times over the years.

That first case and that neighborly, friendly encounter were on the first day of my practice that lasted for thirty-six years. The four years I spent in practice in Memphis rounded out forty years. Private practice in both areas was a wonderful experience. It was an enjoyable, busy, stimulating, rewarding, and often trying practice. I consider myself to be one of the most fortunate people to have ever been blessed with the opportunity to care for the lives of so many wonderful people.

Since being forced to retire at the end of 1987, following quadruple, coronary artery bypass surgery, followed by a minor heart attack some few months later, there has been time to reminisce and realize what a wonderfully full life I have had. I now realize what a splendid, caring family God has blessed me with. I continue to thank him every day of my life.

This is my story - a story of love, care and compassion - both given and received - a story of trials and triumphs - a story of pain and pleasure. The memory of it inspires me every day, and I hope it will inspire you. If so, I will have achieved my purpose in writing.

"Miss Dee"
Our Mother

Maderia Ann Barton Wilson was born March 13, 1880, to Martin Jasper Barton and Mary Marsh Barton. She was one of ten children born to this union. "Miss Dee" was the third of six girls and as Dad often said, "The most beautiful of all six." At age seventeen she met Thomas Decatur Wilson, her teacher. For "Dee" it was love at first sight.

Mama was a brown-haired beauty with fine features, soft brown eyes, a perfect figure, standing five feet one inch tall and weighing 100 pounds soaking wet. Dad was then twenty-one years old, of slender build, five feet eight inches tall with black, curly hair and piercing black eyes that were like two magnets pulling Mama to him. Tom had ambitions to become a physician and was teaching in a temporary position to earn enough money to realize his dream. Little did he realize how strong love was, and it soon overpowered him, and a serious courtship began. He had trouble concentrating on his work because "Dee" kept getting in his way. He resisted for four, long years before love won out. Meantime, Tom had enrolled in medical school and knew that he would realize that dream. In early 1902, Tom and "Dee" were married. She was then twenty-one and he was twenty-five.

After marriage, Dad went back to medical school. As was the custom in those days, mama went to live with his parents, where she became housekeeper, maid, etc. The years spent there were not too pleasant for Mama as she worked long, hard hours all day and into the night. She had a good relationship with Grandma Wilson, but Grandad Wilson was hot-tempered and unpleasant, making life miserable at times. Mama was tough and survived until 1905 when Dad graduated from medical school, then they moved to their own home.

In 1903, babies started arriving on a regular basis until 1923 when her twelfth child was born, and Mama was forty-three-years old. During the ensuing years she survived three miscarriages, typhoid at age twenty-five, endometritis (child-bed fever) at age forty-five, plus cancer of the uterus at age fifty-five, and still lived to nearly age eighty. She died from postoperative complications in October, 1959.

I remember Mama as a spirited, ambitious person who was always busy doing something for her family or someone in the community. She was very intelligent and always encouraged each of us to learn as much as we could about everything we did to improve our position in life. She kept us busy. That kept us out of mischief most of the time. By the time we were three years old, we would be assigned small chores "to help Mama." She knew this would help us develop good work ethics. Mama was also a strict disciplinarian and a hard taskmaster. When we did misbehave or fight, we were punished accordingly. I have never forgotten the "switchings" after a fight or the way she "knuckled" our head for a lesser incident of misbehavior.

Mama had many "bywords" that also had a lot of meaning to all of her children. Some of them I recall (when exasperated or disgusted), "plague take it" or "rotten on it" or "you good-for-nothing thing" or "sorry as fish gut" (for someone who wouldn't work). "She/he moves so slow that dead lice wouldn't fall off of him/her" (for someone that worked slowly). "I'll stripe your legs" (meaning she would use a switch on you for misbehaving), or "I'll knuckle your head" or "you'll get a limmin" (also for misbehaving). Although we were disciplined strictly, we all knew that Mama loved us, and that love was returned in kind.

As a small child I thought Mama could perform miracles—and she almost did. Rearing eleven children, almost alone, was a miraculous feat within itself. During the school year, she would see that we did our homework and special assignments. If we did not understand, she would always find time to tutor us until we did understand and could recite it back to her or solve a math problem to her satisfaction. We would have spelling bees, read aloud to her while she listened, closely correcting when a word was mispronounced and enunciating the proper way to sound the word. We had math classes at times also, but she wasn't the best teacher in math. Nevertheless, she tried and learned with us. She was always challenging and teaching so her children might be able to excel in life.

Mama was a wonderful cook. She was also an excellent seamstress, making the clothes for all the children, even denim shirts, overalls, and jackets for all us boys. Mama was a whiz at growing flowers. She supervised the vegetable garden. She harvested, canned, and preserved the fruits and vegetables as they were harvested. In later years, the task was made easier when freezing of all these came into being. She also had a beautiful alto singing voice. She sang in the church choir and with a special quartet at times. At home, she played the pump organ and often we children would gather around to sing hymns and ballads as she played and sang with us in her beautiful alto voice. Those memorable times we still cling to as the years rush swiftly by.

At the age of forty-three, Mama delivered her twelfth child. She had been sick for several days just prior to delivery with fever, chills, and general aching all over. Within a few hours after the baby was born her temperature rose to 103 degrees, and her condition became critical. The baby was also sick when born, and it was touch and go for both for several days. Dad called in three of his most trusted colleagues for consultation. After that, they took turns staying with Mama night and day for three or four weeks. They also made his calls and "deliveries" so he could be at Mama's bedside at any moment. During this time, we were not allowed in that part of the house, not allowed to make loud noise anywhere in the house, and never allowed in the room to see her. I was five years old and very dependent on our mother for love and guidance. I was really scared and upset, thinking Mama was going to die. I would sneak off and cry a lot, thinking, *Please God don't let Mama die. She's the only one we have to love us.* When Dad would come out of her room, I sometimes asked him, "Is our Mama going to die?"

"No, Son, she isn't going to die. God will take care of her," he would say.

That made me feel better, "But then why can't we see her?" I asked.

"She's too weak now—maybe in a few more days" he replied.

This went on for two or three more weeks—Dad staying home, a lady keeping house and staying with us, neighbor ladies helping with cooking and washing. We were all still scared to play or make noise, afraid we would upset our mother. She began to improve, and after another week or so, we were able to see her. What a glorious day! We were all shocked! Mama was real thin, her cheeks were prominent, her eyes were sunken in deep sockets. She was as pale as a ghost and very weak. When she spoke it was barely a whisper. We all tiptoed in and out looking at her, and barely spoke in a whisper as we told her we loved her and to please get well. I barely paid any attention to the new baby because at that moment I was thinking it was his fault that Mama almost died. Then we all crept out of the room with our thoughts and went our separate ways: probably each to cry mixed tears of sadness for her being so sick and tears of joy that she would soon be well again. It took her several months really to recover from that illness. The newborn was ill, and Dad spent many hours caring for him for the next six months while Mama was recovering. By that time, she was able to begin caring for him and soon had the full responsibility for his care. One other time Mama had to leave home when the measles swept through the household. Mama never contracted measles during all these years, and Dad was afraid for her to take the risk at her age. so Mama had a neighbor and close friend who invited her to stay with them. Mama packed up and left for the duration of about four to six weeks. Measles were tough on us and about twice as bad because our mother was not there to care for and soothe us. After everybody finally was no longer sick, Mama was allowed to come home. What a great day that was for the Wilson household! Looking back, I'll bet Mom was wishing she was still at the neighbors' with nothing to do. Soon she was back in the old routine working from 4 a.m. to 12 midnight, cooking, cleaning, canning, refereeing sibling fights, holding classes after supper, darning socks, and patching overalls. All these things a mother does to keep a houseful of children fed, clothed, and happy. We all grew up soon enough for her, and before long began leaving home to seek another life. With a mother of the type we had, we should have all been prepared for a life of any kind. She had taught us self-reliance, independence, and persistency. Thank god for such a mother. She was a blessing.

Soon, I was the oldest child at home. I was able to spend more time with Mama and to get to know her better. We talked about all the years she had spent rearing a big family while her husband was gone so much seeing patients. As I "managed" the farm for four or five years, I was home in early evenings when Mama and I could talk alone. (Usually Dad would be asleep or away on calls.) We talked of her early childhood and growing up on a small farm with five sisters and four brothers. Her brothers were coddled by their father while he made the girls work the farm, doing everything except clearing new ground for fields and plowing them to grow crops. They chopped the corn, hoed the tobacco, helped to build fences, worked the garden, helped to harvest the grain, hay, etc. They also did the household chores, helped do the washing, ironing, cooking, and milked the cows. While they did most of this the brothers would play the guitar or banjo as they sat on the front porch and sang (so my mother told me). A note of bitterness crept into her voice as she reminisced about her teenage years at home.

Mama also reminisced about her early years of marriage as she lived with Dad's parents as housekeeper while he was away in Nashville finishing medical school. Those were hard and lonely times for her: doing the housework, not feeling a part of the family, and not seeing her husband

Doctor From Bugtussle

for weeks on end. It was almost unbearable for her. Then in 1903, the first baby was born, adding to her burden and woes, but she stayed with it. Before Dad finished medical school Mama found herself pregnant again about four months before he graduated. This was another big blow. Soon after graduation they moved out to a small house in Salt Lick, some six or eight miles southeast of where she had been living. From there, Dad began his practice, and Mama was more alone than ever.

I was full of questions. "What did you have as you began housekeeping?"

"Not much at all, a small amount of furniture given to us by relatives. Pa (her father) had also given me a milk cow, a brood sow and a ewe sheep. Dad bought a horse, on credit, for transportation to practice. It was hard but we made it. Pa's foresightedness assured us of milk and meat. I raised a garden and canned extra food so we had plenty to eat, but not much else. the hard work, loneliness and endless pregnancies was sometimes more than I could bear."

"How soon after you moved was your second child born?"

"About four months."

"Was the baby a boy or a girl?"

"A beautiful little girl that was the spitting image of my mother. We named her Mary Eliza for her grandmothers."

"Was she healthy?"

"Yes, until I came down with typhoid about six weeks after she was born."

"What happened then?"

"A Mrs. Jones came to take care of me and the children, and she let the baby's milk sour. The baby became ill with bloody diarrhea and vomiting. They were not able to control either of them. She had a high fever, became dehydrated, and we lost her."

"Had you nursed the baby while you were sick with typhoid?"

"Yes, up until we knew the cause of my illness."

"Who treated you and Mary?"

"Dr. Smith from Gamaliel, Kentucky."

"How long did Mary live after she became ill?"

"About three weeks."

"Don't you think, Mama, she might have had typhoid also?"

Doctor From Bugtussle

"She might have. The Lord only knows. I almost died myself. Then losing the baby on top of that; for a long time afterward I wouldn't have cared if I had died from the typhoid too."

As I listened to her voice I could feel the sadness in her heart that had been there all those years from the loss of her baby girl. I never questioned her again about that time in her life.

Mama talked to me about how hard she worked, of the heavy burden she had with all the children to feed and care for day and night, of not eating full meals for two or three days at a time; of sitting up with sick children night after night with little or no sleep, afraid that she might lose another one. In earlier years she would wash, card, and spin wool to make thread so she could knit clothing for her family. (This wool came from offsprings of the one sheep given to her as a wedding present by her parents). She knitted sweaters, socks, and mittens from that yarn so her children could have warm clothing in the wintertime.

As she talked of all these things during the earlier years of her marriage, I noted bitterness in her voice. She felt cheated throughout those years because her husband was away most of the time instead of being there with her as a companion and helpmate.

There was both tragedy and comedy in her years of marriage and motherhood—first the loss of her infant daughter, which I related. Second, the near loss of her third son at the age of nine when he fell from a loaded wagon, and the rear wheel ran over his left shoulder and neck. When rescued, he was unconscious and bleeding from the nose and both ears. He was barely breathing, and his older brothers thought he was dead.

"How was he treated for this injury, Mama?," I asked.

"By prayer and watchful waiting. I don't know how he lived. He was near death for several days and then, miraculously, regained consciousness and revived. It must have been the work of the Lord; that is the only reason I can see that he lived."

That son proved to be the best of all of her surviving children. He lost the use of his left arm which hung useless by his side. He refused to be a "cripple" and could do most everything anyone with both arms could do. He was a blessing to the entire family, inspiring us by his hard work and success.

Another near tragedy struck a few years later as Mama and her friend were traveling in a buggy. As they were driving along, the horse was frightened and bolted, causing the buggy to overturn. Both Mama and her passenger were thrown from the buggy, but neither of them was seriously injured. Mama was three months pregnant at the time and suffered a miscarriage resulting from the accident. She had no complication and soon was back to her daily routine.

The third incident occurred when she was near term with her seventh pregnancy. It was peach harvesting time in August, and she climbed up into a peach tree to shake the fruit off. As she did so, she had a sudden pain in her abdomen, followed by a gush of water. She realized her "water" had broken (the membranes had ruptured). She hurried down from the tree, hollering constantly for the "hired girl" to come to her as she went into the house and got into bed. As she told the story, she laughed until she cried and said, "I barely made it before he was born." (Today, August 22, 1993, that brother celebrated his 81st birthday). I'm sure there were many more of these incidents that Mama endured, or enjoyed, that have never been related to anyone.

Throughout the college years, I "managed" the farm during summer vacation, continued to "court" the country girlfriend and earned enough from my arrangement with Dad to pay my tuition and for some used textbooks. At the same time, I would continue my evening chats with Mama to learn more about what she had been through and how she felt about her life of hard work, drudgery, and loneliness over these years.

"Were you happy with your choice of a husband?" I asked.

"Oh, yes! He was the only man I ever saw that I was the least bit interested in from a romantic standpoint. He stirred feelings in me that I never knew existed. I thought he was the most handsome man I had ever seen. It was love at first sight. I still feel the same way about him after all these years." As she talked about Dad her eyes sparkled, and she smiled with remembering the early years of their courtship and marriage.

"Did you know then that he aspired to be a physician?" I continued.

"Yes, but secretly, I was hoping he would change his mind. Of course, he didn't, but I married him anyway because we truly loved each other."

"Have you been sorry that you did?"

"Not really. Over the years, there have been times that I hated the profession he chose and the lifestyle we had to bear, but I have never been truly sorry of the choice I made thirty-five years ago. If you are lucky enough to find a woman that loves you enough to sacrifice another lifestyle to be with you, count yourself blessed and keep her by your side for life."

"Mama, you know that I've made the decision to study medicine?"

"Yes, I know, and I admire you, but it will be a hard life. If you want to do that, and are sure of your decision, we will support you all the way. That doesn't mean there will be money enough for anything you happen to want. You will have to be careful and try to find jobs to help pay your way."

"I realize that, and I think you know I'll be willing to work if anything is available. I expect to have it rough for those years."

"Just remember what we have always taught you: stick with your decision, do your best, be honest and truthful, and you can reach your goal. It will be a hard row to hoe, and there will be times you want to quit. When those times come, I want you to remember one thing: there is always someone you can turn to: *GOD* will always be there when you need HIM." (I never forgot that conversation and advice). Mama and I continued our evening chats throughout the summer of 1938 and grew closer than ever before.

In September, I enrolled in my last year of college with more determination and desire to achieve my goal. That was due in great part to my mother's counsel and advice during those summer-evening chats. I was very busy each day, but at night I missed out talks. Visits home were few and brief.

Mama was always glad to see her children come back, and she made sure to have the foods they especially liked. When we would leave there was always some special package from Mama tucked in the suitcase.

Mama was sixty years old when I left for medical school. She had only a little gray in her hair, her eyes were still "alive," her mind was "keen," she still sang in the church choir and special quartet, did all of her work at home, grew flowers, canned and froze foods, pieced quilts, and still found time to write letters to her children away from home. She had seven daughters-in-law by that time, and all said that she could work circles around any one of them. During the next three years, I saw her briefly at Christmas time and in June. However, halfway through school there was a break of two weeks when I was able to be home. She was still full of life and advice.

"Don't fall in love with some girl, now. Wait until you get through school. Then you might be in a position to get serious about one."

"Don't worry about that, Mama. I'll be too busy to think about such things."

"Pshaw! Men never get too busy not to think of young women. Just watch your step."

I was very aware of the meaning of her advice.

"Okay, I will," I assured her.

Mama and I had two or three long, evening chats that were pleasant and enlightening. She seemed content and happy and sang as she worked, and I was pleased that she was able to enjoy her later years of marriage. After that visit, I was able to visit only three more times until I graduated from medical school. Mama was her same lively self and still full of her motherly advice. Just a few months before graduation I had met *that* girl Mama had warned me about, and six weeks from graduation time, we were married. When I called home and told my parents, they were not too happy about our plans.

"Of course," Mama said, "You didn't listen to a word I said, did you?"

"I guess not," I replied, "but you will love her once you meet her."

Dad asked, "What are you going to live on, Son?"

"Love, I guess. What do you suggest?"

"I'll send you a note to sign, and the bank will loan *us* enough for three months, and by then you will be earning enough to get by," he said.

Mama said, "Wendell, I thought you had more sense than to marry now. What were you thinking anyway? I don't think you have a lick of sense about such things."

"Maybe not," I said, "but I love this girl. Also, it seems I remember some people I am real close kin to that did the same thing."

"Yes, you do, and that is the very reason I am upset with you," she retorted. "That poor girl is in for a lot of trouble for the rest of her life."

"Aw, Mama, we'll make it all right," I assured her. "She is a wonderful person and smart as a whip. I just know you will like everything about her."

"Well, maybe so," she confessed. "I'll let you know after we meet."

Mama had her opinions and never minced words expressing them. At that moment, she was not too happy with either one of us.

"Dad, I appreciate what you're doing," I said. "I'm selfish enough to think it will be one of the best investments you ever made. Thank you from the bottom of my heart."

The first of March, I took my bride of one month to Middle Tennessee to meet the Wilson "clan": my parents, eight brothers, two sisters, and seven sisters-in-law, plus a few grandchildren. Almost all the way from Memphis, Jessie quizzed me as to who belonged to whom, etc. When we were about fifty miles from Nashville she stopped talking, stared straight ahead, and remained silent. I knew what the problem was: "Honey, everything will be all right," I said, "Every sister-in-law went through the same thing. Don't worry about it."

Doctor From Bugtussle

We made it ok and arrived at my parents' home in late afternoon. By then Jessie was more relaxed and responsive. Mom met us at the front door, and I knew by her facial expression that she was as happy as I was with her new "daughter."

"Mom, this is 'Bessie'" (the nickname I had given her).

"You ought to be ashamed to call this beautiful girl such a name," she said. Then Mom opened her arms and kissed Jessie on the cheek. "Welcome to the Wilson family. I hope you can survive the weekend."

As Mom and I embraced, I whispered in her ear, "Isn't she everything I said she would be?"

"Yes, I like her," she whispered back.

Dad came through the door with a quizzical look on his face that quickly turned to a smile. "Dad, this is Jessie, your newest 'daughter.'"

"Welcome to our home, Jessie." As he kissed her on the cheek, she smiled and returned the kiss. I knew then that she felt a part of the family.

Mom said, "Wendell, don't let me hear you call this child Bessie anymore. That certainly is not a very flattering nickname for any woman, much less this pretty thing."

"Come in this room, Jessie, so we can talk some and be away from these two doctors," I heard her say. "Now tell me about your family." I knew then everything would be fine. Jessie's family meant so much to her, and she loved to talk about them.

We stayed two days. Most of the family came to meet and approve of the new member. She scored high marks in everything but one; she was not from Macon County and not even from Tennessee. She was a "furriner" from Indiana, by the way of Missouri and Louisiana. But they forgave her for that and welcomed her to the clan.

When we were alone, I asked Mom how she liked the new daughter-in-law. She replied, "She is a beautiful lady and very intelligent. I think she will make a wonderful wife and mother. I really like her. I feel sorry for her being married to you because of your chosen profession. Now don't you ever mistreat or neglect her."

"I will never mistreat her and hope to never neglect her either. But you know I will have to be away from home a lot, Mom?"

"Yes, how well I know, but don't use that as an excuse to mistreat her in any way."

"Ok, I promise, Mom."

When we left the next day, Jessie and Mom shed a few tears as they embraced for a long moment and kissed goodbye. I'm sure they were kindred spirits.

"Come back to see us as soon as you can, Jessie," she said.

"We will, bye," said Jessie as we left.

We returned to Memphis, I finished medical school, and Jessie went to work. I took the examination for State Boards, was licensed to practice, and on April 1 started an internship. Visits home were a "no no," and we did not see Mama until December, 1943. She was the same lively self but leery of what would happen when I had to go on active duty in the Navy.

She was loving and free with advice: "Don't forget my advice when everything seems unsolvable; God is there for you."

Fortunately, I was on duty only seventy miles from home. We visited frequently, and Jessie and Mama became closer. She taught Jessie many things that were practical and helpful to sustain a marriage and rear a family.

Soon order came for me to report for duty in Rhode Island, some 800 miles away. I left in October of 1944, and did not see my parents again until May of 1946. Dad had aged much more than Mama, who was still alert, active, and working as usual at age sixty-six. She aged slowly and maintained good health until Dad had a small stroke in the early 1950s and gradually deteriorated and succumbed to his illnesses in 1957. After that Mama lost her will to live and constantly said she was ready for the Lord to "take her home" to be with her loved ones. Her personality changed. Where once she was a chronic worrier, she didn't seem to care what happened anymore. This happened after she too suffered a "mini"-stroke in 1958. After that, her physical endurance was gone. In October, 1959, she had emergency surgery with post-operative complications that caused her death two days after surgery.

Mama died with a smile on her face, and I have always said she saw heaven just before she departed this earth.

I couldn't grieve for Mama because she had wanted to "Go home to Glory" so determinedly. She had lived to see all thirty-two of her grandchildren and some of her many great grandchildren be born and was also able to enjoy them. Not many wives and mothers had accomplished nearly as much as did our mother, "Miss Dee," in her lifetime.

"Doctor Tom"
Our Dad

Thomas Decatur Wilson was born March 20, 1876, to George Hamilton Wilson and Eliza Tucker Wilson. He was one of nine children and the fourth of six sons born to that union. His oldest brother "Bud" became a physician and inspired Dad to follow in his footsteps. Dad attended "prep" school somewhere in Monroe County, Kentucky, to obtain a teaching certificate in order to save money to enroll in medical school. While teaching he fell in love with Maderia Ann Barton, one of his students, whom he married in 1902 during his second year of medical school. He was able to continue school and graduated in 1905. In that era most medical graduates did not take post-graduate studies, and Dad went into private practice in the rural area near where he grew up in Macon County, Tennessee. He remained in practice there until 1950 when he was forced to retire due to ill health.

By the time he was ready to begin private practice he had become a father and was without money to set up practice. A family friend loaned him enough money to buy a horse with a saddle and bridle, some necessary drugs and a few basic instruments. He was in business. There were very few telephones in rural areas in 1905, and he had to rely on word of mouth to inform the public of his being in practice. His practice, as well as his family, grew and grew until he was so busy he was away from home at least half of the time. In those years he fathered three daughters (one of whom died in infancy) and nine sons, only one of which was to follow in his footsteps and become a family physician.

For many years "Dr. Tom's" only mode of transportation was his faithful horse. The first one was Nell, a "saddle" mare, meaning she had a gait that was such that it was smooth and easy for the rider to be comfortable for many hours of riding. She foaled three colts over the years, and they too were "saddle" horses. The first two, King and Joe, were excellent "saddlers" who could also "rack" and "pace." Dad rode both intermittently, but his preference was King, whom Dad trusted to take him anywhere in any type of weather, any time, day or night, through the darkest night when Dad could not see the roads or "pigpaths," King would take him home. Many times there would be streams so swollen that King would have to swim to get across. Pausing, Dad would put his "saddle bags" across his shoulder, hold his small bag shoulder high, put his knees on the saddle, hold to the horn of the saddle with the other hand, and urge King to go ahead. Seldom did they fail to cross a stream to get to an expectant mother or a critically ill patient. In winter months, the weather was bitter cold and Dad dressed accordingly; long thick underwear, white shirt and black tie, woolen socks, woolen suit, heavy shoes, high top overshoes, leggings, a heavy topcoat, scarf, ear muffs, and gloves, or thick, woolen mittens (knitted by our mother). Sometimes while he would be dressing, one of the older brothers would saddle the horse so he would be ready to mount as soon as Dad was fully dressed. Sometimes during those winter nights after riding a few miles before arriving at a patient's home or back home from a house call, his feet would be frozen to the saddle stirrups and had to be broken loose by someone so he could dismount. From the beginning of his practice until the early 1930s almost all of his mode of travel was by horseback. He did buy a "T" model Ford car in 1915 or 1916, but because of road conditions was unable to use it from mid-November to about May 1. By 1936, he was able to buy large, high "mud wheels" which made it possible for him to use the car year-round. This enabled him to continue his practice because he was then sixty years old and could not tolerate the "night-riding," as he once had done.

I can see "Dr. Tom" now sitting astride his faithful horse, King. He is wearing a dark-gray Stetson hat, a white dress shirt with a stiffly starched collar, and black tie. His suit is of a dark color, which he wore the year round. There is a frown on his face as he squints into the sun. He was a legend in our part of the country, loved and respected by everybody far and near. He feared no man but was scared to death of snakes and strange dogs.

I recall Dad as a gruff, intense man, always on the go as a busy country doctor, visiting the sick in their homes or attending the ones that would come to our home in the earlier years, or to his small office in the corner of the front yard. Most of the time he would be gone from home by early morning until late afternoon, making his rounds on the ill, or sometimes, the "pretended" ill. Because of Dad's being absent most of our waking hours, most of the rearing was done by our mother, who in essence was, overall, more aggressive than our father was.

Dad had the reputation of being the best "baby" doctor and the best "pneumonia" doctor in Macon and surrounding counties. His first love was obstetrics, and difficult deliveries were always a challenge to him. His colleagues would call him anytime they were in trouble for consultation, and together the problems would be solved. Because of this reputation, he was said to have delivered more babies than any one of the other ten to twelve doctors in the area.

In spite of his being busy with practicing medicine, he had some time to do other things. In early spring, he would plan the work for each week to prepare for the planting of crops. This was dreaded by us, since it meant cleaning out the cow barns and horse stables, hauling and spreading the manure on the fields that would later be plowed up for planting corn, etc. Sometimes, he would even show us how to "turn" a new field or "lay off" a row to plant the seed so it would grow properly. As the crops were tended, he would sometimes pay a surprise visit to the field to inspect our work (such as "chopping corn"). If it was a sloppy piece of work, the "culprit" would have to do it over. As Dad sat on his horse and watched, he would offer constructive criticism. When Dad was satisfied with the work, he would leave. This kept us on our toes since his visits were always unscheduled.

Dad was an avid fisherman and squirrel hunter. During squirrel season he would take the old double-barreled, .12-gauge shotgun and a good supply of shells and head to the woods, saying, "Don't call me unless there is an emergency." (The "call" for an emergency meant Mama would ring the dinner bell two, three, or four claps for each degree of the call, with four claps being the most urgent. At these times Dad meant the four-clapper type only!!). His fishing was for guaranteed results. He was very good at spear fishing and would stay with it for hours when he found trout or other game fish to spear. I have seen him spear a moving trout at twenty feet many times in his prime of life.

The other type of fishing was "seining." This was mostly in springtime or late summer when the streams would rise and become muddy after a rain. He always kept a "dip net" on hand, plus four or five teenage boys to be sure the nets could be manned. We knew how Dad loved to eat fish, so we willingly went along, even though we usually dreaded the one-half mile walk to the creek and a much longer one back after an hour or two of hard work at seining. The net would be wet and heavy: six to eight feet long, four to five feet wide, suspended between two "poles" with "floats" at the top and six four-inch "sinkers" on the bottom strand of heavy cotton twine. This sometimes required two teenage boys (weighing 100 to 115 pounds) to carry the seine on their shoulders for that distance.

But we went—had fun, got scared, sometimes thought we would drown, and were too tired to eat when supper was served. But we went because we knew Dad loved fishing and—we loved Dad. We also enjoyed watching him eat those fish we had worked to catch. Dad usually did most of the fish cleaning, as he wanted to save the head for Mama to make the "fish-head soup," which he considered a delicacy. The next day or two, Dad feasted on the delicacy of fish-head soup while we ate other foods. We watched and were fascinated as Dad consumed the entire large bowl full of fish heads, including the eyes, which he sucked from their sockets as we looked away and snickered. Dad liked squirrel and "squirrel-head soup" almost as well as he did the fish and its soup, and feasted on both as often as possible as years went by. As I reminisce about those years of growing up, watching Dad as he "wore two or three hats," I have a much better understanding of his lifestyle. I also realize he did what he enjoyed most in life, practicing medicine, attending local medical society meetings, attending church and Sunday School, taking part in the proceedings and practices of his Masonic Lodge, visiting with old friends, and, of course, the infrequent times of fishing and hunting.

Life as a country doctor was not an easy one by any stretch of the imagination. Transportation was a problem in the earliest years of practice. Getting paid for what he did was another, larger problem. In rural regions, incomes were largely non-existent to very small. Some few had good, consistent incomes that kept it flowing enough to keep the family together. During the Great Depression of 1929-1933 nobody had money, including our family. Factories closed, banks failed, people were issued script in lieu of money and because of all this, suicides increased by the thousands, and people moved from cities to rural areas and farms. There was also an increase in Dad's practice as a result of the depression. In spite of this, his income did not grow accordingly. Dad treated the sick, knowing they had no money to pay him. When his income was practically nothing, he borrowed money, bought drugs, and continued treating them as though they were paying cash. His charges were minimal: house calls $2, suturing lacerations $2, extracting a tooth $.50 (no anesthesia), and delivering a baby $20. Dad had a large barter practice in those days and we boys (Dennis, Prentice, and I) were the collectors, which we did on Saturdays. He would be paid in sorghum molasses, hay, corn, fodder, pigs, calves, sheep, and sometimes a mule. We soon learned to be selective in our collections as a farmer would give us the scrub calf, the nubbins rather than the good corn, etc. There was strength in numbers, and since we had a three-to-one-ratio, we bargained and got what we wanted. I was usually the spokesman.

"Mr. Hunnicutt, didn't Dad give you the best treatment you could get?"
"Yeah, I guess, why?"

"Well, then I think he deserves the best corn you've got. Not all, but 75 percent at least."

"Ok, I guess you're right. Let's finish loading from this other crib."

"Thank you, Mr. Hunnicut, this is much better. I'm sure Dad will appreciate it, too."

We continued to do that but sometimes ran into an argument, but we usually won using the same tactics each time. Occasionally, Dad would ask: "What happened at the Smiths or the Joneses when you boys collected from them? Sam said you were hard to deal with."

"No, Dad, we just asked him to treat you like he expects to be treated, that's all."

Dad just smiled. "That's good, ok."

The Depression years passed, his practice grew, and he continued at the same pace and the same charges. His cash flow improved as the Depression years left. Soon all the older brothers were gone from home (most of them to work for the DuPont company in Old Hickory, Tennessee), and I found myself to be the oldest at home. I also had to assume responsibility for managing the farm at the age of seventeen. By this time, I had become more interested in medicine or a related field, and felt it would be in my best interest for future years to stay home and, when possible, make calls with Dad and increase or lose my interest in medicine. As the summer passed, the interest grew as I had made more house calls with Dad. Each Sunday afternoon and weekdays, when rainy, we made calls together. This lasted throughout most of my high school and some of my college years as I spent the summers working on the farm. During all of those many months Dad never encouraged, nor did he discourage me, to study medicine. I guess he felt that my mind was made up. He didn't say: "Son, I think you would make a good doctor" or "I don't think you should go to medical school." He just kept setting examples by teaching me the "how" of practicing medicine.

By the time I had finished the third year of pre-medical education, I had found how skillful Dad really was. I had watched him deliver babies with the mother covered so she would not be exposed to the many family members, both male and female, that filled the room. Most of the mothers never had a tear from the delivery. Also, most mothers had no anesthesia or much analgesics. He handled infants, small babies, and young children with equal skill, as he did adults. He taught me how to talk with the families of the sick and dying. Also, I was not to boast of my abilities or accomplishments. Dad said, "Son, show them what you know and what you can do, and your work will speak for itself."

Not only did Dad work at his profession, he also worked at his other interests just as diligently. He was the chairman of the deacons of his church, superintendent of the Sunday school, and chairman of the pastoral selection committee. He was Grand Master of his Masonic Lodge and chairman of the local Republican Committee. He was really a leader in his community affairs.

Once I asked him why he didn't start his practice in a small town or city. "Dad, you are a better doctor than any of the others I know in this county and would be successful anywhere you choose."

"Maybe you are right, son, but remember this: It is better to be a big frog in a little pond than a little frog in a big pond."

I have never forgotten those words of advice given before I became a physician.

Dad kept up his busy practice until he was past age seventy, at which time he began to have problems with his prostate. In mid-August of 1947, he was hospitalized in Lebanon, Tennessee, with urinary tract obstruction from benign prostatic hypertrophy. It was a week before anyone called me in Memphis about his problem. I called his attending physician to find out his condition.

"Dr. McDougall, this is Wendell Wilson."

"Yes, I've been expecting your call."

"I'm calling about Dad. How is he?"

"He is not doing so well. He is obstructed and will have to undergo a prostatectomy, but I'm sure he can tolerate surgery very soon. Can you get away to come down for a day or two?"

"Yes, I'll be there tomorrow about noon."

"That's good, I'll be looking for you."

The next morning, Friday, I flew to Nashville. My brother, Harold, met me at the airport, and we drove to McDougall Hospital in Lebanon to see Dad. I had not seen him for six moths and was really shocked when we walked in his room to see a thin, pale father with sunken eyes and cheeks. He seemed too weak to move.

"Hi, Dad, how are you?"

"Not very good right now," he answered in a weak, hoarse, hesitant whisper. Tears came to his eyes as he whispered again; "If you don't do something for me pretty soon, I won't last much longer."

Just at that minute Dr. McDougall came into the room. "Hey, Dr. Wendell, it's good to see you. How was your flight?"

"Good, but too slow."

"Now, that this young fellow from the big city is here, we'll get some action. Let's go into my office and check his records."

"We'll be back in a few minutes, Dad. Just relax and take a nap. Harold will be with you. Dr. McDougall and I will take care of everything."

We went into Dr. McDougall's office for consultation and a complete check of Dad's medical records, which were not good. He was anemic (hemoglobin of eight), blood urea nitrogen markedly elevated, and serum electrolytes abnormal. In addition, his urine analysis showed many white cells and much bacteria present, and this was only the beginning.

"He's a very sick man, Dr. McDougall. I'm very concerned about his overall condition. I, like you, feel that he might not survive surgery until his infection is under control, his dehydration is clear, and his BUN and creatnine come back to some degree of normalcy."

"I agree with everything you've said, but he'll have to have the prostate surgery regardless. Tell me about the new procedure they are doing in Memphis now."

"Ok, it's called retropubic prostatectomy. It lessens the operative time by 50 percent. There is much less blood loss, and the post-operative recovery time is cut in half. I'm sure you would be pleased with the procedure and start doing it on your patients."

"Sounds good. I'd like to observe one. Maybe I can do that when your father has his surgery."

"Then you agree that it's best to move him to a medical center?"

"Oh yes, I certainly do. Let's go back and break the news to 'Dr. Tom.'"

We went back to Dad's room.

"Dr. Tom, we have some good news for you. We think you should go back to Memphis with this son of yours so they can do a new type of surgery for your problem."

"Is that ok with you?"

Dad seemed to brighten up, and his voice was stronger. "Of course it is if both of you think it's the thing to do. I'm in yours and the Lord's hands now. Let's go."

"It will be Sunday before we can make the arrangements to fly you there. You will be ok until then."

"I'll take care of everything here, including a copy of his complete medial records and a cover letter," Dr. McDougall commented.

"Thank you, Dr. McDougall. I will be back tomorrow, and we will talk some more regarding all of this."

"Come to my office as soon as you get here tomorrow."

"I will, and thanks again."

I turned to Dad. "You look better now," I said. "How do you feel about all of this?"

"Much better now that I know what has to be done. I think everything will turn out well."

"Good. Now, I need to go and have a long talk with Mama. She needs to get her things ready to take that trip to Memphis with you on Sunday."

Someone stayed with Dad, and someone else took me to Macon County to be with Mama and to make arrangements to fly her to Memphis on Sunday. She was happy to see me and to know that Dad was to be transferred to the hospital in Memphis. "I was afraid they would let him die at Lebanon," she said.

"No, I don't think they would have done that, but Dr. McDougall was relieved that we were taking him to Memphis. It lifted a big burden from him."

"Well, I'm glad he's going and you can see about him."

"He'll be in good hands. All of the people caring for him are good friends of mine. I would trust any of the family members to them. Now, you should start preparing for the trip, and a month stay at our house to boot."

I spent the night with Mama, and the next morning we went back to McDougall Hospital again. As we walked in, Dad brightened and held out his hands to Mama. When she kissed him on the forehead, I saw tears glistening on his cheeks. When Mama said, "You look a lot better today," Dad smiled a bit.

"How do you feel today, Dad?"

"Some better."

"Do you think you can stand a plane ride to Memphis tomorrow?"

"I think so, if Mama's with me."

"Oh, she'll be right beside you all the way."

"All arrangements have been made here and in Memphis, too. Don't worry a bit, we will take care of everything."

That afternoon I called St. Joseph's Hospital and reserved a private room for Sunday. I also talked with both of my senior associates, Drs. Pearce and Grobmyer, who said they would help in any way possible to take care of Dad. Then I called Jessie to tell her of the arrangements and our arrival time at the Memphis airport. Everything went well. We transported Dad to the Nashville airport by ambulance where he was carried aboard the plane by a wheelchair. Mama and I soon boarded the plane and an hour later we arrived at Memphis. We were met by Jessie, and she had an ambulance waiting for Dad. Jessie took Mama and our two small children to our home, and I went with Dad in the ambulance to be admitted to St. Joseph's Hospital. That afternoon, three brothers and four or five of their friends arrived to donate blood since Dad would need multiple transfusions. These men had driven from Nashville, over two hundred miles away, to be sure the blood was available. What a gesture of true friendship!

After a week or more of hospitalization for evaluation by the urologist, a cardiologist, and an internist, plus daily intravenous feedings and two transfusions, Dad looked like a new man. He was taking solid food, was ambulatory, and had a sparkle in his eyes once more.

"Well, Dad, are you about ready to have surgery?"

"Yes, I'm ready whenever the urologist is ready."

"Good. Dr. Allen will be in soon and will give you the word."

Later that day, Dr. Allen called to tell me that the surgery was scheduled for 8 a.m. in two days. When that day arrived, there were about six family members in the surgical waiting room, plus some friends that had arrived that morning. One of those people arriving early that morning was Dr. McDougall, whom I had called two days before. Of course, I introduced him to Dr. Allen, and Dr. McDougall was invited into surgery to scrub and assist or to be an observer. He chose the latter. I was also an observer and reported to the family at intervals. All went well during surgery, which lasted about three hours. Dr. Allen talked to the family and reassured Mama that Dad would be fine, but would be hospitalized for a week or two. Dad stayed two weeks, recovered well, and was ambulatory with help. His catheter was removed two days prior to dismissal, and there were no apparent problems. He had a three-week recuperative stay at our home under the care of two excellent practical nurses, my wife, and his. He was "babied" the first few days, and then they made him "toe the mark."

Dad soon began to eat well and regain strength and weight. At the end of the second week, he was seen by Dr. Allen who dismissed him to the care of Dr. McDougall. At home, he improved rapidly and within another month began to see patients in his office, which was fifty feet from the house. Not too long after that he would make an occasional house call to a home nearby. He had stopped delivering babies a year or so before he had surgery, so that was no problem. We visited him at Thanksgiving so we could observe and report his progress to Dr. Allen in Memphis. Both Jessie and I noticed that he tired easily, moved more slowly, and had lost much of his vigor. Although Dad had slowed from every standpoint, he was still able to recall many things that had occurred in his years of practice.

We encouraged him to tell us some of the hilarious or comical ones since it seemed to stimulate him more. After the three-day visit, we felt good about his recovery and returned to Memphis to report to Dr. Allen and resume the busy, growing practice which was only five months old. Dr. Allen was pleased with the report and wrote Dad a letter to instruct and encourage him.

From the time of his prostate surgery, Dad began to age more rapidly but kept his small practice going, which was then at the office only. He was now seventy-three years of age and should have stopped practicing, but I knew it helped him to see old friends, to talk to and advise them as they would reminisce. He kept going, but by nature was slower physically and mentally. Although his heart and blood pressure remained normal, by the age of seventy-six, he had the first of three or four mini-strokes, each of which disabled him more. I made several emergency nighttime visits to evaluate him and each time came away knowing that Dad would deteriorate more and more, finally needing long-term care in a nursing home that provided total care. Our mother could not do the care at home, even though she had help of a non-professional around the clock. After a family consultation, it was finally decided to move him to a nursing home in Nashville where I personally felt he would get the type of care he would best respond to, and near enough that the four children living in the area could visit easily and quickly. Even with the good nursing care, and good medical attention by colleagues, Dad continued to deteriorate in general and to have repeated low-grade infections. He developed a tracheo-esophageal fistula, could not tolerate food by the oral route, developed pneumonia, and in spite of continuous intravenous feedings and vigorous antibiotic therapy, "Dr. Tom" succumbed to the pneumonia in early May of 1957 at the age of eighty-one years, almost exactly fifty-two years from the day he graduated from medical school.

When news of Dad's death was known, the funeral home was crowded with mourning friends, former patients, and relatives.

Two days later when dad was laid to rest at his beloved Enon Church Cemetery, the church was filled to overflowing. Many of the people stood outside, filling the churchyard; the parking lot was filled, and many cars parked along the roadside for two or three blocks. This was a great tribute to "Dr. Tom"—our Dad.

The Early Years

She awoke at 2 a.m. with an urgent need to use the bathroom. It was pitch black, and she wondered what time it was; then she heard the clock strike 2. "Dee" Wilson had gone to bed early that night because she was "dead tired." She was pregnant with her tenth child and near term. All of the other children were asleep, and Tom was away attending one of his many patients so she looked forward to a good night's sleep. Now this had to happen! When she became fully awake, she realized why the pain had awakened her from a deep sleep. She got out of her bed without waking her husband, who had come home at midnight. She went into the kitchen, lit the kerosene lamp, and began timing her pains. They were coming every five minutes and much harder. She knew that she would soon be ready to deliver this baby. At 3 o'clock she woke her husband.

"Wake up, Tom. Come on, wake up!" She shook him awake. "Get up, the baby is on the way."

"Huh, what? Are you in labor?"

"Yes, and it won't be but a few minutes 'til it's here."

When Dad became fully awake, he instantly went into action as the doctor. He watched her closely, examined her from time to time, checked the baby's heart rate and her blood pressure, and was satisfied with her progress. By 4 o'clock it was delivery time. The membranes ruptured, and the baby came in a rush with the "bag of waters." There was instantaneous crying and squirming. "This is a lively one, Dee!"

"Is it another boy?"

"Yes, I'm afraid so."

"I hope it's the last one. I'm so tired of having babies every year or two, I don't know what to do."

"I know — *maybe* it will be the last one."

"You know what to do. You're the doctor." He had no reply to that as he went about the duties of the doctor, delivered the placenta, tied and cut the cord, gave her an injection of Pitocin, did the cleanup, and then asked, "Are you all right now, Dee?"

"Yes, I'm just tired and worn out."

He even became gentle for a few minutes. "I know you are, Honey. Have you thought of a name for this one?"

"I like the name Wendell, like the physician poet and statesman Oliver Wendell Holmes. You can add the middle name."

"How about Winfred? That sounds good to me."

"That's fine. They go well together and keep the WWW initials in the family tradition."

"Thank you, 'Dee,' I love you." She was sound asleep as he kissed her forehead.

Little did my parents realize that deciding to name me for a famous man as they did might have an influence on my destiny in life. They could not foresee that, like my father, I would choose to study medicine, marry before graduating from medical school, and become a family doctor. Neither were the circumstances under which I was born a good omen. It was in the early morning hours of April 24, 1917. A thunderstorm was brewing and within minutes afterward lightning flashed, thunder rolled, and the rain came in sheets, as was usual this season of the year. I have always thought this influenced my hyperactive lifestyle.

I was the tenth child and eighth son born to Dr. Thomas Decatur and Maderia Ann Barton Wilson, who lived in Macon County, a poor rural area of Middle Tennessee, located two miles from the Kentucky border in the Enon community. At the Tennessee-Kentucky state line was Bugtussle, Kentucky, so named when a farmer riding his mule along the dusty country road on a warm summer day, paused to watch as two "tumble" bugs wrestled over a small ball of fresh horse "droppings."

Bugtussle's business was made up of two general stores, Charlie Gass in Kentucky and Arthur Crabtree's in Tennessee, a blacksmith shop, and four or five homes.

One mile south of our home was another rural business community. This section was Pumpkintown; so named when a farmer had a super bumper crop of pumpkins one year, so many that the ground was almost completely covered by the large pumpkins. At "Punkintown," so pronounced by "us" natives, was a general store, a grist mill, a blacksmith shop, and a garage. There were a dozen homes located near this business, which was a busier place than Bugtussle.

The family into which I was born was very busy where everybody from the age of three was assigned a small, daily task. Newborns would sleep with the parents from birth to about six months. After that time, they would be put into one of the two cradles in the parents' bedroom where they stayed until they were weaned from the breast. They would then sleep away from the mother, and by the age of two, they would be moved upstairs where an older sibling would be responsible for their care. That sibling would be a surrogate parent until the child could survive independently from the older brother. However, the child would look to the older one for teaching new words, assigned tasks, etc.

I have never forgotten an incident that occurred when I was three or four. My task was to carry in two sticks of "stove-wood" twice each day. As I was doing so, under Harlin's watchful eye, I "stumped" my big toe. I started screaming at the top of my lungs— "Harlin, I've killed my toe." Harlin picked me up to see the damage. The nail was almost completely off, and the toe was covered with blood, but he could see that the nail hung by a small corner at the base. Holding me on his lap to soothe me, telling me what a big boy I was and how the toe would be ok, he distracted me, and I stopped crying.

"Let me take you into the house so we can fix your toe, so it'll be ok."

"I didn't 'kill' my toe?"

"No, you didn't. We'll make it well."

"Ok."

Inside, all was well as Harlin had the bandages and held me on his lap again, all the time talking to me until I was mesmerized. He knew the nail had to go and with my being distracted again, he suddenly jerked the nail off completely. This started the wailing and weeping all over again. After finally getting a bandage on, I eventually stopped crying but had to be carried around for several hours to make me feel cared for, and I had a long recuperation with a lot of attention.

I have never forgotten losing that toenail and am reminded of the incident every day when changing my socks, because there is only a small sliver of a nail on the inside corner of my left big toe.

During the formative years we were taught honesty, integrity, truthfulness, forgiveness, independence, and respect for our elders. We also respected, loved, and obeyed our parents. We were reared in a Christian home by parents who believed in and feared God. They read the Bible and prayed daily, saw that we attended church and Sunday School regularly into our teen years, or until, as Mama said, we reached "the age of accountability." After that we were supposed to be responsible for all our actions and deeds the remainder of our life.

As we grew older, we learned from older brothers, their friends, and schoolmates: the bawdy songs, dirty jokes, "cuss" words, plus slang words and expressions for certain conditions, people, and situations. Not only did we learn those things, but we also learned helpful and useful things for everyday living, such as the many types of birds. We learned to recognize them by their songs, type of, and where they built their nests, the different materials used in the nest, etc. We learned the difference between a poisonous and a non-poisonous snake by the shape of the head and tail. We came to know the difference between an edible and non-edible berry, plant, nut, mushroom, or fish. We also learned to milk a cow by the way you squeezed the teat as you gently pulled downward to make the milk flow; how to bridle and saddle a horse by the age of eight—to harness a mule and then hitch him to a plow by the same age. By the age of ten, we learned to use a "bull-tongue" plow, to lay off (plow a straight row) for planting corn. The toughest of all the plowing was the breaking of ground with the hillside "turning" plow. The land would be too steep to make furrows up and down the hill, so it had to be plowed by going back and forth across the hill to prevent washing. When I was fourteen, Dad assigned me that job.

"Wendell, it's about time you learned to use the 'hillside' plow. I want you to plow the Adams field. Take Banty and Red. They're slow and sure-footed. Take your time, rest when you need to, but don't take all day. I know the plow is heavy but you can handle it all right."

"I'll try Dad, but that thing weighs more than I do. Is it hard to flip over?"

"Na-a-a-h, all you have to do is kick that lever beside the wing and swing the plow handles just right, and it'll kick into place, ok?"

"Yeah, I think so."

"No, I think so. You *just do it*."

To the hillside field I went, with the old mules barely moving. That suited me as I was dreading to start anyway. Finally we arrived. Nobody told me to start at the bottom of the hill, so I started at the top. Practicing a few "flips" of the plow to get the hand of it I started plowing, throwing the dirt up hill. The first cut wasn't too bad, but by the time we had made the third round, I saw my mistake. As I plowed, the dirt kept falling into the furrow, making it harder to work the soil, but I kept on. By the time two hours had passed, both mules and I were ready for a rest. Flipping that ninety-pound plow with my ninety-pound body was really wearing me out. A fifteen-minute rest and a drink of water did wonders for all three of us dumb "mules."

"Let's go, fellows," I clucked, but nothing happened. "Come on Red, let's go." She looked back at me with a 'grin,' nodded her head, nuzzled Banty, and they took off at a snail's pace.

"Come on, get up, you two, we'll never get through. It's 9 o'clock, and it's not sundown until 7 o'clock."

Oh well, I have all day, why hurry. At 11 o'clock, Red stopped at midfield, bawled twice to let me know that it was near noontime. She repeated the act thirty minutes later, and within another fifteen minutes the dinner bell clanged three times, the signal to "take out" for lunch. Going back at 1 o'clock, I remembered Dad's words: "Now don't take all day." Well, it would be all day before I could finish. During the afternoon that old plow seemed to get heavier with each flip, twice with each furrow, and by 6 o'clock I was literally "flipped out." Thank God we finished that hillside. I hoped I would never have to plow that field again—and I didn't!

Besides plowing, there were many other tasks to do. We had to build and repair fences, buildings, clean fence rows, barns, chicken houses, and cow sheds. To build new fences we, like Abe Lincoln, had to split rails and make pailings (pickets). This was hard work and also required skill, particularly when it came to making pickets and shingles to roof a building. The latter was called "riving," which required two special tools: a sixteen-inch maul made from a select hickory tree, four inches in diameter—the handle and head each were eight inches in length (this tool was made by an expert wood craftsman and was to be used in only certain types of work), and a second tool was called a fro. This was made of forged steel shaped by a blacksmith. It consisted of a fourteen to sixteen-inch blade at one end and a ring had been formed from the same steel as the blade. This blade was four to six inches wide, one-fourth inch thick at the top edge, forged and hammered down to a thin cutting edge so precise that we wondered how it could be done. A foot-long handle was fitted into the steel ring so the craftsman could easily gauge the thickness of each shingle as he deftly "rived" an almost perfect shingle, minute by minute as we watched, open-mouthed, noting that each one was thicker at one end than at the other.

As all of us learned these things, there would be someone with us to help and guide when they were needed: older brothers, tenant farmers, friends, craftsmen, hired by Dad, even one of the ministers that would go with us to the woods when we split rails or made pickets. He loved young people, and we in turn liked his company. He was a big help as he worked alongside us, plus one other thing—he kept the conversation clean and made us appreciate him more.

Other things learned was the care of the farm animals, how they interacted to other types, such as horses to cattle, sheep to hogs, etc. We observed their courtships and breeding habits, how most of the females would at first fend off the advances of the males, and when it seemed that he might be losing interest, she would be very submissive, seeming to invite him to perform the mating. It was interesting, educational, and intriguing to observe their differing techniques and peculiarities as they went about procreation.

After the procreation, we would watch each bred female, observing her eating habits, reaction to the males, changing of her body shape, resting and sleeping times, and then try to figure the time it would take for each to have its young. We kept up with all of them, the cats, dogs, pigs, sheep, cattle, and horses. Sometimes, we would ask Dad how long each animals gestation period would be so we could observe. Whenever Bossie had her calf or Lucy dropped her colt, someone would be there: "Look P'John, the colt is coming. See the front feet, there comes his nose, now watch his body come out next—see, there it comes, now his hind legs are coming, watch him kick!! Look his mama is cleaning him off. Look, Wendell, he's trying to get up. Now he's really standing. See that? Yeah, ain't that great? It's hard to believe he can stand so soon."

When Bossie calved, we watched as she had pain. She would turn in circles, hump her back, and moo in a low tone. One could almost feel her pain. Calves came much like the colts, front feet, head and neck, body, and then the hind quarters. The mother would clean and lick the calf, take care of the afterbirth, then lie down with her newborn. Pretty soon she would stand, nuzzle the calf, and instinctively it would stand and nurse. We would marvel at all of this, and then run to the house to let everybody know that we had a new calf or a new colt.

We always found Mama first. "Mama Lucy had her colt, and we watched it being born, too. It's a girl colt. Can we name her Mama?"

"Sure, it'll be fine with me. What do you want to call her?"

"Let's call her Tinkerbell."

"No, Wendell, that's not a good name. I'd like to call her Jenny Lind."

Then we argued about it until Mama intervened. "If you boys are going to argue about it, I'll name her. Let's call her Nellie. Do you like that?"

"I think it's a pretty name, don't you P'John?"

"Yeah, it's ok, but I like mine better."

Mama said, "We'll take a vote tonight, ok?" The colt was named Nellie.

We watched the dozens of kittens, several puppies, a few lamb, and many litters of pigs come into the world, but none of them held the fascination of the colt and calf coming to life.

Doctor From Bugtussle

As we grew a bit older, we learned other things—such as how to swim, how to whistle in three different ways, the normal way when you purse lips and through your teeth and with two fingers in your mouth. I could never master the third method. Then at about the age of nine, I noticed my friend, Hooper Harwood, whistling real loud not similar to that when others did it with two fingers in their mouth.

"How do you do that, Hooper?"

"Oh, just curl your tongue up on each side and blow. Like this." As he demonstrated, I watched his tongue curl and did mine the same way, and blew and out came a clear note. Of course, I went home and bragged to everybody about how I could whistle without putting fingers in my mouth. Then I would demonstrate to anyone that would stop to listen, showed them how to curl the tongue, and told them how easy it was to do. Two or three tried but could never whistle that way. What an ego trip that was for me (now at the age of 77, I can whistle best in that manner, but not much by puckering my lips).

By the age of seven or eight, we were taught to swim by our older brothers. The "teaching" was done by the throw-in method. An older brother would get in the creek's swimming hole, another older brother would take you to the water's edge and push you in—or if you resisted, would pick you up and throw you in. If you stayed afloat by kicking and "dog paddling," you were on your own. If you struggled and went under twice, someone "rescued" you. By that I mean, they would pull you out of the creek, take a look at you, and if you were not blue and breathing on your own, they left you alone to settle down, and then literally gave you hell for not being able to swim to shore. If one did not respond quickly, there was a mad rush to his side with someone pumping his chest to revive him. These were anxious moments and no one drowned—thank GOD! Neither did anyone ever tell a parent about these situations.

Here is the scene: Five or six naked boys from eight to sixteen-years old swimming in a creek without a care in the world, whooping and hollering. On the bank, three or four feet above are five piles of clothes, shoes, socks, shirts and overalls—no underwear! Some were standing, afraid to go in because they couldn't swim or afraid that an unthinking brother would "duck" him and hold him under just long enough to scare him to death.

The unthinking one: "Come on in, 'Duck' (Dennis). Are you a coward, 'Scrub' (WW)?"

"If you don't come in, we will throw you in."

Old high-tempered me: "I'll hit you with this big rock, too. Just let me alone, and I'll come in when I'm ready."

33

This was repeated many times during summer months. As I recall these scenes, I sometimes wonder how we escaped some real tragedies, but we did. Now my brothers and I sometimes laugh as we reminisce about what we did during those years.

Being sent to the fields at the age of seven to work alongside older brothers might seem very harsh treatment to some, but not to us because we had been taught to accept responsibility from the age of three. In the fields, we had the companionship of an older brother who taught as we worked. To us this was what we wanted, help and company. We didn't mind our daily routine too much. At least I didn't. We expected it. This was our routine: get out of bed before sunrise. Get dressed, wash up.

If above the age of seven, we would help at the barn or in the kitchen. By 6 a.m. we sat down to a breakfast of country ham or fried chicken, hot biscuits, milk gravy, jelly, jams, and preserves.

At each end of the long table was a pitcher of cold milk and a small pot of coffee, the latter for the adults. After the blessing, everybody ate to his heart's and stomach's content, and then made ready to start the day's work. If it was raining, we worked in the wood shed or barn. During the spring and summer months, we would hitch a team to the wagon, load it with plows, hoes, boys and our faithful dog, Shep, and head for the creek bottoms. There, we plowed and hoed 'til noon and then headed home for lunch. At about 1 o'clock, we headed back to stay 'til sundown and then called it a day. After getting home, there were other jobs: milking cows, feeding stock and hogs. After that a hearty supper, and we were off to bed for some sleep. This routine lasted from mid-April to mid-July when crops were "laid by."

Each year before planting and cultivating time, we had the worst chores to do. Cleaning out the horse stalls and the cow sheds topped the list of the bad ones. This usually lasted for a week. For us, that was "hell week." Using manure forks, shovels, and hoes, we literally dug out the cow sheds. After a full winter of droppings there was a lot of cow manure to wade in, dig out, and haul to a field, then spread by the same tools since we did not have a mechanical spreader. After each day of doing this everything smelled like cow manure. It seemed to pervade your whole body, including the lungs and taste buds. During that week, we had to undress in the wood shed, take a bath in a wash tub with lye soap, rinse off in another, and then put on clean clothing before Mama would allow us in the house—then under protest. By the time that week was over, the entire neighborhood smelled like cow manure. Everybody knew the source of the odors—the Wilson farm.

Grubbing sassafras bushes was the next worst task we had to perform. It was hard work for a ten-year-old to swing a grubbing hoe for six to eight hours a day for three days in a row. To me, it was demeaning and pure drudgery. But the humility we suffered through in the formative years of our life made me, personally, humbler and more appreciative of many things throughout the years that followed. Working as we did developed an ethic for work that helped greatly when times were hard and the going was tough. I know it helped me to try a little harder instead of losing hope or giving up. If one ever had an incentive to better one's lot in life there was no better one than working long, hard hours doing something you thoroughly disliked.

Farming as a youngster, and into my early twenties, certainly gave me that incentive to improve my lot in life. Early on as I chopped corn with my brother, Barton, who had the use of only one arm, I was inspired to do something to help my fellow man. Looking at him, I wondered what he would be doing later in life.

"Are you going to college, Barton?"

"I'll have to get my high school diploma first. Why?"

"I just wondered. You should do something besides farm."

"Oh, I don't intend to farm for a living."

"Maybe you'll be a school teacher. You're such a good person that all the kids would love you. I know I do."

"Well, thank you. Maybe I'll teach a while. But I'll have to get my AB degree first."

"What is an AB degree?"

"It means Bachelor of Arts."

"That's backwards. It should be B.A."

He laughed. "Either way is ok, but you have a good point. Are you going to college too?"

"Yeah, but I ain't gonna be no school teacher. I'm going to be a druggist, like Uncle 'Wes' or maybe even a doctor like Dad. Only, I would live and work in town."

"Those are mighty high ambitions for such a little boy. I'm proud to know you are so ambitious, though. Better start studying real hard to do all of that." We hoed on and on as I daydreamed of what I would like to be later in life.

As we chopped weeds mechanically, I was oblivious to all surroundings as I saw myself dressed in a white shirt and tie, wearing a white coat, standing behind a counter and showcase filled with bottles of medicine. I was pouring medicine from one bottle to a second one that was already half full, then shaking the bottle to mix them. Then I saw myself as a doctor, wearing a long, white coat. A stethoscope was hanging around my neck, and I was examining a frail, older woman. I was really in a dream world at that moment.

Then I heard Barton say, "I guess we're all done for today. Are you ready to go home?"

I didn't answer him because I didn't want to let go of my daydreaming. I never did really let go of that dream from that time until it became a reality.

❖   ❖   ❖

The years went by swiftly. Older brothers became restless and wanted to get away from the farm and its drudgery. Most of all they wanted to make some money and improve their lifestyle. Only two of the five oldest boys finished high school. As they would leave, a younger one would step up to fill their shoes. Only one of the five attended college. Barton finished one year at Tennessee Tech and then taught school for a few years before going on to better things. By the time my two brothers, Dennis and Prentice, graduated from high school, they too had the need to make money and left home soon after that. I was then sixteen and the oldest boy left at home. I had the responsibility of the farm over my head and expressed this to Dad. "Am I going to be responsible to make decisions about the farm management now?"

"Not all of them. We'll do it together. But in an emergency, if I'm not here, you'll have to. Think you can handle things?"

"I'll do my best. That's all I can promise."

"Oh, we'll do ok."

For that year and the first three years of college, I was the farm "manager" during the months I was not attending classes. It was good for me in that I learned something about the business side of the farm and also learned to deal with people that Dad hired from time to time as temporary help.

I missed the older brothers' companionship and advice, and would reminisce many hours about the things we had experienced together, such as Prentice and I having chicken pox at the same time. As we played inside the fenced front yard and the neighborhood "playboy" came by riding a fancy horse, he teased us about the chicken pox and asked Prentice his name. Prentice said, " 'Pence Gagn Wilson.' " "Oh, P'John," he repeated it as he rode off. An older brother heard this and began to call him P'John, which has stayed with him these many years, and he will soon be seventy-nine years of age.

Another thing I recall was the time one of us stuck a small tree branch in a yellow jacket nest in the ground and then pulled it out as we ran for home a hundred yards away. We were caught by the whole swarm just before reaching the front door. You can imagine what havoc was caused by that dumb trick, and we paid dearly for that, too.

❖   ❖   ❖

Another one of our "tricks" was the time our older brother brought his new bride home to meet the family, and we threw a dead cat from under the house as they were walking up the front walk to the house.

When P'John and I were six to eight years of age we had many extra "chores" to do. One such was requested by our Mother on the same day our oldest brother was to bring his bride home to meet the rest of the family.

Mom had noticed a foul odor coming from under the house which seemed to be near the living room area. She felt it was from a dead cat which had been missing for a day or two. About two hours before the newlyweds were expected to arrive, she called us to the kitchen with the "good" news: "Prentice, I want you and Wendell to go under the house and get that dead cat out before your brother gets here with your new "sister."

"Aw, Mom, do we have to? It stinks real bad. It will make us sick."

"No, it won't make you sick, and yes, you have to get the cat out. Now go on and do as I say!"

We dawdled around like Tom Sawyer and Huck Finn (in the famous Mark Twain story) in hopes that we would go unnoticed. No such luck — Mama saw us.

"Didn't you boys hear me? Now get under the house before it's too late. *Go on now*!"

We knew Mama meant business but we really dreaded that task. But we dreaded her wrath even more. So under the house we went, our noses and mouths covered with thick handkerchiefs, holding our breath as long as we could as we got nearer and nearer the culprit. As we reached our goal, P'John grasped the "body" and we crawled another few feet real fast. As we were crawling a car drove up, the door closed, and we heard people walking as we got far enough to throw the dead cat out, which happened to be at the same moment the couple was walking near to the house. As the cat sailed through the air, an agitated female voice said, "Oh, my, what was that?" Our big brother didn't answer as our parents were welcoming the new bride into the Wilson household.

P'John and I sniggered softly as we quietly and slowly crawled from under the house at the other end, glorying in our "timely" escapade. We didn't mention anything to Mama about the incident for a long, long time. Our brother never did.

❖ ❖ ❖

About two years before leaving home, Dennis, Prentice and I were in a fight about a work assignment that Prentice was refusing to help with. This took place in the living/bedroom after we had come home from school. We, Dennis and I, were going to force him to go. It didn't work, and as we tussled back and froth, knocking over chairs and tables, our older sister was screaming, "Stop, you're going to get hurt." That brought our mother in from outside to break up the fighting with a long apple tree sprout ready to "thrash" all of us. P'John was nearest so he got his "limbin." Dennis and I sneaked off because we thought we didn't deserve a switching. Mama vowed that she would switch us when she caught us. She kept her vow, too.

Dennis and I avoided her that night and went to bed thinking we were home free from the punishment. Before going to sleep, I recalled Mama's words, "You'll get your whipping yet." Waking up early the next morning, I jumped out of bed into my overalls, latched the door from inside (we didn't have door knobs), and put my shoes on and stood behind the door. Just then I heard Mama's footsteps coming up the stairs to the doorway. She slipped a "case knife" under the latch and opened the door. Dennis' bed was just to her right, and he was sound asleep in the "raw." She jerked the sheet off Dennis and began to strike him with the switch as she said, "I promised you this last night." Dennis came to life with a shocked look on his face, his eyes wide open, and screaming as loud as he could. Mama struck him only four licks and was turning to me to vent her wrath further. Before she could strike me, I ducked out the door, flew down the stairs, went to the grape arbor, and stayed until time for school, then joined the others as they walked to school. I never did get that promised "limbing."

One other episode: From the time I could recall, I could not stand to be teased. As I reached school age, the teasing was worse. I had a terrible temper, and my older brothers played on that. From the age of six, I thoroughly disliked girls so they teased me about the ugliest ones near my age. They also chose to tease me while we were eating and when Dad was away from home. At lunchtime one day, as our young sister-in-law was eating with us, Dennis chose to tease me about the girls. He sat at one end of the table and I at the other end. As he began, Mama asked him to stop, but he didn't. Then she stated: "Dennis, if you don't stop you may be sorry."

Then I was really mad. "That's a lie, 'Duck,'" I said. At the same time, I threw my fork the length of the table, nine or ten feet, and it struck Dennis squarely in the middle of the forehead, stayed there momentarily, then fell into his plate, leaving four bloody tine marks that trickled blood from each one onto his eyebrows and nose. Our young, teenaged sister-in-law sat there in stunned silence, pale as a ghost, eyes and mouth wide open, not believing what had happened.

Mama said: "I told you to stop Dennis, but you didn't. Now I hope you're happy. Maybe you'll listen to me next time." The meal was finished in shamed, sobering, silence as all of us realized it could have been tragic had the fork struck Dennis in an eye.

❖ ❖ ❖

In the hill country of Middle Tennessee and Southern Kentucky there were many illegal "moonshine" stills. These were a livelihood for those people engaged in making good corn whiskey, which was a high grade and potent whiskey. By government standards it was about one hundred and ten proof. Because of its strength and potency it was known as "white lightning."

This whiskey was plentiful and in great demand. The competition was also keen and the price was right (a pint 50 cents; a quart $1.50). On weekends the "white lightning" flowed freely as the natives gathered in homes and public places to socialize. Among them were some of my older brothers, who indulged some at these parties. I recall how they came in very happy and a bit loud, or sometimes barely able to make it to bed as they fell into a deep sleep to wake up next morning with a "hangover," which took most all day to overcome.

By the age of twelve I realized what was happening when their friends and cousins of the same age would gather at our house to tell of their escapades, play "pitch" or poker in the garage or barn as our parents would not allow those sinful card games to be played inside the home. During the course of the evening they would move from one place to another for a half hour, then reurn to their game. Each time they would seem a bit more bright eyed, flushed of face, more talkative and loud. I was curious and decided to spy on them. On the next visit to the garage I followed behind and hid in the shadows to watch and listen.

About eight of them, seventeen to twenty years of age, were gathered in an area where they were not seen by people passing along. "George" had a quart fruit jar that was almost full of a clear liquid. He unscrewed the lid, took two hefty swallows, then another.

"C'mon George, don't drink it all. How 'bout passin' it around?"

"Ok, here!"

"Boy! That's good stuff. Shore hits the spot, too."

Jim took the jar and shook it. Holding it up to the light that streamed in, he nodded his head and spoke: "It must be the best 'likker' made hereabouts, look at them beads. That's a sure sign of good whiskey." He took three "stiff ones," wiped his mouth on his shirt sleeve and passed it on to Paul. At the same time he shook his head. "B-r-r-r, b-r-r-r, that's potent stuff."

Paul followed with a long drink, smacked his lips, nodded and declared, "Boy, that's good! Best stuff I've ever had."

That did it! My curiosity got the best of me. I couldn't wait any longer. I had to taste that *good stuff.*

"Can I have a taste of that 'good stuff' Harlin?"

"No, you can't drink any of this. Where did you come from, anyway? Come on, go back to the house before you get in trouble."

"Why can't I have a drink?"

"You're too young, it might strangle you too."

"I'm twelve years old. Anyway, I want to see if that 'likker' is as good as y'all say it is."

"Dad will skin me alive if he finds out that we let you taste this."

"He won't never know nothin' 'bout it."

"Oh, c'mon Harlin, let the little dare-devil take a drink. Maybe then he will shut up."

"Ok. Here," he said, shoving the jar at me.

I handled the jar gingerly, almost reverently, as I shook it and watched the beading flow upward, thinking, *Boy this is bound to be good.* Then I turned the jar up to my lips, took a small swallow, then another one. I felt the hot, fiery liquid hit my throat, then flow quickly down my esophagus to my stomach where it spread over the upper half of my abdomen as it felt like fire was spreading everywhere. At the same time I was coughing, sputtering, and felt I was strangling on the stuff. Then I was able to breathe again and I knew I was ok. I felt weak, dizzy, and a little faint.

"Had enough? How did it taste? I told you what would happen. Now go on back to the house and keep quiet, you'll be ok. Think you can make it back?"

"Yes," I croaked hoarsely as I walked slowly toward the house, where I could salve my wounded pride.

As I was leaving somebody remarked, "I bet that drink cured him from taking another one for a long time." It did for more than five years, and the memory of that first swallow of "white lightning" still lingers at the age of seventy-seven.

❖   ❖   ❖

As a small child I recall "the Peddler Man" who came every other Tuesday. We could see him for 300 yards away, driving a slow team of mules hitched to a covered wagon. He came so slowly that it was agony as we waited for him to pull up to our front gate. There we waited in anticipation for his arrival so we could see all the many goodies he had in that covered wagon and to get a glimpse of his "awful-looking" right thumb.

Mr. Hale (The Peddler Man) had been born with a deformity of his right thumb which was divided into two from the last joint to the base of the nail, where the two rejoined to make only one nail. This thumb functioned normally but looked "awful" to children. Along the way someone had referred to him as "Mr. Three Thumbs" and the title had stayed with him.

"Mama, Mr. Three Thumbs is here. C'mon, Mama, hurry."

"Give me a minute 'til I get my list, the eggs and hold hens."

We hung onto the sides of the wagon like flies stuck to flypaper as we tried to see the goodies he carried.

"Good morning, Mr. Hale."

"Good morning, Miz Dee. How are you today?"

"Fine, thank you. Here's what I have to trade today."

Mr. Hale took the three hens, weighed them, and put them in a coop in back.

There are six dozen eggs, Mr. Hale. He wrote the numbers, names, weights, and prices on a dirty tablet with a stubby, dull pencil.

"What do you need today, Miz Dee?"

"Here's my list." She handed the paper to Mr. Hale who read each item, muttering and mouthing as he read. The four of us kept pushing and shoving to get closer than the others.

"C'mon, you kids get back, or I'll make you go in the house."

"Here's all ah yore stuff, Miz Dee," as he handed back each item. We held our breath as he handed back the salt, pepper, vanilla extract, etc., hoping that the next thing would be a big stick of candy.

"Is that all you need today? How about a loaf of light bread? It's only a dime."

"Oh, Mama, buy a loaf. It's so *good*."

"Oh, all right, I'll take a loaf."

"Now then, how about a big stick of peppermint candy for all these kids?"

"Get one, Mama, please."

Little sister, Kathleen, looked so forlorn that Mama couldn't say no.

"First, tell me how we stand on the hen and egg money, and what I owe you. Then we'll see."

He got out his tablet and stubby pencil, touched the pencil to his tongue, held the tongue between his teeth and figured. "The hens and eggs brought three dollars and a dime. You bought three dollars and a nickel worth of goods, so you have a nickel to spend. Since you are such a good customer, you can have that big stick of candy for the kids, and we'll call it even, ok?"

"I guess so."

We all jumped up and down. "Oh, thank you, Mama, and thank you, too, Mr. Three Thumbs—uh, uh, uh—Mr. Hale."

"Wendell, you apologize to Mr. Hale." Hanging my head, I mumbled "I'm sorry, Mr. Hale."

He clucked to his mules and looked over his shoulder, "Oh, that's ok, son, I'm used to that."

"I'm sorry, Mama, that's what everybody calls him and when he held up his right hand all I could see was the two thumbs, and it just slipped out."

As he pulled away, we waved good-bye. We watched the wagon as it moved along with heads and necks of chickens sticking up from the coops on back of the wagon, bobbing up and down with every rut and rock in its path.

The peddlers did a great service to housewives in the hills of rural Tennessee in those days as they bartered their chicken and eggs for needed kitchen supplies. I'm sure the wives and mothers were thankful for peddlers.

❖ ❖ ❖

Another service person was "The Rawleigh Man." About once a month Mr. Capshaw would show up at the front door. This man was always dressed in a striped suit, white shirt with a colorful tie, and wearing a Homburg hat. He carried a large square case which exuded pleasant smelling, mixed odors. He always greeted us with a pleasant smile and a cheerful voice.

"Hello there, you beautiful kids (we usually looked like ragamuffins with our patched overalls, dirty, bare feet and legs, and tousled heads). Is your mother at home?"

"Yeah, I'll git her; Mama, Mama, the Raleigh Man is here."

"I'll be there in a minute." Mama would come to the front door, drying her hands on her apron.

"Hello, Miz Dee. How are you today?" smiling at Mama as he removed his hat. "Do you need anything today?"

"Yes, I think so, have a seat there on the porch. I'll be right back."

Mr. Capshaw sat down, opened the large case on the floor in front of him, and waited for Mama. We all crowded around to see and smell the aromas of his wares. Mama came back in a hurry as always.

"You children move back out of the way so I can see."

Mr. Capshaw had several kinds of things: flavorings, spices, condiments, tonics, liniments, perfume, shampoo, face and body powders, body oils for ladies, shaving soaps and after-shave lotions for the men, and always the large bottles of liniment for those sore back muscles. We ogled and listened to his sales pitch as he extolled each one to Mama, hoping to sell her many things. He didn't do too well with Mama. She looked and listened, then usually bought two or three items—vanilla extract, body powder, and a large bottle of liniment, the latter of which she always kept hidden from Dad.

"Wouldn't you like some of this nice-smelling soap, Miz Dee? I'm sure the good doctor would like it."

"You're wrong. He's too busy even to notice me these days, and I'm too busy taking care of kids to care. You're nice to think of it anyway. Thank you."

"Thank you, Miz Dee. I'll see you next month." Then he always gave each of us a small stick of candy so we would welcome him back each month when he came with his large "suitcase" full of nice things for mama.

These episodes I have mentioned are only a few of many that happened in our early years.

Growing Up

When siblings were near the same age, as P'John and I were, it led to much rivalry, particularly since we had similar temperaments. This made us very competitive, leading to many arguments and fights. He usually won all the battles, and I never forgot that point. I made a vow to "whip" him some day. It never quite happened that way, but the battles became closer as we got older. Our last fight occurred when we were sixteen and seventeen. It happened on a Sunday, at home, before Mom and Dad returned from church. It was also fought in the back seat of a car. P'John was first-string catcher on the baseball team of the local "cow-pasture" league, and I was second-string catcher. They were to play out of town, and he wanted to look well-dressed for the game. He needed a new cap to wear and did not have one, but I did . He had gone to our room, got my new cap, left his old dirty one, and was wearing mine on his way to the car to leave for the game.

"Where do you think you're going with my new baseball cap?" I asked.

"We're going to Hermitage Springs for the playoffs, and I need a good cap. Since you don't need yours, I'm going to wear it."

"Oh, no, you're not! We're playing a game at Salt Lick, and I need my cap, so let me have it back. If you needed a new cap, why didn't you pick up chestnuts like I did and buy yourself one? Come on, let me have my cap."

"If you want it, come and get it."

By this time he was in the back seat of the car, and I went after him. As we tussled, slugged each other, and fought over the cap, Dennis and a friend, who were in the front seat, tried to break up the fight. In the heat of the battle, one got his face scratched, and the other had a cut lip. We both were bruised and bloody, but nobody won or lost—and I got my cap back in one piece. I was elated. I hadn't won the battle but had won a moral victory. After that we called a truce and quit fighting.

All was not work on the Wilson farm; we also found time to play. On rainy days, we would have corn-cob battles. This game was played by rules made by the older brothers and could be played by any number from two to ten. Sometimes we would have teams of three or four on each side, which is more competitive. Our one-armed brother, Barton, was the most accurate in throwing, and we had to draw straws to get him as a partner. When someone was hit three times, he was out, and whoever was Barton's opponent usually lost. Sometimes a wet cob would really hurt so bad that one would have to hide out to cry some before continuing. We didn't play that game too often because of the pain inflicted.

Other outside games were baseball, horse shoes, marbles, and ante-over (a ball was thrown over the house to be caught by the opponent; if it was caught three times that was the game), archery (we made our own bows and arrows), and track. We also fished and hunted some. When it snowed in the winter months, we did a lot of sledding as well.

Indoors there was Rook, dominoes, fox and goose, checkers, etc. Since there was a large family, we would have tournaments of the different games to make it more interesting. Again, all of these competitive games taught us to accept defeat, as well as winning each game that was played. This again prepared us for the future battles of life and made me, personally, more determined each time I wanted to accomplish something. Without those early years of trials and tribulations, I might not have been as successful in my endeavors.

Following the growing and cultivating season came the harvesting. Shortly after laying by the fields we had cultivated, blackberries would ripen, and we would take to the fallow fields and fence rows where the thorny vines grew in clusters. We had to wear long-sleeved shirts, overalls, plus heavy shoes and socks to keep from being "wounded" by the thorns. We also filled our socks and underwear with sulfur to keep chiggers off. It helped, but not 100 percent. We still got bit by the "critters." The berry picking lasted two or three days, and we were miserable. It was always hot and dry. The thorny vines would wrap around us, and the biggest, ripest berries were always the hardest ones to get. By the third day, we would be miserable with scratched, sore hands and many chigger bites in the armpits, around the waist line, in the crotch, and around the ankles—all of this in spite of our liberal use of the powdered sulfur and bathing nightly with lye soap.

At about the same time as blackberry picking came wheat "thrashing" (not threshing). I recall the first threshers being horse drawn as they moved from farm to farm. After locating, the power came from a wood-burning engine, which apparently made steam that turned a large wheel connected to the thresher box by a belt. Bundles of wheat were fed into the thresher from each side, into a "throat" that carried this into toothed, revolving drums that removed the grain. The grain fell through a chute and a fan blew the chaff and straw through a long pipe making a strawstack. Wheat threshing was a big day in the environs of Bugtussle and Punkintown, as the farmers surrounding our farm would bring their grain crops there because it was larger and more centrally located. Also, the community threshing was more economical because the travel time was slow and complicated. It also was less costly to each farmer as he paid less in toll (giving a percentage of his grain) for the threshing.

Along with the community threshing came a social event, as the farmers, wives, and small children would come and bring food for the noonday meal. Eating would be done in shifts while the threshing continued as men took turns on every part of the process. Our mother dreaded those times because she had to accommodate for all the extra people. Sometimes the threshing would last two or three days. When finished, there would be two or three different stacks of straw left in the fields, which would be hauled away by neighbors to be used to fill bed "ticks" on which people slept or be fed to animals in winter months. Wheat threshing at our place left many fond memories.

After threshing time was over, then came hay making. Mowing and raking hay was done by horse-drawn vehicles. Mowers had long blades attached to one side of the machine. When not in use, the blade was pulled to a standing position by use of a lever. It was lowered to a horizontal position by that same lever, then "geared in" by stepping on a foot pedal. That sickle blade would mow a five-foot-wide strip of hay each round. How much one mowed in a given time depended upon the speed the team would move. Since I was one that wanted to get things done in a hurry, I kept them going at a fast pace, sometimes to the chagrin of my father.

After two or three days we had to return to the same field to rake the hay. Raking was also done with horse-drawn machinery. This vehicle was pulled by two mules. This machine was six-feet wide, had wheels four feet tall with several curved tines between the wheels and a seat for the driver. A six-foot-long tongue of wood extended in front with a cross bar near the end with a strap on each end of the bar which would be attached to the horses' (mules') collar. To the right of the driver's seat was a lever to raise and lower the long fingers (tines) which gathered the mown hay as one moved along. Again, the driver efficiency was judged by the time it took to rake a field of hay. I never hurried very much with this chore, since the smell of new mown hay was so relaxing and pleasant that it would almost lull me to sleep. It was one of the most pleasing chores on the farm. As one moved along picking up the hay, it was easy to daydream or reminisce about past activities or build castles in the air about your future. Dumping the full load was mechanical as one pulled the lever, dumped the hay, let the lever down, and continued on.

The last part of haying was the toughest. First the long, windrows had to be raked from the ends to midfield, then picked up by hand with pitch forks, loaded onto a hay wagon, trampled into place by someone on the wagon, hauled to the barn, then unloaded with a hay fork, and dumped in the hay loft. The last part took three people to perform the task. One to push the hay fork down into the loose hay, extend and lock the two lateral prongs in place, tell the driver to start the mule to move the load along a track situated inside the barn near the peak of the roof, as the form operator held onto a long, trip rope. The third person inside the barn would yell loudly "trip." Simultaneously, the mules stopped, the hay-load was dumped, and the process repeated until the wagon was emptied. Now you can understand why Dad needed so many boys to operate the farm. It is also easy to understand why all nine of the Wilson boys wanted to leave farm life at an early age.

After haying time came, harvesting was done of the root crops, the fall fruits, the dried beans, and peas sown in the cornfields after the last plowing. The dried beans were stored in the grain shed, along with wheat, oats, and barley, all in separate bins. The dried beans were shelled by beating them with tobacco sticks, then separating the hulls from the grain by hand. This was a long, tedious method, but it kept us busy and out of mischief.

Later on Dad bought a "pea sheller." This machine separated the hulls and grain as the unshelled beans were fed into a hopper at one end as someone else was turning a crank which shelled the beans and peas, then blew the hulls out the opposite end. This was a wonderful invention and again saved us many hours of drudgery.

By the time we had reached high-school age most everything on our farm was becoming mechanized except the plowing. This we still did with mules. Dad felt that it was too dangerous for smaller boys to use a tractor on a hillside farm with several small fields to cultivate. So, in essence, I was a plowboy until the age of twenty. By that time I realized the wisdom of Dad's thinking and also realized that it would be my last year to work on the Wilson farm. It was unbelievable how smart Dad had become that last year I was at home.

The "early years" would not be complete if I did not recount some of the many laughable, happy, and comical, as well as the sad, tragic, and near-tragic incidents that happened. Some I have already recounted, such as the swimming "lessons" and the "dead cat" episode. I also recall an incident of our preteen years as four or five of us were skinny-dipping in the creek, about 100 feet from a little-traveled country road. Our clothes were in separate piles on the creek bank near the road. Suddenly, a giggly female voice got our attention, and we all went underwater, then popped our heads back out to see a half-dozen girls our age standing on the creek bank laughing at us. They had put all of our clothes in one big pile near the road. Boy, were we in trouble. Our leader, Pete West, spoke up.

"Why don't you girls go on home?"

"Oh, no, we want to watch ya'll swim a while first."

"Aw, come on, let us alone."

"No, this is fun. We want to see your big 'muscles.' You're always bragging about how tough you are, so we'll just watch a while. Don't you think they're cute, Mable?"

"Oh, yes, especially P'John with his 'BIG' muscles and his purty black eyes."

"I'll bet he's a good swimmer, too. Let's see you swim, P'John. I dare you."

Prentice took the dare. "Ok, here goes." As he swam away his buttocks came up just above the water. They all screamed, hid their faces and giggled, then cheered.

"Now are you satisfied, Mable? Go on home and leave us be."

"Ok, we'll go. Don't you want your clothes first?" They all giggled again, picked our clothes up, moved them nearer the road, and left. By this time the sun was almost setting, and we were still afraid to get out, and afraid not to, because we all had chores to do once we got home.

The girls just sauntered off, as they looked over their shoulders, giggling of their triumph over us big "men." I don't know how many of the gang remembered that incident as I still do and still laugh about it, too.

Another incident happened to me at age thirteen. By that age, we were allowed to go hunting alone. I chose a cold day in November to take my initial, solitary hunt. All of us boys hunted with the old double-barreled, .12-gauge shotgun. It kicked like a mule, and everybody had bruised shoulders after a hunt or when a big brother allowed us to fire the gun. I knew this and dreaded to hunt with it, but I had to prove that I was man enough to be on my own. Dad was away on call so I had to ask Mom's permission. I waited until she was alone so an older brother wouldn't snicker when I asked. "Mom, can I go rabbit hunting by myself today?"

"Are you sure you can handle that big old gun?"

"Oh, yeah, I've shot it before."

"Did it 'kick' very hard?"

Shrugging my shoulders, I said, "Some, but it didn't hurt much. Can I go?"

"I guess so, but don't stay long. If you do I'll really worry about you."

"I won't. It's 10 o'clock now. I'll be back by 3."

"Make it 2 and I'll let you go."

I wrapped up, put on a stocking cap and gloves, took the shotgun with six shells and went off. I hunted the fields and woods for a half mile from the house where the rabbits usually lived in abundance. By 1 o'clock, I had not seen a single one, so I started back home. As I was walking through the orchard, which was overgrown with weeds and sagebrush, there was a sudden movement and something brown running away. I had my rabbit! I put the gun to my shoulder, caught the brown 'animal' in sight and fired. There was a writhing of agony, then all was still. *Boy, that must be a big rabbit*! I hurried to find the "kill," pulling the weeds back to see—I was shocked. Lying there was one of Mama's fat, brown hens. *Now I'm really stunned! What should I do?* I sat there for at least ten minutes pondering my fate. Should I take the hen home and face the ridicule of all the older brothers or should I just bury her and carry the quilt with me? I decided to face the music and suffer the consequences. I knew Mom would miss that old hen, and I could hear her saying: "One of my biggest, fattest hens is missing. I wonder what happened to her. Have you seen her, Wendell?"

"No, Mama. How many did you have?"

"Twenty-two—and now I count only twenty-one."

"Aw, you probably just miscounted, Mama."

Now my conscience began to hurt and told me to take the hen to Mama, or I would be sorry. So that is what I did.

That 100 yards seemed two miles long. As I walked along very slowly, each foot seemed to weigh ten pounds, and each step I made took a supreme effort. When I got there I hid the hen in the woodshed, went into the house, put the gun away, and faced Mama.

"I have to talk to you, Mama. Just you and me."

"Why all the mystery? It must be awfully serious," she replied.

"No, I just want to talk to you first without other big ears around. Can we go outside?"

"Sure, come on."

We stopped in front of the woodshed. I looked all around, then in the woodshed to be sure no one was in earshot. "I have something to tell you. But first, tell me you won't be mad at me, ok?"

"I promise not to fuss at you. Now tell me before I die with curiosity."

"Uh, I killed one of your hens." Then I gave her a step-by-step account of what happened—and held my breath. She didn't get mad at all. Instead she laughed a big, hearty laugh and asked where the hen was.

"I put her in the woodshed 'til I talked to you."

"That's good. We can have her for supper tonight. I'm proud of you for telling me the truth. It took a lot more grit to do that rather than just burying her and never telling about it."

"Thanks, Mama. I knew you'd understand. I'll be ok if nobody else finds out about this now."

"They won't tonight if it's left up to me."

Somehow they found out. In a few days, Dennis began to call me Dan'l Boone, and I could laugh about it by that time. I'm sure there were many more comical escapades that I can't recall now.

Some near tragedies and two real tragedies occurred in the family during those early years. The second born child died at a few months of age as our mother was recovering from typhoid fever. The third son was critically injured at the age of nine when he fell from a wagon, under the rear wheel, which ran over his left lower neck and shoulder. The two older brothers and two older cousins were with him. They lifted the wagon up off him as he lay unconscious and bleeding from both ears and his nose. They thought he was dead when someone pulled him from under the wheel and noticed he was breathing. They somehow got him home, which was a mile from the scene. Our mother said he hovered near death and unconscious for two or three weeks before he regained consciousness and began to move. When this happened she noticed that he could not move his left arm and hand. As he improved, Dad had two of his colleagues to examine and consult regarding what course to take as treatment of the paralyzed extremity. This tragedy occurred in 1917, when major surgery and general anesthesia were both very, very risky to life. It was, however, considered, and Barton was told of the possibilities and given a choice. He was resolute in that he refused to consider amputation of the arm.

"Son, your arm and hand will be useless the rest of your life."

"No, it won't, you'll see."

"Whatever you want to do, you'll have a lot of pain and suffering for a long time. But if you think you can stand the pain, I agree to watch and wait. If you change your mind in future years, surgery will be less risky by then."

Barton went on to recover over a period of many months. During that period he learned to do everything necessary for day-to-day living with his one hand. By the time we younger siblings realized he could not use the left arm and hand he was helping us learn those routine chores and living habits. Throughout the growing years, I marveled at how fast and accurate he did things. He could shoot a gun faster and more accurate than most of us. Dressing was nothing to him. He could tie his shoes, button his shirt, and tie his tie as quick as a wink. Barton loved sports. He fished, hunted and trapped game. He played baseball and basketball, pitched horseshoes, played marbles and anything that came along. We never thought of him as being handicapped. With all this, he was a successful businessman. At one time he owned two businesses, ran a dairy farm, and "oversaw" another farm. I admired and almost idolized Barton.

Some of the near tragedies also had comical twists. One brother, Harold, was kicked in the chin and mouth by our workhorse, Dan. The horse moved slowly and as Harold turned him loose into a pasture, he slapped old Dan across the hind quarters with the bridle. As he did, the horse retaliated with a lazy, soft kick that landed on Harold's chin and knocked him to the ground. He was stunned, but not badly injured or unconscious. He learned a valuable, painful lesson. Never trust a lazy horse. That same brother had a terrible case of poison ivy in his early teens. It involved his lower body and extremities to the point that he was unable to wear pants. Mom solved that problem by putting him in dresses for a two- or three-week period. Of course, all the brothers and his close friends "ragged" him constantly. We thought it was a payback for the constant teasing he was guilty of doing to us younger ones.

The second oldest brother, Harlin, suffered a ruptured appendix in his late twenties and was critically ill just before and for several days after he had emergency surgery. He spent a two-month recovery period at home with our parents keeping close watch over him. He was fortunate in that there was an excellent, board-certified surgeon and a good friend of our father's that lived and practiced in the small town of Scottsville, Kentucky, only thirty-five miles from our home. Without his knowledge and surgical skills, Harlin might not have survived.

There were no other critical illnesses or injuries in the family that I recall, or had related to me by my parents or older siblings. However, we had our share of minor illnesses and some surgery. An unforgettable trip to Dr. Graves' Hospital in Scottsville, Kentucky was made on a hot August day in 1933 to have our tonsils out. The trip was made in an open Model A Ford over dusty, unpaved country roads. Dad drove at a steady speed of thirty, never slowing down for ruts, mud holes, chickens, or dogs. The dust boiled up and into the car, filling our eyes, nose, and mouth. It was so bad that one could not see fifty feet behind the car. We arrived about 8:30. Dr. Graves came in soon after to examine us. He looked at our throats and commented on our "rotten" tonsils—then listened to our heart and lungs, then pronounced us okay to have surgery.

"What's your name, Son?"

"Wendell Wilson."

"Who gave you that name?"

"My Mama did. don't you like it?"

"Not particularly, but I don't like mine either."

"What's your name?"

"Lattie. Sounds almost like a girl, doesn't it?"

"Mine does, too. So I guess we're even."

"Well, names don't mean much anyway. Now let's get on with the tonsillectomy. First, we'll do a little lab work. Julie will be here in a second."

No sooner had he left than a beautiful brunette came in with the lab tray filled with syringes and needles, small bottles, and test tubes. I was so struck by her beauty that I hardly noticed when she drew blood. Then she spoke. "There, that wasn't so bad, was it?"

"Humh? Nn—no, I hardly felt the needle." I was so mesmerized by her that they could have done the surgery while she held my hand. Then I came back to reality when an elderly nurse came in.

"Are you Wendell Wilson?"

"Yes, Ma'am."

"Ok, I have a pill for you here."

She gave me a small white-and-yellow capsule which I recognized as being 50 mgs. of Nembutal. I was afraid to take it. "Do I have to take this."

Looking down at me over her glasses, she put her hands on her hips and said in a clear, firm voice, "Yes, you do, and with only one small sip of water, too."

I swallowed the pill while she scowled at me to be sure I did. Within a few minutes I felt drowsy and was ready for a nap. Not yet. In came that same nurse. "Let's take you to surgery. Here, get in this wheelchair." Getting up I almost fell as I got into the wheelchair and rode into the operating room. "Let me help you into this chair," she went on.

This was a special, operative chair for doing ear, nose, and throat surgery as the patient sat in a semi-erect position. I was so drowsy and weak that

I was not able to sit erect. Then Dr. Graves came in with his white cap, mask, and gown on. Everything was a white blur to me. He spoke to me in a voice from a distance, "Are you ok now, Son?"

I mumbled a slurred "Yessir."

He grabbed my shoulders and pulled me erect. "You'll have to sit up now so we can get these tonsils out. Now open your mouth and keep it open."

My world was still a blur—I was s-o-o-o sleepy. Then the stern, faraway voice said again—"Sit up there." And someone jerked me by the shoulders. My throat didn't hurt at all, it was filled with instruments and blood. He had removed my tonsils! I didn't care; I just wanted to sleep.

Pretty soon, I woke up. My throat was killing me. Then I saw Hallie in the bed next to me, sound asleep. The next thing I knew Dad was shaking me awake. "Come on, Wendell, it's time to go home."

Somehow we got into the car and started the long two-hour trip back home in that same hot, open car. We took off in a cloud of dust. Within twenty minutes the nausea and vomiting started. Dad kept up that 30 m.p.h. pace, as we leaned out and let go of our bloody stomach contents.

"Please stop, Dad. I need a drink of water."

Hallie said, "My throat hurts, too."

"Ok, we'll stop at Hayesville store. We'll need to get some basins, if you throw up again."

The water was wonderful as we drank the cool liquid from a dipper. It soothed our raw throats and made it possible to continue the trip.

We took off again with each of us holding a shiny tin wash pan. They came in handy too since the nausea soon came back. We fought and fought, but we lost the battle, and we also lost all of that cool, sweet well water we drank just a half hour before. We endured the torture for another hour as Dad sailed over those rough, unpaved country roads while the dust boiled behind us, the chickens flew up in front of us, and the dust engulfed us, burning our eyes and nostrils and filling our lungs. We arrived home at 4 o'clock, barely able to speak or walk. Hallie recovered within a week, but I continued to bleed some and could take only bland liquids in small amounts for another two weeks, plus another two weeks doing nothing before recovering. That tonsillectomy was a sad, destructive experience, one that will never be forgotten.

Dad took care of our minor surgery problems such as lacerations that required suturing, boils and abscesses that had to be surgically drained, as well as the many stone bruises that also had to be drained. This latter problem was a bit more complicated since it was a deep abscess of the heel. With the hard, thick, tough skin of the heel it could not drain (rupture itself as "boils" often did). These occurred during late summer and fall after going barefoot for long periods and bruising the heel. They would really hurt, so much that the tough brothers cried and stayed awake nights from pain. We all tried to hide it from Dad as we knew the surgery was imminent if he saw us walking on our toes to avoid the pain. He always caught the "victim."

"Prentice, do you have a stone bruise?"

"Yeah, just a little one. It don't hurt too much."

"Come here and let me see." P'John lay across the bed as Dad examined him.

"Is this were it hurts?"

"No," answered P'John.

Dad put more pressure on the spot, and P'John pulled his heel away. "Does that hurt," asked Dad?

"Yeah, that hurts when you mash so hard!"

"You need that abscess drained or it'll get worse. Wendell, get my instrument bag, also the alcohol and merthiolate. Dennis, get a pan of warm water and soap. You stay where you are, Prentice. Scrub his heel, put some alcohol and merthiolate on it, and we will drain it."

During this time, he had "sterilized" a scalpel in a solution of bichloride of mercury.

"Now Harold, you and Dennis hold his legs and feet. Now, grit your teeth, Prentice. Get the gauze sponges ready, Wendell." All did his bidding and waited breathlessly. With one swift, sure movement of the scalpel, Dad opened the abscess so quickly that P'John felt no pain until the purulent fluid came rolling out. Then he yelled and tried to kick as tears rolled down his cheeks. Dad slipped a small rubber drain in the incision. We applied a dressing, and P'John hopped off as he wiped away his tears.

This surgical procedure was done on all nine of us boys at some time in our growing years. It may sound barbaric, but it was the only way to relieve the pain and prevent complications from the abscess. Within a day or two the "patient" would be walking normally again. (No antibiotics had to be given.) Mama did most of the treatments in our family; she used the home remedies as her medications or treatments: cool-water soaks for acute strains an sprains, mustard plasters for pleurisy, three or four drops of coal oil on half a teaspoonful of sugar for coughs, oil of cloves in a hollow tooth to relieve toothache, calomel to "purge" us with our spring sickness followed by a "round" of sulfur and molasses and warm, sweet oil for earaches. Dad didn't always agree with her treatments, which they sometimes argued about, but her results were as good as his. She had no disastrous complications, and we lived to be full-grown.

There were some special events in our lives on the farm. Some I have mentioned and others are unforgettable, which I will describe. One in particular has been deeply etched in my bank of memories. That one is ... "Hog-killing" time in Tennessee.

This event always took place in the coldest days of winter, usually November or December. To prepare for this, we would select the hog to be slaughtered a week or so earlier and move it to a smaller enclosure to add more weight by feeding larger amounts. As the day for slaughter came closer, Dad had been preparing for the event. First, a three-by-six-foot trench was dug about eighteen to twenty inches deep; four two-inch-wide strips were laid across the trench about sixteen inches apart. These supported a heavy metal pan which was longer than the ditch, three feet wide and two feet deep. A platform of heavy oak plank four feet wide was built on each side of the "scalding pan." About six feet from this stood a cedar post that was six inches thick and eight feet tall. Three feet from the top, there was a "lift" pole, angled so the short end extended three feet from the post and the longer end touched the ground where it was anchored. The night before the date of slaughter, a fire was laid under the pan between the platforms. Before daylight on hog-killing day, the fire was lit and the long pan filled with water. Within an hour or so the water was hot, and the butchering crew gathered. Dad was usually around, along with two or three older boys and two sharecroppers who were well experienced in this. The mode of transporting the hog's carcass had been made ready (a mule-drawn slide) and the hogs were feeding, unsuspecting of their fate.

The butchers went into the pen armed with a heavy ax and a small rifle. If possible the hog was knocked in the head and killed; sometimes the rifle had to be used. The hog was then dragged to one side to have the throat (neck) slit with a large butcher knife to allow all blood to drain from the body while it was still warm. Since all of this was being done before time for school, we were allowed to watch the proceedings. When the bleeding stopped each hog was loaded onto the mule-drawn sled, two at a time, and moved to the scalding platform. By now the water was near boiling and ready for the next step. Heavy chains, anchored on one end, lay across in the pan. The hogs were lowered into the pan, then rolled back and forth by men as they alternated pulling and loosening the chains. As they were rolling the hog, an experienced person would check from time to time to see if the hair was loosening. When it was ready, the chains were anchored on the opposite side, the hog rolled onto the platform on that side, and the men would scrape the hair from the carcass with butcher knives. Each man usually had his own favorite knife for this job.

After all the hair was removed, a slit was made in each back leg just in front of the tendon and a two-foot long, heavy hickory stick, sharpened at each end was inserted beneath the tendon and the carcass removed to the hanging pole. There the long end of the pole was raised, to lower the opposite end. The carcass was hoisted up to the desired height, the hickory stick placed in a notch of the pole, to suspend the hog carcass head down, for the next phase of butchering to begin. First, the carcass was rinsed thoroughly with warm, then cold water. Next, the belly was opened its entire length, ending at the cut made in the neck at the time of actual killing. The entire small and large intestines were removed and discarded. The urinary bladder and kidneys were removed and saved. The kidneys were used for some special food, and the urinary bladder was thoroughly cleansed so we younger children could insert a small reed into the neck and blow it up, tie a string around the neck, hang it out to dry, and have a balloon to play with for several days. The liver was removed and saved for food.

The carcass was then lowered to a table, the head removed, the chest opened, the heart and lungs removed, thoroughly irrigated; then the rest of the body was cut into the usual cuts of hams, shoulders, bacon (known in the country as "sowbelly"). Dad and one of the sharecroppers were expert trimmers of these parts of porkers, and they trimmed closely. These trimmings were put in separate containers to be ground into sausage. Ribs and backbones were separated with axes and heavy knives, and usually eaten shortly after hog-killing time. Excess fat trimmed from the hogs was separated and cooked in a big black kettle outside over an open fire. This was known as "rendering lard." This was used as cooking oil when beans, corn, and other vegetables were cooked, and also used when frying meat, fish, and poultry.

The "hog killing," with all its afterkill procedures, lasted for a week or more. There was one part of the hog considered a delicacy—the brain. Getting to this part was not a delicate procedure. However, only our father and his trusted sharecropper friend, Ollie Rush, were allowed to do that. It had to be done with heavy butcher knives and an ax, removing the jowls and ears before the skull was opened to remove the brain.

The sausage grinding was done by hand and lasted for several days because it was an after-school chore and would last into the night hours. Every part of the hog possible was used or preserved for food. Hog killing was usually done at two different times because of the family size. The second butchering time was not so exciting as we remembered the hard work and long hours spent at the different tasks. Each of these times, eight to ten hogs were butchered. That meant that every year, during our childhood and teen years, we would spend two weeks of the year butchering hogs. It's no wonder I have never forgotten those days.

Other big events each year were July 4th, Thanksgiving, and Christmas. We actually celebrated more on Independence Day than either of the others. I have always felt it was because our parents had heard so much from their grandparents regarding that era in their lives.

We would become excited a week before that day since there was always a picnic and a fish fry. The neighborhood families would gather at a certain home about mid-morning. The fathers and older sons would go fishing with spears and arrows. By noontime they would come in with their catch, usually enough to feed everyone there. But there would be fried chicken, country ham, and other meats. There were vegetables galore, homemade breads, cakes and pies in great numbers, and everybody ate to their heart's content. Afterward the men would talk about the fish they caught for dinner, and the women chatted about families, and the children would play games. Later, we sang hymns and patriotic songs before each family returned to their respective homes.

Thanksgiving was not as large a celebration as the 4th of July, but a day that we set aside for celebration and relaxation. There was a bountiful feast with all the family there to enjoy together. There were no turkeys in the Tennessee hills, but chicken was plentiful, and it was served baked, fried, and cooked with dumplings. We also had country ham and sausage with hot biscuits and homemade sourdough bread. To all of this was added vegetables in abundance, plus jams, jellies, and preserves, to say nothing of cakes and pies. Most of all, the traditional pumpkin pie was all spiced and topped with a thick meringue made with rich cream. That day and that meal were always fit for a king.

Christmas! What a glorious day it was. We would start counting the days and marking the calendar about two weeks before time. There were some pre-Christmas events at school and a community Christmas tree at our church. There we had a day for decorating the tree, then a ceremony on Christmas Eve with some gifts for small children and recitations and singing followed by speeches—then a prize for the best recitation. Once or twice I won, which really inflated my ego.

That night at home we would try to find out what we would receive from Santa, and how he could make it down the chimney without getting burned.

Deep down we knew who Santa really was, but we played the game and went to bed early so we could wake up to catch Santa in action, but never did.

There was not always a tree and often not many gifts. We always hung our stockings on the mantle with our names pinned on each, hoping to get them filled. They always had an apple, an orange, some candy, and sometimes a banana. Those things were hard to find, and we counted our blessings when "Santa" left them in our stockings, and cherished the memory of those gifts. During the day, we played games, sang Christmas songs and hymns as Mama played the old pump organ and sang with us in her beautiful alto voice. That was the most enjoyable day of the year for the entire family.

After the celebration came the Christmas dinner. It was something to behold. The table was loaded with food: two or three kinds of meat, vegetables of all varieties, three kinds of breads, jams, jellies, preserves, pudding, cakes, and pies covered a sideboard near the table. It was a meal beyond comparison.

Birthdays were made into a special event, particularly for the honoree as they would be granted a special request for their favorite cake or pie for dessert on that occasion. Sometimes tricks would be played on the recipient. I recall the older brothers doing this to our older sister, Hallie, in late November just after "hog-killing" time. She was a teenager at the time. An older, trusted brother presented a covered dish to her after the meal. "Hallie, since you're the oldest girl in the family, we want you to have this special gift from all us boys." Then he set the dish in front of her. She looked at the plate, then back at Harlin, saying, "Thank you, Harlin." Then Hallie uncovered the dish. Her face fell and took on an anguished look. I saw her eyes fill with tears and wondered why. In the plate was a pig tail. At the same time, the older boys were singing "Happy Birthday," clapping their hands and laughing. Hallie's face was flooding with tears as she left the table screaming, "I hate all of you awful boys." The laughing stopped as they regretted their little joke that spoiled their sister's birthday.

Birthdays usually ended on a happy note with the honoree getting a light spanking, being struck the same number of times as his birthday and "one to grown on." After this he would be put under the bed for five minutes, and the ritual was over. These rituals continued through the years until we all grew older and stopped because it ceased to be fun anymore. It was always something for all of us to remember and recall some of the incidents that happened at birthday times.

One of the most memorable things that occurred in the Wilson home was going to school for the first time. Everyone was excited to attend that first day. We younger ones would see the older ones come in from school excited about something that happened that day, telling Mama about it. It aroused our curiosity and made us *want* to start as soon as possible.

"Mama, when can I start to school?"

"When you're old enough."

"How long will that be?"

"Oh, in another year or two."

"That's a long time yet. I want to go now."

"You'll just have to wait until you are at least five. Now run on and play."

We'd sulk a bit, then soon forget all about school until another exciting event we heard about. It still gave us something to look forward to every year.

All of the Wilson clan attended Enon School, the only one in our vicinity. The building was about fifty to sixty feet long by thirty to forty feet in width, all in one room. There were two doors in front, separated by about fifteen feet, one for the smaller children and the other one for the larger ones. There was a row of windows on each side of the building, but none at either end. The building was heated by one large pot-bellied stove that sat in the exact center of the building and was used only in the coldest of the winter months. At the rear end of the room, which the pupils faced, there was a long blackboard that accommodated the entire building. The building was filled with school desks of various sizes for the eight grades that would attend. All eleven of us Wilson children attended this school. There was a spacious playground, large enough for baseball and basketball, and a croquet court. Water supply for Enon School was from a well near the building. There were two buckets and two dippers, one for the girls and one for the boys. Toilet facilities were available for the girls as a large, outdoor toilet, northwest of the building. I do not remember a "privy" for the boys, but I do recall our using the wood southeast of the building for "nature's calls."

There was not a separate dining space in the building so families as large as the Wilson gang would gather inside and have lunch together. Lunch usually consisted of meat, bread, vegetables, and dessert, with extra food for some more unfortunate pupils that had no lunch. Weather permitting, we gathered outside on a flattened log with our two baskets of food, where we had an uninvited guest or two to enjoy the fried chicken or country ham with us. Our parents expected this of their children, and we enjoyed having guests, as well. Mama always inspected the baskets after school, then asked, "Well, who did you feed today?"

"Oh, Tim Holloway didn't have any lunch, and he looked hungry, so I asked him. Was that ok, Mama?"

"Yes, of course, it was. It's not his fault that he had no food. It's because his daddy is too lazy to work." She never stopped sending extra food as long as we attended Enon School.

Going to school regularly for the first time was a thrill. It meant we were growing up. We could also be away from home all day, play games at lunch and recess times each day, and be with friends every day, too. I entered the first grade at age six. I recall very little of that first year, but because of an incident that occurred in the second grade, I have never forgotten that year of school.

As we sat in class late one fall morning, Tim Holloway came in and sat down beside me. He smelled dirty and looked unwashed. Then he started scratching, and I noticed a rash between his fingers that looked like scabies, and moved to another seat. Our spinster teacher, Miss Hattie Harwood, really got angry with me and spoke harshly: "Wendell Wilson, you get back in your seat. Just because you're the doctor's son you think you're too good to sit by Tim!"

"No ma'am, I ain't too good to sit by him or anyone else, but he has the each (itch), ma'am and I'll get it."

"No, you won't. Get back in that seat or I'll paddle you."

I didn't want the "itch" and neither did I want a paddling. I decided to take my changes with Tim. That was a *bad* mistake. That night I told Mama the story and she was so mad that she called "Miss Hattie" and blessed her out. "If he gets the itch, I'll hold you responsible because all the other kids will get it, too. You knew better. Why didn't you use a little common sense instead of exposing the whole class to this filthy stuff. I ought to get you fired."

Mom was right. In four or five days I began to itch between my fingers, under my arms, and other places. Pretty soon two or three brothers started the same thing, and scabies was in full swing at the Wilson home. Every night for two weeks all of us would be treated. First, we filled a wash tub half full of water, scrubbed the entire body with lye soap, then rinsed in cool, clean water in a second tub. Then we applied a mixture of lard and flowers of sulfur to make a paste. We applied it to the whole body and would sleep between clean sheets every night. Each of the beds was stripped each morning, bedding was washed in lye soap and boiled for half an hour in a big black iron wash kettle and hung on the line to dry. Our clothing was treated the same way. At the end of two weeks the itch was gone. I never sat by Tim again. Neither did Mom every forgive "Miss Hattie."

During the first four years of school we had two teachers. Miss Hattie taught first and second grades, and Mrs. Lena Birdwell taught third and fourth grades. Miss Hattie was a very good teacher but used some poor judgment concerning her pupils, as I have related.

Mrs. Lena was an excellent teacher. She was redheaded and had a fiery temper that made us fear and respect her. She was a strict disciplinarian. She did an excellent job of teaching the basics of readin', writin', and 'rithmetic; sometimes "to the tune of a hickory stick" (as the song goes). We had spelling contests, reading drills, and exercises in problem solving ('rithmetic) at the blackboard. Her methods really gave me an incentive to learn and a good basis for understanding the higher grades. Unexpectedly, she would call out a name. "Wendell, come up here and spell the work 'understanding'—then pronounce it correctly by each syllable." She would say: "Raymond, come up here to the blackboard—now let's add 12 and 16." Most of the time he was not able to solve simple, third grade math problems. He was a slow learner and two years older than his classmates, much larger and had a hard time reading. I was his private tutor in reading and spelling. He, in turn, was my buddy and bodyguard. Nobody picked on me. Raymond wouldn't allow that. Reading and spelling were my strong points, and Mrs. Lena bragged on me just before spelling bees, and we usually won, giving me an ego boost.

By the time we reached fourth grade, Mrs. Lena was teaching that grade also. Then she took on the fifth grade the following year. So our education followed the same pattern, which was much better for the students because of the continued method of teaching.

By the time I had reached the sixth grade, students started dropping out of school for various reasons, and classes became smaller and smaller. By the seventh grade, we had only one teacher, my eldest brother, a math whiz. Not only was I under my brother in the seventh grade, but the only student enrolled in that grade. Fred expected perfection from me, which was impossible since math was my weakest subject. His tolerance level was low when it came to my not understanding mathematical problems. He literally "gave me hell" for this weakness and punished me for not doing math problems assigned as homework. His method of punishment was either to stand at the blackboard for five minutes with your nose in a ring, or stand facing the classroom for five minutes while holding a geography book with your arm extended. It was real punishment too; I know by having been through both. Neither seemed to improve my math skills.

Covering both seventh- and eighth-grade subject matter that year was challenging, but it kept me busy and out of mischief. It also taught me to accept and meet a challenge head-on. I did well; made better grades than eighth graders on examinations in everything, except math, in which I only made Bs and Cs. Since I did so well overall, it boosted my ego and increased my desire for learning. As the school year was near closing, Fred asked me to stay after school. I just knew that he was planning to get after me for not doing better in math. I was prepared for anything. He surprised me.

"Wendell, would you like to take the eighth grade examination that is given by the county superintendent and go on to high school next year?" he asked.

"Yes, I'd like to take the exam, but I don't think I want to go on to high school this fall," I said.

"Why not?" he continued, "You know the subject matter really well, and I think you'll do fine on the examination, even math."

"That's not the problem," I explained. Dennis and Prentice will both be leaving next fall, and I will be needed more at home. Besides, I had just rather wait another year to start with my own age group. I think I'll do better with another year of maturity. Can I still take the examination even if I still won't go?"

"Sure you can," he said.

So I took the examination and passed with flying colors. I even did *very* well in mathematics. That exempted me from the next year's examination. That was in 1931. That April, I turned fourteen and was the oldest full-time boy at home. I also was five feet two inches tall and weighed 100 pounds soaking wet. Regardless of that size, I felt my "oats," strutted my "stuff," and shaved my face to show that I was a man to be reckoned with. Boy, what a fool I was!

Late spring and early summer came too soon. We had a daily routine as in earlier years, but I had to be the responsible one. Getting up at 4 a.m. to do the chores, back to the house for breakfast, and then to work a ten- to twelve-hour day was not easy to look forward to every day.

With all the hard work and well-learned lessons of working the farm, other things were also learned, such as how to survive a drought, which occurred in the summer of 1931 and '32, when streams dried up and crops failed, as did the economy. Along with this came the Great Depression, followed by bank and business failures, resulting in many, many suicides and bankruptcies. Hunger and disease were rampant, followed by increased numbers of ill people as the death rate soared. This directly affected our family, as our father's workload increased sharply, and his income fell drastically.

Because of these conditions, foodstuffs that we grew and livestock we raised for meat supply were also scarce. The drinking water supply also ran low, and that became a critical situation. The fruits and berries did not produce and in early fall, Mama sent P'John and me to the woods in search of wild berries or grapes. The only thing to be found were the small "possum" grapes that grew high up in the trees, where only the opossum would climb to get them. We devised a way to beat the wily possum. Tying a long rope to a bucket handle, then to his body, P'John climbed the tree as high as possible, sometimes tying himself to a tree limb, picked the grapes, then lowered the bucket of grapes to me as I waited on the ground. That was both difficult and dangerous grape picking. But the rewards were well worth it and appreciated by the whole family that winter as we ate that delicious "possum jelly" with hot, buttered, homemade biscuits.

The scarcity of drinking water almost resulted in a tragedy. In late summer Dad decided that we should dig the well a few feet deeper to have a larger supply of water. Since it was solid rock, it was necessary to blast it out with dynamite. Our sharecropper, Hubert Shoulders, took on the task. By the end of the second day he and Dad decided that a blast would be set off at the end of that day, then uncover the well for the night, then begin to remove the rock and debris the next morning. The blasting was successful, and the well was opened for twelve hours to allow it to "air out." Hubert arrived early the next morning and prepared to go down into the well. As he came up, someone spoke to him and asked if he thought it was safe yet. "I don't know, but we'll soon find out," he answered.

"It still smells bad. You had better be careful or somebody may be hauling you out of there."

Dad came in then and said, "You boys get ready for school. I'll watch and talk to Hubert, and I'll call if he has a problem."

Pretty soon we heard Dad calling every few seconds. Then his voice became urgent, then almost frantic. We all ran the few steps to check: "What's wrong, Dad?"

"Hubert doesn't answer, and he isn't tied to the cable. See?" The cable and a five gallon bucket were hanging there as a stark reminder of Hubert's peril.

Without any hesitation P'John said: "Lower me down." Dennis grabbed the windlass handle as P'John stepped into the bucket and we rapidly lowered him the thirty feet to the bottom of the well. No voices!

"Are you ok, Prentice?"

"Yes, pull us up as fast as you can."

Dennis and I were really pouring out adrenalin by then and brought that 250 pounds the thirty feet in a few seconds. P'John had tied a rope around Hubert, lashed him to the cable, stood in the bucket, hugging the victim, all the while trying to pump his chest. When they surfaced, Dad grabbed them both. We took Hubert outside and noted he was very pink. Dad commented, "Carbon monoxide," and as we laid him on the ground and pumped his chest three or four times, he began to breathe on his own. Dad was trembling from head to toe as he shook his head.

"I sure am glad you boys were still here. We might have had a dead man to get from that well."

"It's all over now, Dad, and Hubert will be okay," I said. "Is it all right if we go on to school now?"

"Let me settle down a bit. Then take Hubert to the porch, in the shade, before all of you leave."

Without a word, we did his bidding, each deep in his own thoughts about what it might have been without us around. I was also thinking how brave P'John was.

Very little was ever said about incidents of that type that happened at the Wilson home. I suppose it became commonplace over the years and not mentioned for that reason. I have really never understood why.

As the drought continued in its second year, things worsened. By the end of that summer we could not wear our old shoes from the year before. We had grown out of them and besides, they were too worn and "holey" for wintertime wear. Our clothes had been patched over and over again, plus being handed down to smaller brothers more than once. Our parents were in a dilemma as to how they would solve the problem. I heard them discussing it.

"Dad, school will be starting soon, and the kids don't have shoes to wear."

"I know, Dee, maybe they can go barefooted until things improve. Our money has run out. I'm having to buy medicine for these real poor people that are sick. They have no job, very little food, and no prospects of things improving. On top of all that, I am buying everything on credit now. Don't know how long I can continue that."

"Oh, Dad, something has to improve soon, or we'll all go to the poor house. I guess the Lord will provide a way; He always has."

"I hope you're right, Mama. Let's trust in Him and pray that He answers our prayers. Now let's try to get some sleep. I don't know about you, but I'm worn out."

With that they became silent. Then I heard snoring, like the sleep of the exhausted.

Sleep didn't come to me for a long time that night as I lay awake and thought about the things our parents were so concerned about. The next day it was haunting me, and I *had* to talk to Mama about it. I approached her as she was in the "meal" room mixing biscuit dough.

"Mama, can I ask you something?"

"Yes, if it isn't too hard to answer."

"Are we going to the poor house?"

"No, of course not, why?"

"I heard you tell Dad last night that if things didn't get better, we would end up in the poor house."

"Oh, that's just a saying when times are hard. We'll be ok. Don't you worry."

The next day or so Dad came in with a worried, tired look, which Mama noticed immediately. "Are you all right, Dad?"

"Yes, I'm just tired and concerned about all these poor people. some of these babies are so badly undernourished that they have no resistance and are likely candidates for infectious diarrhea, strep throat, or meningitis. I have two or three right now that are really worrying me, and there's not much I can do about it. My caseload is growing by leaps and bounds since so many people have moved back to the farms. All I can do is to keep trying."

Dad was gone most of the time during the drought and Depression years. He came home only after making his daily rounds to several homes to care for the many people with various and sundry ills, plus delivering babies or repairing wounds. He seemed to thrive on the busy life and I could see a sparkle in his eye when we asked about some friend who was ill. That seemed to stir something inside of me as I listened to him and saw his reactions. I was *very* interested in his work, thinking, *Maybe I would like to be a physician.*

The following late fall and winter months the rains came regularly in amount enough to break the drought. People's spirits were lifted as they once again felt relief from the drought and looked forward to bountiful crops and plenty of food at harvest time. Also, further hope that the Depression would be over with the election of a new president, Franklin D.

Roosevelt, who had begun many federal programs to guarantee jobs for the thousands of unemployed citizens of our great country. These programs were in effect in 1932. Banks and businesses reopened, new goods were being produced, and prosperity was beginning anew. The world sang the praises of President Roosevelt, referring to him as a saviour of our country.

With the "New Deal" came improvement in schools, roads, public transportation, recreational facilities, such as parks and playgrounds, and by 1936 electric power was brought to our rural areas by the Rural Electrification Administration. This changed the "world" for us Tennessee country folks. Now we could have radios, refrigerators, lights in every room, electric well pumps to afford water to the entire house—even a toilet and bathroom right inside the home.

By that time all the older brothers had left home; most of them were married with families. I was a freshman in college and leading the "Life of Riley." My goal was set, and I intended to pursue it to the end. I'll have to admit, I missed all the fun and games, the brotherly competition and advice, particularly about girls. I also missed their helping hands with the farm work the year round. With this situation, it was lonely sometimes, and I would recall the many things we did together as we grew up. Some situations and happenings I will relate as they were pertinent to our early years of everyday living.

High School

In the fall of 1931, I entered Macon County High, the only high school in the entire county. That year our older sister, Hallie, was a senior; Dennis and Prentice were sophomores. With four of us in school, Dad felt it would be best that he buy a second car so we could drive back and forth to save time and get home earlier from school. This was fine in the fall but when winter came things were different. To reach the school ten miles away, we had to cross two streams, neither of which had a bridge for vehicles. The smaller one near the school was not a problem. the one nearer, a mile or more from home, was another matter. It was larger and in early spring and during the winter would be swollen by heavy rains and unable to cross by car.

When this happened, we had to park the car on the school side of the stream, cross on the swinging foot bridge, and walk home. In wintertime it was worse as snows came, streams rose, and freezing weather followed. At these times, we parked the 1932 A Model Ford by the roadside, drained the radiator, walked the mile home in whatever weather, and repeated this until the creek went down enough to cross. That winter, Dad worked on his political friends to get school-bus service to our house. He had had enough.

High school was a big change for me. It was a new life away from home. There were many new friends to make, challenges to meet, new activities to participate in, and new organizations to join. I was a joiner and became involved in everything possible to learn about them.

One extra-curricular activity I became involved in was football and soon learned it was a mistake. At the age of fourteen I stood five feet two and weighed 106 soaking wet. The first day I reported, Coach Osteen looked at me very quizzically, "Son, do you think you can play this game?"

"Yes, sir, I think I can. Ask my brother, P'John."

"Ok, if your brother says you can, we'll give you a try."

"I think he can, Coach. He's tough."

"Ok, then we'll put you at deep safety position."

"That'll be fine, Mr. Osteen. Thank you."

As I trotted down the field to the deep, deep safety position, someone yelled, "Go get 'em, Scrub." From that day until many years after that, when old friends saw me anywhere in Lafayettte, they greeted me with a friendly, "Hi, Scrub, good to see you."

Because the coach was doubtful of me I was very determined to show him I could play football. Soon after the practice sessions began, I had the opportunity to do the proving: the fleet halfback eluded all tacklers and headed downfield toward the goal line. Getting a good angle on him I made a diving, shoestring tackle on him and brought him down. The entire squad cheered, clapped, and hollered, "Atta boy, Scrub." Boy, was I a hero! I felt six feet tall, I had stopped the star of the team. As I got up something ran down my face. When I wiped it away, my hand came away bloody. By now I realized that the heroic tackle was not so smart. The coach took one look and sent me to find a doctor. Looking in the mirror I saw that my right eyebrow was lacerated and bleeding. I dressed and headed to the drug store nearby, where our older brother, Harlin, worked. He greeted me with, "Well, what happened to the big football player?"

"Have a little cut over my eye. Think you can fix it?"

"Come to the back and let me take a look." He cleaned it up and took a good look.

"Oh, yes, this will be easier than fixing your big toe when you were three years old."

He pulled it together with adhesive tape, put a band-aid tightly over that, and in a week's time I was back at *deep safety* once again. I remained on the football squad during the four years, and by the third year was playing substitute center on offense and guard on defense. By then I weighed 130 pounds. By my senior year I was playing first-string center and still at guard on defense. My inflated ego was greatly injured as we lost eight of the ten games we played that year.

Football was not my only interest in high school. I sought recognition in all curricular activities also. During the third year, we formed a chemistry club and a drama club, since they had added speech and drama classes to the curriculum. That same year I served as president of the Future Farmers of America and was active in school plays and public speaking. All of these kept me very busy and out of mischief. With all of that my grade average was better than the first two years.

As the senior year began, I was eager for school to start. Working on the farm that summer made me really realize that I wanted to do something different in my life. While at home, I made house calls with Dad on weekends and really looked forward to this routine. He did soften the work a bit since he never asked me to go with him at night. When school started, so did football practice. We had a new coach that year, and he let us play the position we chose. Of course, I chose to play at center again, this that is where I stayed. Classes were easy that year, and I was able to stay with all the other things I was involved in before, plus noticing how pretty the girls had become during the summer vacation.

I noticed the beautiful, slender, red-headed, speech teacher with whom I soon became infatuated. I was also "in love" with a slender brunette with deep-blue eyes and soft tan skin. She flirted with me as we rode the bus each school day. Although I was more aware of the opposite sex, they occupied very little of the hours we spent in school. In addition to playing football, I was a member of the livestock judging team, had the leading role in the senior-class play, won the school "declamation" contest, and was voted best all-around student by "popular" vote of the student body. Boy! Was I riding high!

Then I was brought down several pegs. First, the speech teacher was married to the man of her dreams. The sixteen-year-old flirty brunette, ran off with the thirty-two year old teacher and also married. To top off my problems, the faculty met and decided that I did not deserve the honor awarded me by the student body and awarded it to a female classmate who was an excellent student, and just happened to be the girlfriend to a son of our high school principal. Had I been older it might have discouraged me, but I had been used to losing other types of battles, so I survived the heartbreaks and learned some valuable lessons about people. The action of the school faculty lowered the other student's respect for them and elevated their respect for me. I still count that year a successful one—even if we didn't win but two football games.

One other thing occurred in the senior year that was very valuable to me and other members of the class. Our class in agriculture started a pig project to raise money and to be recognized by the county leaders and other schools nearby. Three of us bolder ones approached our teacher concerning the project. The other two wanted me to be the spokesman so we went to his office. The door was open, and Mr. Hix sat at his desk. "What can I do for you boys?" he inquired.

"May we come in for a minute, Sir?"

"Yes, come on in and sit down."

"Thank you. We have an idea and want your opinion."

"Ok, let's hear it."

"We want to start the pig project that was mentioned last week and have been talking about it, and most everybody in class is interested in joining the 'club.' Here's our idea: we buy young, purebred gilts that are with pigs. When they farrow (have pigs) then each club member will sell two from that first litter, put that money together, and pay off the debt.

"That's a great plan, but where do you get the money?"

"We'll borrow it form the local bank. Mr. Parker has always said he would support us in any sound, worthwhile, progressive project. Now we can find out if he really will."

"Sounds good to me. You have my full support. You may not get the money, but you have nothing to lose. Good Luck!"

Mr. Hix got us excused for our trip to the bank, and away we went with our spirits buoyed by thoughts of success. Arriving in the bank's foyer, we were greeted by the receptionist/clerk. "good morning, what may I do for you?"

"Good morning, ma'am. We'd like to see Mr. Parker. I think Mr. Hix has spoken to him regarding the visit."

"Just a moment, I'll ask Mr. Parker. Have a seat." Within two minutes she came back. "Mr. Parker can see you now. This way, please," she said.

We looked at each other, raising our brows in disbelief. Feeling more confident than ever we followed Miss High into the inner office.

"Good morning, fellows. What can I do for you?"

"Good morning, Mr. Parker. I'm Wendell Wilson. This is Clyde Coley, and this is Harris Hix. We'd like to discuss something with you concerning a project we have in mind."

"Here, have a seat so we can talk. Now let me hear about your ideas."

"We want to start a pig project, and here's our plan" (and we proceeded to outline it in detail—then wound up by saying that we knew he would help, because he had said he would be glad to help with any progressive, worthwhile endeavor).

"Yes, so I did. but you know that banks have to have collateral to loan money."

"But, Mr. Parker, the pigs will be collateral."

Mr. Parker was a hard-nosed businessman with a reputation of being tough to deal with, but we could see that he was softening up to our ideas. Then he leaned back in his chair and launched a lecture about what a risk it would be to the bank by loaning money without a viable collateral—how hard work, honesty and integrity were the basis for success. Then he said, "I think you young men are honest and have integrity, but I don't know how hard you'll work. I'll talk to Mr. Hix today, and he'll let you know what our bank can do."

We thanked Mr. Parker and left in silence. I couldn't contain myself but a minute.

"What do you think, Harris?" I asked.

"I feel like we'll get the loan. How do you feel, Coley?"

"Same as you do."

"That makes it unanimous. Hot Dog! Let's get back to school," I shouted.

We had to wait until classes were out for the day, and that four hours seemed like four days. Then Mr. Hix called us in. He had a big smile on his face that told us what we wanted to hear.

"Well, boys, I don't know what or how you did it, but Will Parker is going to loan us enough money to buy the bred gilts."

All of us jumped for joy, thinking we were real entrepreneurs.

"Mr. Hix, how are we going to decide who gets the gilts, and when will we be able to see them?" I asked.

"Ok, first things first. We'll see them tomorrow afternoon. I have arranged for a field trip on a school bus to Mr. Long's farm. While we are there everybody will take a look at the gilts and make up their mind as to which they would choose. After that, we will have a drawing. At that time, I'll choose the method."

The next day we left school at 1 o'clock and arrived at the pig farm half an hour later. There they were, about twenty beautiful, young, purebred, Duroc-Jersey gilts, each already with pigs (expectant mothers). The dozen or more boys bailed out of that bus in a hurry to admire and judge the merits of each one. Then decided which he would choose for the project.

"Ok, fellows, come on over and let's have the drawing," Mr. Hix said. He took his hat off, placed several small pieces of paper in the hat, and explained. As he mixed the papers, he was saying, "There are numbers on each paper to match the number of boys to draw. Whoever draws number one gets first choice, number two gets second choice, and on down the line. Fair enough? Now line up and draw. Here, Wendell, you can be first. After all, you were the big mouth that started all of this."

I pulled out the first piece of paper I felt, took a look, and was shocked. I had picked number one! That meant I would have first choice of a gilt. My heart was pounding so I could hardly breathe when the drawing ended.

"Does everybody have a number now?"

"Yes, sir," we hollered in unison.

"Ok, who has number one?"

My voice was shaking as I held up the paper. "I do, Mr. Hix, and I know which gilt is the best one."

"Congratulations. Now show us which one is the best for a brood sow."

I walked to the pen, put my hands on the gilt that had all of the physical qualities that the livestock judging book had described for producing good pork, and to have large litters. "This is the one. She's perfect, and I bet she'll have ten or twelve pigs every time."

Somebody spoke up, "She's not quite perfect, Scrub, look at her right hind leg."

"Oh, that's nothing to worry about. She'll be the best. Anyway, she hardly limps." Everybody chose their gilt, and most of them were happy with their choice, but worried how they would get them home. Mr. Long came to the rescue by volunteering to deliver them free as a way to help our project.

The pig project was a big success. The loan was paid back by selling the new pigs. Mr. Parker was happy and praised us, plus we got recognition from other county schools, some of whom started their own projects. For me, it was a good lesson in business and public relations.

The sow proved to be as good as predicted, farrowed twice a year, delivering ten to twelve piglets each time. From that experience, I was able to make enough money to register for college classes for nine months.

Graduation time came in late April just after my eighteenth birthday, and I felt ten feet tall and was eager to enter college in September, 1935. After graduation, I worked on the farm, as usual, but with a different role, the leader and often the decision-maker. I bargained with Dad for two things: to have a corn crop of my own, on shares (in essence I was a sharecropper). Second, that he would pay my lab fees, organization dues, and for my text books and board, and I would pay for meals and social activities. It was a good deal for both. The summer went well in every phase, and we were together on weekends as I made house calls with him. My "pot" of money for college was fattened some more when we sold pigs on two occasions. When crops were laid by about mid-July, I again ran into more good luck.

While visiting in Red Boiling Springs, we went by the local general drug store for a coke and to visit with the owner and his employees. While talking to the owner, Mr. Chitwood, he mentioned that he could use an extra hand for the summer, if he could find somebody willing to work.

"You're looking at one right now. Would I qualify?"

He looked me up and down, looked away to the back with a quizzical expression. "How old are you anyway?"

"I'm eighteen, sir."

"Are you willing to work ten hours a day?"

"Yes, sir. I've been working that much or more on the farm. I'd like to try the job. But I'll be going to college in September. I plan to take pre-pharmacy or pre-medicine, so this job would help both of us."

"Ok, I'll give you the job. Remember, it'll be ten hours a day and six days a week, plus two free cold drinks and one ice cream cone each day."

"Sounds good to me. It'll sure be better than following a mule all day plowing corn with a double shovel."

Mr. Chitwood laughed a deep belly laugh. "You'll do all right, son. I've heard what you did in school. We'll get along fine."

"Thank you, sir. I'll have to get Dad's permission. Can I call you tomorrow (Sunday)?"

"Sure, call me here about 2 o'clock."

Back home that evening, I asked Dad about the job. "I'd like to work there the rest of the summer. Since crops are laid by and the grain has been threshed and stored, surely they can handle everything else."

"How much will he pay?"

"A dollar a day, six days a week. Dad, that's *six dollars*!"

"Where will you stay?"

"Aunt Mertie said she could give me room and board for two dollars a week. I can save three-and-a-half dollars every week. By the time college starts, I will have thirty more dollars. That will help a lot."

"I guess you can give it a try. It will be a good experience anyway."

In mid-July of 1935, I went to work at Chitwood's Drug and General Store. I dressed in one of my two pairs of good pants, a white shirt, and best shoes. With these clothes, a clean shave and my hair slicked back, I just knew that I would make a good impression on Mr. Chitwood and the public. "Good morning, Charlie. How are you today? Is Mr. Chitwood here?"

"I'm fine. No, Mr. Shade hasn't come in yet."

"Is there anything for me to do yet? Maybe you can show me around so I'll know where some things are."

"Yeah, that's a good 'idy.'" He showed me all about the soda fountain, the dry goods, then the hardware department, and finally the drug department. He explained that sometimes ladies would come in to buy piece goods by the yard, and we had to do the measuring of cloth to get the needed number of yards, etc. By the time the owner came in, Charley had oriented me to the whole store. He also told me that there would be a little bookkeeping each day. This I wasn't ready for but was something I really needed to learn.

Pretty soon Mr. Chitwood came in the back and greeted both with a cheery good morning and asked Charley if he had showed me around.

"Yes, we've been through the whole place, and I think he can handle most everything that comes along, Mr. Shade."

"That's fine. Wilson, you are directly responsible for the soda fountain from cleaning the place to ordering supplies. The salesman will come on Tuesday each week and will help you. Charley or I will explain anything you don't understand."

"Yes, sir. I understand. I'm sure there will be questions."

Things went well and before long I was making milk shakes, ice cream sodas, and occasionally a banana split. Working the soda fountain became an embarrassment shortly after beginning my job as a "soda jerk."

About 10 a.m., a well-dressed lady came into the store with her two teenage daughters, fifteen to seventeen years of age. The mother and older girl had their noses up in the air, but the younger one was friendly and flirty. She was also pretty and dressed in a blue dress that matched her big blue eyes.

"Come in, ladies, what can I do for you?"

"Do you serve ice cream and milk shakes?"

"Yes, we do. Have a seat please. Now what would you like?"

Mama ordered a dish of vanilla ice cream. Big sister ordered a chocolate soda, and the pretty little sister ordered a strawberry milk shake.

I served water, and napkins were placed on the table. I made the chocolate soda, and put Mama's ice cream on the dish—then mixed the milk shake and while it was in the mixer I served the soda and cream. Now the strawberry milk shake was ready, and I poured it into the glass, placed it on a tray to serve it in style. Just as I got to the table the tray tipped a little as did the shake. Some of the strawberry shake spilled onto the beautiful blue dress little sister was wearing. I was mortified. Her dress was ruined, as was my reputation. "I'm sorry Ma'am, I don't know what happened, let me get a towel." Mama was mad enough to kill me and as I came back to the table she grabbed the towel from me.

"I'll clean the dress off, *young man!*"

"I'm s-s-sorry, Ma'am, I'll make you another shake," which I did.

Little sister seemed to enjoy the shake and actually smiled at me as she drank it. Mama scowled and big sister was silent as they prepared to leave.

Doctor From Bugtussle

I apologized again as did Mr. Chitwood who said there would be no charge.

Little sister hung behind Mama and waved bye at me as they left. When they were out of earshot I apologized again. Mr. Chitwood had a big laugh about it and said not to worry about it. "That's not the first time it has happened and it won't be the last," he added.

Soon after that I was watching as he filled prescriptions, and he called me to the back.

"Yes, sir?"

"Would you like to learn to do this?"

"Yes, if you think it's all right."

"Sure it is. You won't be able to fill narcotics, but anything else is perfectly safe. Start right now. I'll watch you for a few days—then let you know if you are capable enough to be on your own."

Pretty soon I was filling non-narcotic prescriptions on a regular basis. I felt a little uncomfortable doing so, but continued until I left to enter college.

Working there was very easy compared to farm work. I was also clearing three or four dollars each week and having fun, too. I learned how to measure cloth for the ladies, to get the correct size plow points for the farmers, to almost get the exact pounds of different-sized nails for the carpenter.

As much as I enjoyed my job it was not something I wanted to do for the rest of my life. So when the time drew near for entering college, Mr. Chitwood and I set a date for me to leave. When that day came I dreaded to go to the store because I might become emotional and shed tears (and grown men don't cry). There was a lot of banter filled with an undercurrent of sadness. I was glad to know that Dad would soon be there to help hide my feelings.

"Thank you, Mr. Chitwood, for letting me work with you and Charley these weeks. I can truly say that I enjoyed every day I spent here. I learned a lot and had fun at the same time. I especially appreciate your interest in my future and all the encouragement you've given me."

"You've been a big help to me, too," he said. "I know that whatever you do for the rest of your life, you'll give 100 percent of your time to the task. I feel you will also be successful in whatever you do."

"Thank you, Sir."

About that time Dad drove up. I waved to Charlie. "Bye, Mr. Craighead, take care of yourself and watch what you eat and drink." I shook

Mr. Chitwood's hand again and walked out the door, fighting back the tears that were filling my eyes. Another short chapter in my life was closed.

College Years

In mid-September, 1935, I made a giant step forward, enrolling in college. Early that morning, my father took me by car to the county seat in Lafayette, Tennessee, to board a bus to Nashville, Tennessee. This was the beginning of my journey to college in Murfreesboro, Tennessee, thirty miles south, to enter Middle Tennessee State Teachers College, which is now MTSU. The night before I had packed the family suitcase with my meager belongings, and after a fitful night's sleep, I was ready to go by 6:30 a.m.

About 6:30, Dad said, "Come on, Son, it's time to leave."

"Ok, I'm ready to go. Good-bye, Mom."

Mama and I embraced and as she kissed my cheek, she said, "Be a good boy now and don't forget to write." I jumped in the car with the old suitcase and was on my way to a new world.

As we pulled out of the drive, Dad asked: "How do you feel about all of this?"

"I'm a little scared but thrilled at the thought of going to college. I'm also grateful to have this privilege to be able to go so I can meet new friends, and most of all, to learn about new and different things in this big world. Maybe this'll help me decide what I really want to do the rest of my life."

"Uh-huh, I see."

We drove the rest of the twelve miles in almost complete silence, each deep in his own thoughts. I was thinking: "How will I know what courses to take? Will there be someone to counsel and guide me? Will I make friends that will be of help?" My thoughts were interrupted as we arrived at our destination and went into the drugstore/bus station where an older brother worked.

"Hi, little brother. On your way to college, huh? Good for you; enjoy it."

The bus driver came in. "How many passengers do we have, Harlin?" he asked.

"Just one. This scared little brother of mine. He's on his way to Nashville and then to college in Murfreesboro."

"Good. Going to make a teacher, I guess."

"Not on your life. Maybe a pharmacist or even a doctor, but never a teacher!"

"Want a ticket?"

"Yessir, how much to Nashville?"

"Two Dollars."

As I handed him the two dollars, I was thinking of how much it was going to cost to get into school—and would I make it? By then he was taking my bag to put on board. I shook hands with Dad and Harlin and, not looking back, climbed aboard the big, nearly empty, Greyhound bus and headed for my destination. Nobody could see the tears in my eyes, or know the fright inside me as the bus pulled away from the curb to take me on my first trip alone into a new world.

Aboard the bus and alone with my thoughts, I hardly noticed the countryside. I did not pay attention to the infrequent stops for people to board until we reached Gallatin, Tennessee, and several passengers left, as others boarded the bus. After that there were no more stops until we arrived in Nashville, and I noted the tall buildings along the streets. Soon the bus slowed, turned twice, and came to a stop. The bus driver called out: "Nashville, all out for Nashville." As I left the bus and picked up my suitcase, Mr. Knight said, "Good luck in college."

"Thank you, Sir."

Inside the bus station everything and everybody seemed to be in constant motion.

"One ticket to Murfreesboro, please."

"Round trip or one way?"

"One way. Thank you."

"That will be two dollars, please."

I gave him the two dollars as again I thought, *God, this is getting expensive*! Within fifteen minutes the PA system blared out: "Attention, all passengers to Murfreesboro and Chattanooga, your bus will be leaving from gate four in ten minutes. Start boarding now." I grabbed the battered suitcase and hurried to gate four. A black porter stood beside the bus.

"Where are you headed, Sir?"

"Murfreesboro." He jerked the bag from me and slung it into a compartment under the bus. My eyes and mouth flew open. I started to say something but I was interrupted with—*"Yore bag will be okay, Sir!"* I looked and there it was with all of its scratches and scrapes, staring back at me as if to say, "I'm fine, get on board, let's go to college." We took off on time and after more frequent stops than before, within an hour the driver announced, "All out for Murfreesboro."

A little chill passed through my entire body as I realized we had arrived at *my* destination. I soon came back to reality, took up my faithful friend, the family suitcase, looked at it, and said, *"We are here."* With *it* in hand I started out to really find where I was. As I was looking around, a car pulled alongside me, and a friendly voice said, "Looking for the college?"

"Yessir, I am. Could you show me which direction to go?"

"I happen to be going that way. Hop in. Put your old suitcase in back" (he didn't show *our* suitcase any respect!).

"Thank you, Sir."

"Are you just starting to college?"

"Yes, sir. We register tomorrow."

"This your first time in Murfreesboro?"

"Yes, it is. I like the looks of it too."

"You'll like it more when you stay awhile." He turned into a drive, and I saw the buildings with the tree-studded campus. It all looked beautiful to me. We stopped in front of the largest building with large, curving steps which seemed to reach upward to two beautiful, wide-open doors that were saying, "Welcome, come in and join us."

This was the place I wanted to be. I felt as though I had come home.

"Here you are, young fellow, right in front of Old Main. Good luck. Enjoy The College."

"Thank you. I appreciate your help, your kindness, and the ride."

I glanced to the right and thought, *that building looks like a dormitory, maybe it's Jones Hall. We will see.* Lady luck was still with me. As I walked toward the entrance, there above the door was Jones Hall in bold, golden letters. Inside I saw an office sign and knocked on the door. A pleasant, female voice answered, "Come in."

"Good afternoon, ma'am. I'm looking for the house mother."

"You've found her. I'm Mrs. Freeman. My husband and I are the house parents."

"I'm Wendell Wilson. I'm supposed to have a room here for this quarter. Am I on your list?"

"Let's see. Yes, you are. You'll be in room 215, and your roommate will be a Mr. Baker that is supposed to arrive today also. Why don't you sign in—then we'll go see the room."

After signing in, making the deposit, and getting a key, Mrs. Freeman showed me the room, explained the house rules, and gave me a map of the campus. I felt like exploring and looking around the area, then returned to the room, unpacked, and claimed my half of the room. Someone then knocked on the door, which was open, and with a good Southern drawl said, "May I come in, Suh?"

"Yes, come on in. I'm Wendell Wilson. Just call me Wilson."

"I'm James Baker, and you can just call *me* Baker." We shook hands, smiled at each other, and were instant friends.

"Where are you from, Wilson?"

"Bugtussle." His eyes opened wide, and then wider.

"Bugtussle? Never heard of that place."

"You're kidding me, aren't you?"

"Well, yes and no. I'm really from Enon. Don't tell me you've never heard of that either?" He really looked puzzled by then. I thought it best to explain to him at that point. "By the way, where are you from, Baker?"

"Flat Rock. Now don't tell *me* that you have never heard of *my* hometown?"

"I'm not sure that I have. Where is it?"

"Just about eight miles south of Nashville, but still in Davidson County."

"Well, Baker, you're not far from home then. I guess it's up to us to put our hometowns on the map."

The next day we both registered and started classes two days later. As luck would have it, we had no classes together. His aim was to teach and mine was different. Each of us was assigned an advisor, and mine happened to be the assistant professor of chemistry.

"Hello, I'm Mabel Green, your advisor and counselor."

"I'm Wendell Wilson. Glad to meet you, Miss Green. I certainly will need your help and advice."

"I'll be glad to help in any way possible. What are you interested in?"

"The sciences and possibly a pre-med course. However, I am very weak in math."

"But you'll need some math in that course."

"I had rather not take it this first quarter."

"Let's give it a try and see how you do."

"If you insist. I'll do my best."

That was my first mistake.

The second was signing up for French.

Both were tough and boring. By the fourth week I was ready to drop both because I knew that I was failing math and maybe French too, but I decided to stick it out until mid-term exams.

About noon, two days before exam time, my abdomen began to hurt. First, the pain was in the pit of my stomach, then around my umbilicus (navel), and then all over. By 4 o'clock, the pain was much worse, and I felt some nausea. By this time, I had to lie down as I had also begun to feel dizzy. About half an hour passed, and I dozed a bit. Soon Baker came in.

"What's the matter, old buddy, are you sick?"

"I don't feel so hot. I've got a bellyache and feel queasy. I'm not going to the cafeteria. Maybe I'll feel better not eating anything."

"Ok, I'll see you later."

The pain eased a bit, but when I moved it worsened and never stopped. About midnight I had some vomiting. After that, the pain settled in my right side and then to a smaller area in the right lower quadrant. There was no sleep for me or my roommate. By 6 a.m. "Dr." Baker gave me his diagnosis.

"You know what's wrong with you, boy, you've got appendicitis."

"How do you know, Baker? You're not a doctor."

"No, I'm not a doctor, but I've seen some people with appendicitis, and I say that's your problem. I'm calling the house mother and school nurse right now."

"Ok, Baker, you may be right. Go ahead and call."

Baker notified Mrs. Freeman who called the nurse. Within ten minutes the nurse arrived, took the history, and made a cursory examination.

"Mr. Wilson, I agree with Mr. Baker. I'm calling the school doctor now. I'll be right back."

Five minutes later she was back. "Dr. Goodman will be here soon. He wants you to have an enema immediately. Will you help me, Mr. Baker?"

"I'll be happy to, nurse."

"You'll have to go to the bathroom for this procedure."

"Come on, Wilson. He helped support me as I barely moved along, holding my right side. By the time we arrived the nurse was there, holding a large, red rubber bag in her hands."

"You'll have to take off all your clothes, Mr. Wilson. Baker helped me take off my pants and shirt. I hesitated. "Your underpants too!" I was mortified. I had never undressed in the presence of a female and a complete stranger.

Baker said, "Come on, Wilson, let's take them all off." He did that gleefully.

"Now lie on the floor on your right side on this towel and curl up. I did as she commanded. I had never been in this position before. Lying on the floor, completely naked, with a female standing over me ready to do mayhem.

"That's good. Now let's give the enema. You just relax. It won't hurt a bit." Then while my roommate watched, as he snickered and made snide remarks, the nurse proceeded with the procedure. I saw her holding the bulging, red bag in one hand and the end of a long tube, attached to the bag, in the other hand. The end was gently curved and glistened with Vaseline.

"Will you hold this bag for me, Mr. Baker? Thanks."

Now relax. Then she gently inserted the tip in my rectum. "Raise the bag slowly, Mr. Baker." She let the warm soapy water flow in. It felt good, and I *did* relax. Then the abdominal cramps started, and I felt that my colon would explode. I moaned. She removed the tubing tip, which helped some.

"Relax! Don't move and hold this enema for two minutes." That seemed like eternity.

Now you can sit on the commode and expel the solution." I barely made it as the smelly and explosive "results" filled the commode. "Good, now let's get back to bed so the doctor can examine you." God, it was really painful to move now, as Baker half carried me back to bed. A young, well-dressed man came into the room.

"Hi, young fella. I'm Dr. Goodman. Tell me about your bellyache, when the pain began and what the course has been since."

I recited the whole thing: the when and where of the pain, then nausea and vomiting, and the present state of everything.

"I see. You're a good historian. Now let's take a look at your abdomen." He checked the abdomen closely, pressing gently at first and then more firmly. When he touched the right lower quadrant, then quickly let go, the pain was unbearable, and I had to bite my tongue to keep from screaming.

"Ok, that's enough. We need to get you to the hospital right away. You're in real danger of your appendix rupturing."

That really scared me. *Here I am all alone, facing a life-threatening problem. I have no identification, no money, they are unable to reach my family, and I am not legally able to sign a permit for surgery, and my appendix could rupture any minute. What am I to do?*

"Dr. Goodman, let's take him on to the hospital now," the nurse said. "We'll keep trying to reach his family. I'll call Dr. Robinson to see him immediately so he can get this boy to surgery right away." Luckily, Dad called before Dr. Goodman got away. He found out how serious the problem was and said he would be here as soon as possible, but they should go ahead with the surgery.

We arrived at the hospital in record time. The nurse put me in a wheelchair and then in a room. "This is Dr. Robinson's patient. He has acute appendicitis."

"We have been expecting him. The doctor will be here any minute."

As I lay there waiting, still all alone, my life flashed before me. I recalled all the many bad things I had done such as cursing, lying sometimes, as well as the few times I had cheated in school. Then my present life again reared its head, and I became more frightened. I had never prayed before, but I did now. "Dear God, please watch over me; You are the only one with me right now, and my life is in Your hands and the doctors. Please, God, forgive all my past sins and watch over me through this surgery, and throughout this illness." The silent prayers made me feel more secure and that all would be well. I was ready to go into the operating room. The nurse came by to say Dr. Robinson was here to see me; in walked a distinguished man of about sixty years of age.

"Hello, young man. I'm Dr. Robinson. They tell me that you have a bad bellyache and probable appendicitis."

"Yessir, I sure do have a bad bellyache."

"Let's take a look. Just relax now, so I can check your tummy." His expert hands moved over my entire abdomen, smoothly and quickly. He located McBurney's point in a few seconds, pressed gently and released quickly. My abdominal muscles contracted, and my entire abdomen became rigid. "You have a classic case of acute appendicitis, and you are a very sick boy. I don't think the appendix is ruptured, but it is probably gangrenous by now. We need to get you to surgery right away before the appendix does rupture. I have talked to your father and he agrees. The operating room is set up and all is ready for us. The nurse has a shot you will need to take before you go to sleep."

"Thank you, Dr. Robinson. I'm ready to get rid of this problem."

The nurse said, "Turn over and let me give you this shot in the hip (It was really painful). "Oh, by the way, there is someone here to see you before you go to surgery. In walked my roommate Baker. The tears flowed freely, running down my face. As we silently shook hands, I managed to blubber, "Thanks for saving my life, 'Dr. Baker.'" Then we had a good laugh, and I thought the appendix would surely rupture.

"Didn't I tell you that you had appendicitis, boy?" He laughed again. "Now don't you worry none. Everything will be ok, but I'll just stick around a while to find out."

"Thanks, Baker, you're a prince." I gave him the thumbs-up sign as they wheeled me into the operating room. As we arrived, the entire room was brilliantly lighted, and a very large light was suspended over the operating table. There were three nurses and three doctors all clad in white gowns, caps, and masks. All were completely silent; then a strange, faraway voice spoke: "I am Dr. Sleepingood. Let's get you on this table." Two pairs of hands grasped me gently and moved me onto the operating table. Boy, I was sleepy! Then the faraway voice spoke again: "Now let's take a nap," something was placed over my face, and I must have drifted off for a short nap because the next thing I knew somebody seemed to be standing on my belly, but I couldn't move or yell "Get off me, you're killing me." Then I went back to sleep. Sometime later I heard Dad's voice from a mile away. "He's beginning to wake up now. Wendell, can you hear me?" I tried to say yes, but no words came out. Then Dad said, "How do you feel now?"

"I'm hurting real bad; ask them to give me something for pain."

"Not yet, Son, it's too soon. You need to wake up more before you're given any more medication." I drifted off again—then soon was more awake.

"Have you seen Dr. Robinson, Dad?"

"Yes, we've talked."

"Was the appendix very bad?"

"Yes, it was. The entire appendix was gangrenous and ready to rupture."

"Thank God it didn't. Dad, have you met my roommate?"

"Yes, I did," Harlin spoke up, "Baker told me the whole thing, and he probably saved your life. He also helped me get your things together and took me to the dean's office to clear your records. He's a true friend."

"Yes, he's solid as the Rock of Gibraltar."

The next two days passed without incident, and I felt much better. I asked for food and was refused. "Could I please have some water?"

"Maybe just a sip or two, but no more. You're still getting IVs, you know."

"How about letting me sit in a chair, Nurse?"

"Absolutely not. You won't be allowed up for another week."

The next morning Dad and Harlin came in to announce that I was doing fine, and they both needed to get back home to their jobs. "Someone will be in to see you in two or three days. We'll call every day to check on you." Again, I was all alone to paddle my own canoe. That didn't bother me too much because I felt I was lucky to be alive. In 1935, there were no antibiotics, no sulfa drugs, and one had to rely on their natural resistance to infections. I must have had a very strong immune system because I recovered normally. However, I suffered through dehydration, very little to no food, three or four catherizations, no bowel movements for six days, and all this time I was still in bed and weak as a kitten. I was also getting mean, cranky, and weaker.

"Nurse, please give me something to eat. You're starving me."

"I'm sorry, but not until the doctor orders it."

"Ok, then I'll ask him tonight." When Dr. Robinson came around that evening, I was ready for him. He checked me, then the chart, mumbled, said "Uh huh," and then said, "Looks like you're doing all right."

"Then I can have some food, right?"

"Well, we'll start you on a liquid diet tomorrow."

"Oh, gosh. Right now I feel like I could eat a horse."

"Liquids tomorrow and then maybe soft food the next day."

"I'll settle for that. How about letting me up, then maybe I can pee. I can't while a nurse or an orderly stands over me watching while I strain and nothing happens."

Dr. Robinson laughed and said, "You're a gutsy little rascal. Ok, we'll give it a try."

The next day I got *very thin* Cream of Wheat, chicken broth, and half of a baked potato. Boy, they were good! I felt better the next morning and asked for more food and for bathroom privileges. To my amazement, Dr. Robinson agreed to both. As soon as Dr. Robinson left, I called the nurse.

"What do you want, Mr. Wilson?"

"I want to go to the bathroom."

"Ok, I'll send the orderly in to help you."

"I won't need the orderly. I can go without help."

"No, I'll send him in, and don't you get up until he gets here."

I tried anyway and found out I was too weak to walk without his help and barely made it back to bed, as I almost fainted. Cold sweat engulfed me as I lay there faint, weak, and short of breath. From then on, I listened to that nurse.

For the next three days I was allowed up in the chair three times a day and to the bathroom with help, and I needed assistance for both. This was my eleventh hospital day and still no bowel movement. I reminded the nurse of the problem. "I'll ask the doctor what we can do when he makes his rounds tonight." She did and not long after Dr. Robinson left, she came in with that red-rubber enema bag with its attachments. "Doctor is giving you a small, warm, mineral-oil enema tonight and a warm soap suds enema in the morning."

The pre-op enema picture flashed across my memory. I dreaded this process, but I had to open my big mouth. I guess I deserved the treatment. After all, I was still alive. I was not so embarrassed this time. The nurse was gentle, and the warm oil felt soothing as it slowly filled the lower colon. "Now just stay on your right side for the next hour, and don't try to expel the oil. You need to let it stay in the colon as long as possible." That was *my* nurse speaking, and I obeyed her. Within an hour, I expelled the oil and some other material. A good night's sleep helped a lot. My nurse came in the next morning about 6 a.m. with her red bag and the long tube. Conditioned as I was to what was coming, I turned on my right side and curled up.

"You forgot something, Mr. Wilson. Take your underpants off, or do you want me to call the supervisor?" I didn't want to, but I knew that being exposed was part of the dreaded procedure, and I complied. The results were good, which made the nurse and me both happy.

After that I was ready for a hearty breakfast. The food cart stopped by my door, and a cheerful voice sang out, "Breakfast time." She set the covered tray on the table. "Enjoy the good food, Mr. Wilson," and away she went. I could hardly wait and jerked the lid off! I was shocked, it couldn't be *my* breakfast. It was only thin Cream of Wheat, a half-glass of lukewarm milk, and a thin piece of half-toasted bread. This was a mistake. I pushed the call light, and the nurse appeared.

"Yes, what do you need?"

"They've sent someone else's tray to me. I expected some solid food."

"No, you're still on liquids until tomorrow."

"I thought Dr. Robinson was my friend."

"He is, that's why you're still on liquids."

"Ok, maybe I'll get some real food tonight."

On the twelfth day, I had a soft diet that was delicious. I also got something else. When the surgeon made rounds, the nurse accompanying him was carrying a sterile tray.

"Ok, young man, we need to get rid of your skin clips. Let's take your dressing off. Looks fine. It didn't look fine to me. The incision was six inches long. The skin edges were held together by a dozen dull, brassy, curved pieces of metal that had little hooks on each end. I just knew it would hurt like the devil when they were removed.

"Are you going to give me something first, Doctor?"

"Naw, this won't hurt. Let me have the clip removers, Nurse." She handed an instrument to him that reminded me of "hog ringers" we used on the farm. I dreaded this more than the surgery; at least then I was half-asleep before leaving my room. Now I was fully aware and full of dread. He inserted the curved tip of the remover under the "humped" clip, closed the blade, and the clip straightened, the hooks came out, and—I felt no pain. It was soon over with and redressed.

"Do you feel better now?"

"Yessir, thank you, Doctor."

"You should be able to go home in another two days. We will let your parents know. Is that ok with you?"

"It sure is. That's the best news I've had in a long time. I want to thank you now for all you've done for me. I realize that I might not be here without your surgical skills and excellent post-operative care. You've also helped me make a decision in what I hope to do in the future."

He smiled. We shook hands. "I'll see you tomorrow. You do what these nurses tell you to do."

"Don't worry, I've learned my lesson."

For the next two days I counted the hours until someone arrived to take me back home for a complete recovery.

On the fourteenth day of my hospital stay, my father and brother came for me. I was as thrilled as a small child on Christmas morning after Santa had left his/her stocking filled with "goodies." The bumpy ride home didn't bother me at all. When we came in sight of the old house, it looked like a castle to me. When Mama met us at the door, she was definitely a queen in my eyes. They carried me into the house on a "pack saddle" because I was too weak to walk the fifty feet and up three steps. Mama took one look at me and said, "Lordy Mercy, you're half-starved. We'll have to start feeding you right." Those words were music to my ears.

Doctor From Bugtussle

"I'm ready for some of your good food, too, Mama. Thank God, I'm home." Mama lived up to her word. The soups, soft foods, good whole milk, rich desserts, and finally the good staple foods of beans, potatoes, etc., soon had me back on my feet, and I was getting restless for something to do that would fill the idle hours.

Dad had not questioned me about what I intended to do now that I was well. He just observed my progress and sensed that I was restless and needed to be doing something. The next morning he said, "Wendell, I think you can handle some light jobs now. There was a bumper corn crop this year, enough to fill the cribs, and they had to throw a lot of it in the loft. Why don't you start throwing that back from the front a little bit each day? When you get tired, you can stop for a rest and then work a little more. That way you can soon have the corn all moved and at the same time gain strength. Besides, you won't be bored."

"That's fine, Dad. I'll start this morning."

"Don't overdo it the first day."

"Don't worry, I won't."

Later that morning I walked the 100 yards to the barn (which seemed a mile). I rested five minutes and climbed the stairs to the loft. I had to rest another minute as the weakness seemed worse. I surveyed the situation, noting that Dad was pretty sharp. There was at least ten wagon loads of corn piled to the front of the hay loft. Back of that pile was an open space about twelve by twelve feet in size that would hold the corn. Dad knew that would keep me busy for at least a week, since I couldn't last very long at a time. The first time I lasted an hour, working at a snail's pace. I took a fifteen minute rest, tried for another half hour, and had to quit. It took me the whole week to finish the job, but I did it. By that time I had gained some strength. I was eating three full meals each day and felt good. That night I noticed my high school ring was missing. That was my prized possession. It symbolized an accomplishment. Besides, I had saved money made from selling chestnuts picked up the fall before so I could buy the ring. The next morning, I asked Mama if she had seen the ring.

"No, I haven't seen it. Maybe you lost it when you threw the corn back."

"Maybe so. I thought I watched what I was doing. If we don't find it I will have to move the corn twice more and be really careful with every ear that is moved." That I did. By the time the corn was moved, slowly and carefully twice more, I was much stronger. The ring was never found, but it was a blessing in disguise. It helped me to make some decisions: (1) I would never be a farmer, (2) I set a goal to study medicine, and (3) I would re-enroll in college the next quarter and devote 90 percent of my time pursuing that goal, taking courses that I preferred, to make high grades to accomplish that goal.

The next day I announced my intentions to Dad, who only smiled and said, "Good."

In mid-January, 1936, I again enrolled at Middle Tennessee State College. I was determined to make a success at something I wanted to do. I did not ask for an advisor this time, since my mind was made up, but an advisor encountered me anyway. "Thank you, Miss Carr, but I have already selected my courses and am waiting approval of the instructors." All of the chosen subjects were approved, and I settled down to work with more determination. There was no French or math to worry me, and classes were a pleasure. At the end of the first six weeks, As and Bs were on my report cards. At the end of the first quarter my grades held up, and so did my self-confidence. The second quarter went well. Again, the grades were above average, and I felt that my problems were behind me. I had found myself and was back on the right track and intended to stay there.

When the quarter ended, I found myself with a job and had to return to the farm for the summer. Managing the farm had few rewards, but was relaxing and helped improve my physical stamina. Social life was practically nil. There were no pretty, intelligent girls around Bugtussle or Punkin Town and I missed that important part of college life, particularly Catherine, the beautiful, blue-eyed, blonde farm girl from Cross Plains, Tennessee, whom I had "dated" some during the second quarter. That problem was solved toward the end of the summer when a girlfriend of my younger sister came by for a visit and caught my eye as she was leaving.

"Hey, where have you been all of my life?" I inquired.

"Oh, I've been visiting my brother in Washington, D.C. this summer. Why?"

"It must have been fun. You look wonderful. Where are you staying now?"

"At home. I'll be going back to school in a couple of weeks."

"That's good. Maybe we will meet again before the summer ends. Good to see you."

"Maybe, bye." As she walked away she looked back over her shoulder, smiling and eyes glowing. That stirred something inside me, and there was no doubt that we would meet again. A phone call the next day, a date on Saturday and Sunday, which became a habit and a learning process. The days flew by, and soon the summer was gone, and I looked forward to my return to college life.

In mid-September, 1936, I was back on campus at Middle Tennessee State again.

My roommate was a senior, pre-med, honor student this quarter. The Lord was surely looking over my shoulder again. William Chambers was a twenty-one-year-old aspiring to enter Vanderbilt University School of Medicine to become an anatomist. To do this, he had to prove his capabilities since he was not doing his undergraduate work at a school with university status. So far he had a grade average of 4.0, good enough to prove his ability in any school, but he wanted to prove himself more. His schedule included calculus. physical chemistry, advanced physics, and Latin. He was also a student assistant in general chemistry. What a role model I had!

I was awed by two things: his being a senior and his scholastic ability. I knocked on the door: no response. I tried again. The door opened swiftly, and the man standing there had an inquisitive look on is face (saying to me, "Why are you disturbing me?") I had to break the ice. "Hi, I'm your new roommate. Are you William Chambers?"

"Yes, I am."

"I'm Wendell Wilson. May I come in?"

"Sure, come on in. Where are you from, Wilson?"

"Lafayette. Have you heard of that 'Metropolis'?"

"Sure, we're neighbors. I'm from Carthage." That broke the ice. He actually smiled, and I knew everything would be ok.

"Well, guess I had better unpack. Which part of the space do I use?"

"Here's your closet, a 2 x 4 foot open space with a rod for hanging clothes and a shelf above. This' your chest of drawers, and here's your desk and chair. If you need a reading light, you'll have to buy your own. Hope you don't have a radio or many clothes."

"A radio? What's that?" He laughed at that.

"You're ok, Wilson. Ready to go to supper?"

"Yep, is the food still as lousy as ever?"

"It's the best on the campus."

"Yeah and the only one."

I registered for classes the next day, signing up for chemistry, biology, German, English II, and economics. That was eighteen quarter hours. I would be busy.

"What courses are you taking, Wilson?"

"Here's my schedule. Do you think that'll keep me busy?"

"Yep, but you can do the job. If you run into any problems, I'll be glad to help."

There were problems galore, and Chambers was a good teacher. He would explain to me, I would recite back, and this would go on until we both thought the subject matter was completely understood. It must have helped a lot because I earned more As and Bs than expected. Our nights were filled with hours of study with fifteen- to twenty-minute breaks for relaxing and then hitting the books for another couple of hours. Studying this way was not a bore. We were learning together, and he was teaching also, which was what he aspired to do for his lifetime. The year went swiftly as the hours of studying continued night after night. Many times, William came to my rescue as I wrestled with chemical equations, a problem in economics, or a lack of understanding some facts of biology. He would explain and then ask me to recite back. This would continue until we both felt that I completely understood. This proved to be my salvation as my grades continued to improve from quarter to quarter. All was not work. William visited his parents several times during the year. While visiting, he would hunt and trap wild game. On two occasions, he returned with skeletons of a fox and a raccoon.

"What are you going to do with all those bones, Chambers?"

"Study anatomy. This is a hobby I've had for about six years. I'll assemble these into a skeleton of the animal—then identify each bone. As I do this, I'll be preparing for my future goal of teaching anatomy. But first, I will have to go to medical school to acquire an M.D. degree, then go for a Ph.D. in anatomy—then I'll teach medical students somewhere in this country."

"Boy! That's great. I know you'll easily reach that goal. Can I help in any way?"

"Yep, just don't touch the skeleton while it's being put together. Look and ask all you want, but don't touch."

"Ok, I'll watch and you teach."

He would work for an hour or so each night, finding the right bone, fitting it to the next correct one with a special glue. As I watched the skeleton take shape and asked questions, it was fascinating, as well as very helpful, to me in medical school later. One thing he did that I will always remember—each bone was numbered as it was put in its proper place. The number was placed in order on a chart with its proper name. That was his method of teaching and remembering as well.

William was the most disciplined man I had the privilege of knowing in college. He usually went to bed at the same time each night, got up the same time each morning, ate his meals at the same hours each day, and then scheduled the study time each night. On Saturdays and Sundays, he relaxed after school and hunted and fished if at home in Carthage. During the time I knew him, he never had a girlfriend or socialized any. I couldn't stand that type of life and wondered about him. On an occasion or two I asked, "Don't you want me to introduce you to a beautiful blonde? She would be a lot of fun."

"No, thanks. I don't have time for girls."

"They're fascinating creatures to me. They're so different from men that I have a hard time understanding them. Besides, it's an excellent way to study gross anatomy. Boy! It's great. Come on, let me introduce you to Grace. You'll have a great time."

"Not tonight. I'll take a rain check." But he never did.

That didn't stop me. I wanted to learn more about women. I wanted to learn ballroom dancing, the art of socializing, how to greet people correctly, and to improve myself in all the social graces. So I left Chambers with his animal skeletons while I went to classes in dancing, joined the dramatic club, tried out for bit parts in stage productions, met interesting people (mostly girls), and broadened my social life. Doing these things didn't change my goals. I stayed on course, thanks to William Chambers and the prospects of working the family farm at the end of this, my second year of college life. I was more determined than ever.

At the end of that school year, I felt good about my accomplishments from all aspects. My grades had been far above average. I had met some fine, intelligent people that had been good friends, and lastly, met and dated some beautiful, intelligent girls that helped to improve my social graces. With all of this, the professors and instructors had encouraged, helped, and advised me to relax, return to school, and never give up. All of this strengthened my self-worth and determination. I had no choice, and after exams, prepared once again to return to the farm for the summer.

As we were packing to leave, Chambers and I both stopped, sat on our beds, and had a chat. "I want to thank you, Chambers, for putting up with me this year. You've been a wonderful roommate. The good Lord was surely looking over my shoulder when I was fortunate enough to become your roomy. You've kept me on track and improved my self-confidence 200 percent."

"Thanks, Wilson. You've been a big help to me, too. My shell is falling off me now. I might just take your advice about women."

"That's great; you'll have a lot more fun and solidify gross anatomy." That was good enough for a deep chuckle from William and made me feel good.

"By the way, Chambers, how did you come out with your application for admission to Vanderbilt Medical School?"

"Great. I'm being admitted on condition that my grade average is as good as last year."

"Well, then, you keep your bags packed and head for Nashville. Congratulations! I'll bet that someday you'll be teaching at Harvard, Yale, or even Mayo."

"Thanks again, Teacher," I said. both of us had tears in our eyes as we shook hands and returned to packing our battered suitcases.

I never saw William Chambers again, but a good friend told me years later that he was indeed teaching anatomy at a large, well-known university in the Eastern states.

We said our farewells and left, he to enter Vanderbilt Medical School, and I, to return home, there to do the lowly tasks of plowing corn with mules, planting tobacco, mowing and raking hay (with mules), harvesting and threshing grains, and milking cows after sunset and before sunrise. It was good for me, it humbled me, as well as making me more tolerant of people who had spent their whole life in doing menial tasks. Farm life again further strengthened my resolve to become a physician. With the hard work I still found time to make house calls with Dad to test my interest in practicing medicine. The interest was greater! I was still on the right track.

Romance was still in my summer agenda as well. The strawberry blonde soon surfaced again, and Saturday nights and Sundays found us together somewhere. A big problem with having "dates" was transportation. the family car was also Dad's mode of transportation in his practice. I had to find a way to see that tantalizing, sexy, strawberry blonde. The only other "vehicle" was the trusty horse. So I swallowed my pride and would saddle Joe to make the two-mile trip. Sometimes, I would hitch him to a nearby tree at the church building and wait for her to arrive with her family or friends. They were usually riding in a wagon that was padded with straw and covered with a quilt to sit on to make the ride bearable. Her "magnetism" pulled me to the wagon so fast that I was there to help her from it. Everybody else was ignored as we held hands, headed for the church, and to the back seat where we sat for two hours as the preacher was quoting Scripture and verse, telling all us "sinners" we were going to "hell" if we didn't repent and seek the Lord before it was too late. This was so common, and we were too smitten with "love" that we hardly noticed what he was saying. We usually, furtively, held hands and played footsies as we endured the two hours of "hell-fire and damnation" Rev. Gooding blasted the congregation with. As we stood for the last song ("Shall We Gather at the River") I whispered in her ear: "Thank God that's over. I'll meet you outside in ten minutes and walk you home."

"I'll wait for you near the wagon. Hurry back so Mama won't fuss at me," she replied.

"Don't worry. I'll be there, waiting breathlessly for you."

As she came out the door, I was by her side. "Hi, city girl. Are you sure you can walk these country roads for two miles?"

"Sure, I could walk ten miles so long as I'm with you."

"Ok, let me get my 'vehicle'."

When I came back, leading the horse, she giggled: "I hope this horse walks real slow."

"He will. He's an experienced courtin' horse."

Marie had a sexy, husky voice and used it expertly. This night was made for lovers. A full moon, bright stars, and a slight breeze made it perfect. Even the horse drifted along as he sensed our mood. We linked arms, walked slowly and close, our bodies touching, longing for each other. We were far behind the family wagon so we could "smooch" as we walked. It was tantalizing for both. "Marie" was blessed with a near-perfect body, beautiful, large, blue-gray eyes, a sultry voice, and a ready smile. Boy, was she ever an attraction for the opposite sex. I had trouble controlling my desires. She aided and abetted them. There was one big problem: she had marriage on her mind, and I didn't. We endured the summer without getting into any 'trouble'. We lingered on front porches until midnight or until curfew time. The trip back home was short and full of thoughts of Marie. As I rode along talking to "Joe," you would think there was a third party with us.

"What am I gong to do, Joe? I can't keep this up much longer, or there will be trouble for sure. You do know that I'm going to medical school, come hell or high water. Guess I'll have to 'ditch' that girl." My hormones said: "Don't do that. You'll be ok. Don't put yourself in too many risky situations." "Yeah, you're right, but what am I going to do, act like a eunuch? Never! It's too much fun. I'll take my chances." The summer was short, I spent less time with Marie, controlled my desires, went with Dad more on weekends, and keep my goals in mind.

That last date was one of reminiscing of the last two summers, promising to write, to be together for holidays, and not forget each other. Tears were shed by Marie, but not me (grown males don't cry). I was relieved but, at the same time, sad to leave.

"You know I have to go, Marie. I've set goals, and it takes years to reach them."

"I know, and I'm willing to wait."

"Don't say that. Marriage is out of the question for me for at least eight more years. Think of me only as a close friend."

"You know I can't do that. I've been in love with you since I was fourteen."

"That's a real compliment, but don't wait for me. You might be an old maid by the time I can ask a woman to marry me. Come on, let's talk about something else."

Mid-September 1937: once again I packed the Wilson family suitcase and left for Middle Tennessee State College. This time there was more determination within. I was more mature, had written my year's curriculum, and was looking forward to classes in each course. The trip to college was much shorter this time than the previous two, and before really realizing it, we arrived in Murfreesboro, and soon onto the college campus. It looked great to me with its giant shade trees of oak and maple, winding sidewalks, and concrete seats strategically placed under shade trees beside the walkways. One could sit and daydream, build castles in the air, or actually sit there with a beautiful coed whom you were trying to favorably impress. At that stage and state of mind, I was actually in love with my surroundings. I moved on to Jones Hall (my second home).

I knocked on Mrs. Freeman's door with a firm rap. As it opened I was saying: "Hello, Mrs. Free"— it wasn't she. Coach Freeman stood there with a stern look on his face. "What's your rush, young man?"

I'm sure he saw the look of disappointment on my face. After all, when you expect to see a beautiful 35-year-old female smiling at you, and you are greeted by a 45-year-old, pot-bellied, balding, thick-lipped, crooked-nosed male scowling at you; who wouldn't be disappointed?

"I-I-I'm sorry, Coach, I just thou—."

He cut me off. "I know what you thought, so what do you want?"

"I'm Wendell Wilson. I'll be staying in the dorm again and was told that a private room was being held for me."

"Ok, let's take a look. Yep, you do. You'll be in room 219, ok?"

"Yessir, that's fine. Second is the best floor in the dorm. Thanks, Coach."

"No problem. Here's your key, hang onto it, or it will cost another two dollars. Next time you show up, maybe my wife will be here," he chuckled.

"I will. Dollars are hard to come by these days." I picked up my suitcase and headed for the stairway, hurrying to room 219.

I registered the next day. My courses were German II, quantitative and qualitative analysis (chemistry), biology III, entomology, and English III. I was a fool to take on that heavy load, but felt I had to. Besides that, I was determined to have some social life also. It was rough and tough. That year I found out what good friends I had made really meant to me. Paul Stewart, my chemistry lab partner, helped with equations. James Baxter taught me logarithms so I could shorten the time calculating chemical equations. I learned to use the slide rule for this to save time and be accurate. How I learned all this, I don't know. After the third day of attending classes, I realized there was not enough time for me to meet this rigorous schedule. Something had to give. What should I do? Then I remembered "Maw Green's" words, "If I can be of help anytime, you know where to find me." I went out of the chemistry lab, down the hall, and knocked on her door.

"Hello, Wendell, come in."

"Thank you, Miz Green. I need some advice."

"What's the problem? Have a seat and let's talk about it."

"I'm taking too many quarter hours and need to drop a course. I need you to help me decide which course to drop."

"What are you taking now?"

I gave her the schedule. "Hmmm, this is a big load. What had you thought of dropping?"

"I had about decided on dropping entomology."

"Yes, I agree. Besides you can take it next year."

"Good. How do I go about this?"

"No problem. I'm still listed as your advisor, and I will speak to Dr. Maynor, the department head. You will get a note of approval to your instructor, and then you will have a clean record."

"Thank you very much, Miz Green. I'll never forget this."

"Glad to be of help. By the way, have you had any more fights?"

She was referring to a fracas I had in the hallway outside her office my freshman year when a fellow student accused me of stealing his chemistry textbook. "I thought you had forgotten that incident, Miz Green."

"I never forget a good, clean fight, especially when it's for a good cause."

"Thank you again, Ma'am."

"Good luck, Wendell. Let me know if I can help anytime."

I left her office knowing that the decision was a wise one. My burden was lifted, and I was relieved.

The days were filled with class work and laboratory experiments and not much else. My brain soon became tired, and I realized I needed to exercise and relax.

I bumped into Ralph Gwaltney, a friend and classmate, who was on the tennis team.

"Hey, Ralph, how are you these days? How is your tennis game?"

"Ok, I guess. I'm still on the team."

"That's great, congratulations . . . are you running any more besides when you practice?"

"Yeah, I run track for half an hour most every morning."

"What time do you run?"

"About 6 a.m."

"Do you run alone?"

"Yes, I do."

"Would it be all right if I joined you?"

"Sure. When do you want to start?"

"How about 6 in the morning."

This started a daily routine. We jogged for half an hour, showered, ate breakfast, and were ready for the day. Near the end of the quarter, my funds began to dwindle, and I was looking for a job and mentioned it to Ralph. "I know one that we could probably get, but you might not like it," he answered.

"Oh, I'll take anything so long that it won't interfere with my class work and labs."

"Mr. Bock is looking for two waiters for lunch and supper six days a week."

"Great, let's apply. How about if we call and make an appointment?"

"Fine with me. Do you want me to call?"

"No, I'll do it, Ralph. After all, I was the one who brought it up."

The call resulted in an appointment that night at closing time. We arrived a little early, which seemed to please Mr. Bock.

"Do you boys want to see me?"

"Yessir, I'm Wendell Wilson that called, and this is my friend, Ralph Gwaltney. We want to apply for the jobs for waiters."

"Have you had any experience at this work?"

We both spoke at the same time. "Yes, I have."

"You both seem like good boys. I'll take a chance on you. When can you start? The lunch hour is from 11 to 12:30, supper is from 4:30 until 7 p.m. I'll pay you $1.50 a day, plus your meals. Is that suitable?"

"Yes, that will be fine, Mr. Bock."

"Can you start tomorrow?"

"Yes, I can. How about you, Ralph?"

"No problem."

"Good, be here promptly at 11:30, wash your hands, and go to work."

The work was good. Our prior experience was a big help to both, and pretty soon the number of customers began to grow, and Mr. Bock was well-pleased. He would walk up and down constantly, just stopping long enough to work the cash register. He was a small man with a pointed chin and thin lips drawn down at the corners. He kept a small half-smoked cigar in his mouth constantly, even talking around the cigar. As we got to know him better, sometimes we would tease him about how he was able to talk and hold the cigar in his mouth at the same time. He actually smiled about that, but I never heard him laugh the entire year we worked for him. The two of us and one girl could take care of 100 customers an hour. We felt he got his money's worth, but wondered if we did ours. Mr. Bock never sounded the "d" in my first name. "Come on, Wenell, move a little faster, you can talk to those girls when you aren't working here. Clean those tables off, people are waiting." "Ok, Sir." And we moved like lightning. As I would pass I ribbed him a little. "Is this fast enough, boss?" Or—"We're going to run out of food, Sir." He would run back to the kitchen and check on the food, then as we would rush by him with a filled plate he would check again. Deep down he liked a little teasing. he was just an "old Scrooge" where money was concerned.

That job lasted the year 'round, and Ralph and I stayed with it. After all, we got two meals, plus $1.50 each day we worked. That was far better than plowing all day with a mule and getting no pay. I got into trouble only one time. The blonde ex-girlfriend came back to campus for a weekend visit. She called for a friendly visit. That night after work we had a very friendly visit and since that was so nice, I asked to see her for a walk the next morning. The stroll was fine. It was a beautiful spring day and as we strolled we reminisced. Time passed too fast, and Catherine casually remarked that it was near noon, and she had to meet her ride in half an hour.

"What time is it, Catherine?"

"Ten minutes to twelve."

"Really! I'm supposed to be at work in ten minutes."

"I'm sorry. I didn't realize you were working today."

"Afraid so. But being with you was a lot more fun and *much more enjoyable* than waiting tables. Mr. Bock will understand." Apparently, he didn't. As we neared the restaurant, Catherine's ride showed up, we held hands briefly, I gave her a friendly peck on the cheek, thanked her for a great weekend, said good-bye, and went into the restaurant. There stood Mr. Bock with a scowl on his face and the stubby cigar clenches in his teeth. I thought, *He really is an old Scrooge. Here goes my job.*

"Hi, Mr. Bock. Sorry I'm late, but I can stay late."

"No, we don't need you, Wenell. You're *too* late."

I looked around. The place was full, the waiters were scurrying around, people looked impatient, some spoke to me, "Come on and bring me some food." I made a decision! "Mr. Bock if you don't need me *now*, you never will. If you decide you do, let me know." I turned and walked out. Mr. "Scrooge" Bock was taken aback, but he was right in what he did. I needed to be taught a lesson, and he did it right there in Bock's Tea Room while 150 people watched and some listened as he did so.

Two days later, Ralph came by my room to tell me that Mr. Bock was asking about me, and said he would like to see me. "Does he want me back to work or just talk to me?"

"I think he wants you back. We're having a hard time waiting on the people. I asked him if he needed you or did he want to get someone else."

"What did he say?"

He said, "I'd druther have Wenell, but he might not come back. I am his emissary. Come on back."

"I sure do need the job, and I know you need the help. Sure, I'll go with you in the morning." During our jogging, we discussed how the situation should be handled and decided that we both act as though nothing had really happened, and I could go on back as usual. We arrived promptly at 11:30 as usual, but Mr. B. was up front.

"Good morning, Mr. Bock. Ralph said you wanted to see me."

"Ah, I did. Get your apron on and get back to work." Nothing else was said about being late that one time and everybody was happy.

That taught me if one accepts a responsibility, he should be responsible at all times. If someone trusts you, be trustworthy. Do your best at all times and never show favoritism. During all the years since that incident I have tried to follow those beliefs.

Working in Bock's Tea Room was not the only job I had during the college years. As a freshman and sophomore, I washed dishes in the cafeteria and took care of a thousand-plus white mice that they were using in a mutation experiment. I did the menial tasks: cleaned cages, fed them every other day, counted the dead and newborns each day. I also kept an accurate daily log. All of this for twelve dollars a week. It lasted for six weeks, and I was able to take part in some extra-curricular activities with that money.

That third year was extremely busy and tough. It was also very fruitful in more than one way. First, my grades were good enough to help me be accepted into medical school when I applied later. I learned to socialize, also learned the basics of ballroom dancing. but the most important thing that occurred was becoming a member of the Sigma Club, an on-campus Honors Society. To become a member, one had to meet high moral, ethical, and religious standards, and also be a student achieving a certain grade level set by the faculty. This really increased my self-worth and confidence.

The chemistry and biology courses were challenging and interesting. We spent many hours in the labs after regular school hours, dissecting small animals and drawing illustrations of dissected anatomical parts of the bodies. Some time was also spent in mounting, staining, and studying slides to learn the microscopic makeup of these parts. Chemistry labs were not only long, but tedious and repetitive, particularly quantitative analysis where everything had to be accurate to the thousandth degree. Because of this part, the classes were small and sometimes the members were called "eggheads." A few were brilliant, but most of us were just determined plodders that made the grade. It was sometimes hard to stick to the set goals as you spent the hours in labs, worked jobs to be able to eat, or have money to register for the next quarter of classes.

It would have been a lot more fun to have taken "crip" courses, but I personally would not have had my self-esteem and worth had I not put forth the effort to achieve the goal I had set and announced to family and friends what I had intended doing. Looking back to the college years, the third one was the most critical for the future. It really was sobering and maturing for me. When the final exams were over, and the adrenalin stopped flowing so freely, I realized how tired and pent-up I had been for that nine months.

Although it meant another three months of menial tasks and reverting to some of the things in earlier life, I was looking forward to this "vacation."

Two days later, I was back on the family farm and ready to relax for three or four days before undertaking the responsibility of running the place for the next three months.

"Hi, Mom, what's cooking?"

"You look half-starved. When did you eat last?"

"About twelve hours ago, and I am starved."

"Supper will be ready in about two hours. You'll have to wait 'til then."

"Ok, I'll take a nap then."

Before I realized it, Mom was shaking me awake and saying, "Your supper is ready. Come on and eat before it gets cold." I looked at my watch, then realized I had slept for more than two hours. When I was fully awake the hunger pains came back full blast. "Ummm, that smells good, Mom. I can hardly wait to sample it."

"I fixed some of your favorite things. Let's sit and eat."

The table was loaded with fried chicken, country ham, hot biscuits, gravy, mashed potatoes, green beans, pickles, relishes, plus jam and jellies. It was hard to wait as Dad asked the blessing. When it was over he said, "We're glad to have you home for a while, son." That sobered me, and I realized that he really did care for me and for what I was planning to do.

"Thanks, Dad, I'm sure glad to be here, too. I hope we will all enjoy the summer together. Mom, all of this food looks great. I'm afraid I'll founder myself. You make me feel like the prodigal son has returned."

"We're just glad to see you. Do you realize that you haven't been home since Christmas?"

"Yes, I do, Mama, and I'm sorry, but I've been really busy. I've had a full schedule of classes, a lot of dissecting labs and chemistry labs. I have also been waiting tables at an off-campus restaurant twice a day. But that is no excuse for not calling or writing more. I'll try to do better this last year."

By the time we had finished, I had eaten so much that I was almost ashamed of myself. "Everything was so good, Mom. I've made a pig of myself. Thank you."

For the next three days, I ate three large meals each day, slept eight to ten hours each night, and by the fourth day I was full and rejuvenated. Again, I was ready to take on the tasks Dad had assigned me. Sunday came, and I attended church with my younger brother and sister. We sat in separate pews from our parents, who also sat in pews across from each other. Dad lead the prayers, Mama sang in the choir, as had been their habit from the time I could remember going to church. While we were there, Marie Abston came in with her family, and we soon spied each other and cast meaningful glances across the aisles separating us. Church lasted about two hours, and the benediction ten to fifteen minutes before we could leave. Of course, Marie and I headed for each other. Kathleen (my sister) came along.

"Hi, Marie, how are you? You look great today."

"Thanks, you look good to me, too. When did you get home?"

"Thursday night. I was worn out and half-starved. All I have done is eat and sleep. I feel great now. Guess I'll hit the road tomorrow."

"Are you going back so soon?"

"Naw, I mean starting the farm work."

"Oh, I see." She turned to Kathleen, asking, "How are you doing today, Kathleen?"

"Fine. I didn't think you even saw me, just my big brother home from college."

"Aw, you know better. I just see you a lot more often. He does look good to me, though."

"What are you doing these days, Marie?"

"Nothing much, and I'm getting bored."

"We'll have to see if we can't do something about that. Do you still have the same phone number?"

"Yes, I do," she said with a very meaningful and inviting look, which said, "please call me."

"I'll call you when everything is settled down. Maybe we can get together soon."

"That will be fine. I'll look forward to your call."

The next day, Dad and I had a long talk about my plans for the summer. We agreed that I should manage the farm and that the two of us should coordinate the work and other activities. We also agreed that he should pay my tuition and books for this last year of college for my working the farm. There should be an allowance of $100 per quarter for other expenses. "What about my social life this summer, Dad?"

"Oh, well, I think you can find time for plenty of that. A little advice first. Be careful of that young lady that you are romancing with or you will get yourself in trouble."

"Oh, I will watch out, Dad. I have too much at stake to go too far and cause the both of us to suffer the consequences."

"Just to be safe go by the drug store and let Harlin advise and supply you with safety materials."

"Ok, I will. Now I'm ready to go to work. Where shall I start?"

"First thing you should do is to have Jack show you all over the farm so you can decide for yourself what needs to be done first."

"Good idea. I know you have calls to make so go ahead and we'll look at the situation."

Jack and I saddled a pair of horses and canvassed the cornfields, the tobacco patch, the wheat and oat fields, then all of the hay fields. "Don't you think we should lay by the corn first, Jack?"

"Yeah, it's ready. It'll take a week. Some of it will have to be done with the double shovel (a two-pointed plow that is pulled by one mule). With that plow we can kill the weeds between rows. You can take the riding cultivator since I need the exercise, ok?"

"Let's go ahead and start about 1 o'clock. It'll take me a few days to get back into the swing of this." Within five days, we had finished the corn plowing, and we were through with it for the summer. The tobacco crop was tilled and cared for by a sharecropper that lived on the place.

"The wheat's not ready for the binder yet, Jack. Let's take a look at the fences and fix them. Let's start with the pasture." That was a bigger job than expected, and by the time we had finished all of them, I had a few blisters and bruises. but I also was not so tired from the work. My stamina was increasing by the day, and I was craving female companionship and needed to expend my energies in a different direction.

Friday night I called Marie. "Hello, beautiful. What are you doing tomorrow night?"

"No plans yet. I've been waiting for that call you promised to make."

"Could I see you tomorrow night about 7? If I can borrow a car."

"Seven is fine. I'll be at my brother's house. Come a little earlier if you can."

Saturday, I saved my energy by just piddling around and laying plans for the evening. During the day I mentioned to Jack that I needed a car.

"You can have mine tonight if you can drive it."

"Good, I appreciate it. I'll fill it up with gas and get it back in good shape."

At 6:30, I arrived at the brother's house. Nobody was there except my date. "Where is your brother and his wife?"

"Oh, they had to go to church at Liberty. He's preaching there."

"Oh, I see. Where do you want to go?"

"Let's just stay here a while. Come into the living room."

"Thanks. You look great and your perfume is wonderful. You are irresistible." As she turned to me with that certain look, we were in each other's arms. Our hungry lips met in a longing kiss as we stayed in a long embrace.

"That was wonderful—you took my breath away. It's good to see you again. You are beautiful to look at. I like your hairdo. Your dress fits just right, and your eyes are shining with happiness."

"I'm happy because I'm with you. Tell me about college life this past year."

"It's been a great year. Class work has been tough, but fun. I have met a lot more friends and a carload of beautiful coeds. they have been teaching me to dance and to make love, but no sex."

"You dog, you'd better not do anything like that."

"Come on, Marie, I was just teasing. Come here." I smooched her again with a torrid and long embrace. Her response was equal to my advances. I had to control myself, or there would be a lot of trouble. When we stopped, our breathing was a little fast and ragged as we both were stimulated. We held each other silently for a few minutes as we calmed our emotions. "We had better stop this, Marie. Let's go for a ride and cool off."

"I guess you're right. Where are we going?"

"Oh, we'll just take off and talk. How about driving by the high school and reminiscing a bit?"

"Ok, that's what I would love to do."

We drove slowly as we talked mostly of what everybody did during the time we spent in high school. The longest time was spent talking about the last year I spent in high school and how I was fooled by Lillian, whom I dated and how she "fell" for a thirty-two year old teacher that divorced his wife that year so he and Lillian could be married. We had a good laugh over that. Then she remembered my winning the public-speaking contest for the school and how proud she was of me when I won. Marie also recalled the student body electing me the "best all-around student" award and how the faculty later denied that honor to me and awarded it to a female classmate, who happened to be the girlfriend of the principal's son.

"Yeah, I remember. I was really hurt by that. I even went to the principal to let him know how I felt. But now I have to laugh about how they were influenced by their children's relationship. That's life for you. Some disappointments do strengthen one throughout life. At the time I was helped by many friends that supported me and let me know that I got a dirty deal. It doesn't hurt anymore."

We drove back toward her brother's house, and by the time we arrived, they had returned home. We went in to see them. "Hello, Thelma, how are you? It's good to see you. How are you, J. C.? How are things with you?" We exchanged pleasantries, they excused themselves, and we were alone again. We couldn't keep our hands off each other.

"Let's be careful, Marie. We had better calm down."

"I know, but it's been so long since we've seen each other."

"We're young, and there's plenty of time for courtin'. Guess I had better go on home." We held hands and talked. Two minutes later, we were in a close embrace again. You had better go now. Wendell."

"Ok, I'm going. See you tomorrow night at church. That is safer. I won't be able to walk you home tomorrow night either. Bye."

The drive home was a thoughtful one. I was in no position to "court" any girl in such a way that she might think seriously of marriage. There would certainly have to be more self-control by both of us, or we would have to stop seeing each other. This was the decision I came to on my way home and vowed to tell Marie of the decision. The goals I had set were my first priority, and I intended to stick to those goals, even if it meant hurting someone I didn't want to hurt, especially Marie. Being with her was enjoyable and helped pass the summer faster and we stayed out of trouble.

In the meantime, the farm work went on. Wheat and oats were combined and later threshed. Hay was mowed and raked. All of this I did with horsepower. I rode the mower and rake for endless hours, beginning as soon as the morning dew left and continuing until sundown. That went on for a full week before finishing. The hay "cured" for four or five days, then was raked into "windrows," and piled into "shocks." We loaded the hay onto a wagon with pitch forks, trampled it down, and hauled it to the barn where it was removed from the wagon by a hay fork and stored there. That was really tiring, as you handled the hay four times before completing the job for storage. I thought there had to be a better way to do this. Finally, the harvesting and storing was all done except the corn crops which would be done in November. I had a lot more leisure time the last weeks to prepare for returning to college life.

During that time, I made more house calls with Dad than earlier on. I found this a lot more interesting than in earlier years and months. It also made me realize even more that studying medicine was really the path I wanted to follow.

"Dad, do you think I can make the grade to get into medical school?"

"I think you can if you concentrate on this last year of pre-med classes and not so much on a 'hot-tailed' girl.

"You're right, and I've begun to realize that. I'm preparing to break off my relationship with this hometown girl when I go back to school in a few days. Don't worry, I'm not about to get into trouble and have to marry someone. I'll wait for that pleasure later."

"Good. I was getting a little worried about your activities. You've been spending a lot of time courting her, and that could be very risky."

"I know what my goal is now, and nothing is going to stop me unless I'm just not smart enough to make the grade."

The next weeks went flying by. Daytime was spent with Dad, plus packing clothes and concentrating on college courses I planned to take this last year. The nights were spent in less time with Marie as a safety measure. Again, the last nights alone with her were not too pleasant. She wanted promises, like writing at least once a week, not forgetting her for other girls, and to come home more often.

"I'll do my best, but I can't promise anything. there'll be a lot of pretty girls to meet and date, but I'll also be very busy in class and lab work. I'll have to find a job. Why don't you socialize more with other people, and we can see each other when I can come home during the year? That will be easier for both of us."

"Are you trying to get rid of me?"

"No, Marie, I just don't want to let this thing get too serious. I'm going to medical school! Don't worry, I'll never forget you."

After a teary good-bye we parted, and I felt relieved. At least I was honest with her, but I knew within my heart this courtship had to stop.

Two days later I was on my way back to college for my last year. Riding on the bus back to MTSC, I wondered what was in store for me. My brother, Prentice, had decided he needed a college degree and was enrolling in the same school and was to room with me. I was a bit leery of this, but would give it a trial first. He had been working for the DuPont Company, and he had been promised a better position if he had a college degree, especially in chemistry. I knew it would be rough on him after being out of school for four years, and he would need tutoring, which I could do since having had three years of college chemistry. We had a double room reserved for us, and I, having gotten there first, arranged everything and was settled in when "big brother" arrived two days later. He came in his own car. He also had a closet full of suits and dress shirts, plus ties to wear. The girls would really make a play for him!

He settled in, met several of my friends, and we went together to register the next day. On the way, I advised him to not take tough courses, such as math or a foreign language. "Oh, I'm not afraid of math. We use it a lot in some of the labs where I work. so I may take chemistry as well."

"Fine by me, but more power to you. You will have an advisor anyway."

As we arrived to register, I spotted Miz Green and introduced them. "Prentice has decided to return to school after working for four years. He will need some advice and counseling."

"I'll be glad to help," the helpful lady replied.

I left them to register for my courses, including more chemistry, and went back to the dormitory. P'john soon came in and threw his schedule on his desk.

"What's wrong, man?"

"I'm not sure I'm doing the right thing. It may be too tough for the first quarter."

"Let's see. What are you taking? Chemistry I, general math, American history, and English I. Oh, you can do it. You'll just have to get back in the habit of studying again."

Classes soon started, and we didn't see much of each other during the daytime hours, but we stayed in at night. He would occasionally ask for help in chemistry or English. He did well in spite of the four years of absence from the classroom. He made friends too easily and, coupled with those that I had made for the past three years, our room was full, usually from 5 to 9 o'clock nightly. We had a talk and decided something had to be done, or we would both be in trouble with our grades.

"How about our putting a sign on the door? Visiting hours 5:30 to 7 p.m. Other hours reserved for STUDY." It worked, and we lost no friends as a result.

The quarter went by quickly as we both were busy. P'john applied himself well and was into the routine of schoolwork and some extra-curricular activities. Class work and extra labs kept me busy, usually until 5 o'clock three days a week. My leisure time was taken up with research in the library, and this left little time for social life. Some nights were spent in ballroom dance, and the Dramatic Club met every two weeks.

The Sigma Club met monthly, and every member was required to attend. Looking back, campus life was really busy. At that age (twenty) my energy level was high, and I had to use up the adrenalin that flowed so freely. So far I had little time for finding a coed that interested me. Then something happened.

About three weeks into classes, they were hazing all freshmen on campus. As we were standing in line in the cafeteria, several freshmen girls came in and stood in line near us. They were all barefooted and dressed in old, long dresses. As I looked, one caught my eye. She reminded me of my mother's pictures at that age. She saw the look on my face and smiled at me. The attraction was so great I couldn't resist walking up for a closer look. I was almost tongue-tied, then I saw her bare feet. They were perfect to me. "Hi, you have beautiful feet. They match the rest of you. If you're having the annual barefoot contest, you should easily win first prize."

She giggled, "Well, thank you. That's quite a compliment."

"Are you enjoying college life."

"Yes, so far it's great..."

"The next three years will get better as they go along. Where are you from?"

"Lynchburg."

"Oh, that's where they make the famous 'Jack Daniels' whiskey and pretty women, too, I see. I also hope to see you around sometime." She wouldn't tell me her name, but the next day I found out who she was and where she was staying, and vowed to call her to try for a date. It took me another two weeks to contact her through a friend. I called the dormitory where she roomed and asked to speak to her.

"Hello, how are your pretty feet? I'm the brash fellow that admired your feet and spoke to you in the cafeteria last week. My name is Wendell Wilson, and I want to apologize for my behavior that day."

"Oh, that was ok. It tickled me. Thanks for the back-handed compliment."

"I'd like to see you sometime and apologize in person. Could I do that?"

"I'll have to think about it."

"Good. May I call you back in a couple of days?"

"Yes, I guess so..."

I waited three days to let her think I was not too eager. When I called she wasn't in, so I left a message, and waited two more days until a Friday evening. I knew by the grapevine that she would be on campus Saturday and might be homesick. She was in that time and very receptive to my call, seemingly eager to talk to me. I knew then that now was the time to ask for that date, so I did.

"How about that personal apology I want to make? Could we meet somewhere tomorrow after lunch?"

"That'll be fine."

"Wonderful. I'll see you then at the dorm."

Would you believe that when I arrived, I was so excited I was shaking. When she came down the stairs, she looked as excited and as scared as I felt. I had to swallow a lump in my throat before being able to speak. All I could say was, "Hi, you look great. Shall we go?"

I had no idea where we would go, but we started walking aimlessly, talking about the campus and how beautiful it was with the big shade trees, winding walkways, and benches beneath the trees so people could rest or just sit and talk. One large tree looked particularly inviting with all of its large branches shading the bench and grass beneath it. I thought, *This is a perfect place to get acquainted.* "Let's sit on this bench for a while, ok?"

"It looks like a perfect spot to me."

"Now, pretty girl, tell me about yourself."

"There's nothing to tell that would interest you."

"Anything about you would be interesting to me. Then I'll go first, but it'll probably scare you away from here."

"Try me first. Then we'll see."

"Well, to being with, I'm from a family of twelve children. Shall I go on?"

"Yes, go ahead. That doesn't scare me. I have six brothers and sisters myself, and that's a fairly big family, too."

"Then you understand where I'm coming from. We live in a rural area of Macon County, Tennessee, so far back that we have no paved roads and have only had electric power for less than three years. We still farm with mules, ride wagons to church, and go swimming in the raw. That's enough about me," I added.

"No, tell me more. I want to know if you're for real, so be honest in what you tell me. I have a way to check on you."

"Do you mean you have been checking on me?"

"Yep, I sure have."

"Then I don't need to tell you any more. You sure are sneaky."

That stopped the interview, and we were having light conversation, bantering back and forth, listening to a mockingbird in the tree and soft music from the nearby dorm as she smiled softly. I was in seventh heaven. Then our beautiful, pink cloud burst as the mockingbird flew to another branch to launch his new songs. While in flight, he sprayed the area with his droppings which landed on the shoulder of the beautiful "princess" and spoiled our romantic interlude. We both were shocked and speechless. Out came my handkerchief, and I tried to apologize as I wiped the offensive droppings from her beautiful pink dress. On her face was a look of horror and pain while her eyes filled with tears. All I could say or do was: "Shall we go back to the dormitory?"

As we walked back in complete silence, I wanted to put a comforting arm around her to let her know how sorry I really was. That was impossible as we both knew how each felt about the incident. At the front steps, I barely murmured a good-by and left. After the accident I was afraid to call or see her for another ten days. Then I accidentally bumped into her on the way to lunch. We talked, and the ice was broken. "May I call you again?" I wanted to know.

"Yes, I wish you would" (the mockingbird didn't ruin our romance after all).

I soon came back to earth and reality. The final exams were facing me in a week, and nothing else mattered except that. I ate and slept chemistry, chemical equations, biology, and dissecting labs, working slide rules, reciting poetry for Ms. Dunn, etc. Women were left out of my life during that period. When I did relax, it was jogging around the track or playing a set of tennis with a friend. That was a crucial time for me. It meant being accepted or rejected on my application to medical school. I must have done the right thing because all my grade averages were great.

The grind began again two days after finals and I needed some moral support. I first went to James Baxter, my math tutor and advisor, and was encouraged by him. "You don't have anything to worry about, Wendell. Why don't you talk to Miz Green also?" I made an appointment for the next day, and at 3 o'clock that afternoon, I was in Miz Green's office, listening to her.

"What in the world is wrong with you, Wendell Wilson? Don't you know you are doing fine? Have some faith in yourself, relax more, have some dates, go to a movie, but just relax for a while. By the way, have you applied to medical school yet?"

"The applications are on the way. I'll need three letters of recommendation for the application when I complete them. Will you be able to write one for me?"

"Sure, I'll be glad to. Who else is sending one?"

"Mr. Edney in biology and also our family doctor and dentist."

"Good, now get out of here. Call your girlfriend and stop that worrying."

"Thanks, Miz Green, you're a real friend." Boy! Was she ever. I never dreamed I would hear those words of advice come from *her* lips.

I heeded Miz Green's advice. I went straight to the phone in our dorm, called "that" girl, and asked if I could see her the next day. Either in a weak moment or a state of desperation, she said, "Yes." After the phone call there was still time to play a set of tennis, and by the time we finished there was barely time to eat, then a quick shower, and a good night's sleep. The next day I felt rejuvenated, was ready to take on the tough courses and challenge my competitor. The self-confidence had returned. The "Green" formula was working.

Within a week the application for medical school came, and I had it in the mail in another week, complete with letters, pictures, and grade transcripts. Now all I had to do was to stay busy, keep up the daily routine of class, labs, exercise, play tennis, jog each morning, have an occasional date, and wait. That way I kept so busy that I was never bored and had no time for worry. By the time the three applications were returned, I was ready to accept anything. Two were accepted and one, the University of Texas, was rejected because of no formal mathematical courses. When I studied (Louisville and Tennessee), I chose Tennessee because it was less expensive and closer to home. I also had the choice of entering in June or September. I called on P'john for advice, and then Dad. Both advised to wait until September and get my B.S. degree since I might need it in future years. I was to find out later how right they were. Before the quarter ended, I knew what my future would be for the next four years. Now I could relax, play more, and get that B.S. degree.

I'll never forget the day that application was returned as approved. After the morning classes, I went by the post office at school, picked up the mail, and saw the official letter from the University of Tennessee in Memphis. I was afraid to open it. I took it to the room where nobody was around and put it in my desk. I sat down in a chair, thinking, *What if they didn't accept me? What will I tell everybody?* I was in a dilemma, *What am I to do?* I knew that it had to be opened, but I waited as long as possible before I had courage enough to do so. Finally, with my hands shaking so bad that I could hardly hold the letter, I tore the envelope open and unfolded the pages. There it was in clear, typewritten letters: "Dear Mr. Wilson: We are pleased to inform you that your application for admission to the University of

Tennessee School of Medicine has been approved by the Committee of Admissions."

I couldn't read any further, the tears were blurring my 20/20 vision. I locked the door as they flowed freely, for joy, for the next five minutes. I wanted to shout to the world. I made it! I made it! Do you hear, I made it! I was nearly insane for a little while. Thank You, God, Thank You, Thank You.

After finally getting myself under control, I read the whole thing through twice to fully understand what it all meant. I finally unlocked the door, washed my face, and looked in the mirror to see if I still looked the same. I waited for P'john and all my friends to tell me that I looked different, or had I seen a vision? I *felt* different, so maybe I would *look* different.

Everybody came and went as usual. Nobody asked if something was wrong. Then a good friend (James Armstrong) saw me and asked: "What in the world has happened to you? You seem to be walking in outer space. Come on back to earth and tell me what is wrong. Has some girl told you she's mad about you?"

"No, nothing like that. I've just received the best news of my whole life. Sit down and let me tell you what has happened."

His eyes and mouth flew open as he sat, gingerly on the bed and stared at me in expectancy, thinking some glorious event had happened.

"Well, *tell* me what it is."

"I have been accepted to *medical school*! Isn't that great?"

"Yeah, it sure is." A big smile came, he stuck out his hand, and tears came to his eyes. "Congratulations, Wilson, I knew you could do it. Boy, I'm really proud of you. You deserve a medal. Now what are you going to do, tell the whole world?"

"I feel like it, but I guess I'll call my parents first if I can find a dime. Then I'll tell P'john. Tonight, I'll celebrate by taking my date to the movie, then we'll split a hamburger and coke. Afterwards, as we walk back to the campus, I'll break the news to her. Won't she be surprised?"

"Yes, she sure will."

"You don't sound too enthused about my telling her the good news."

"Well, you do know how she feels, that all doctors will drink heavily, and work day and night."

"I will never do the heavy drinking, Jim. I don't do any at all now, you know that. Louise bases that on one relative she admired who fell into the habit when he was practicing. I have to tell her. Besides, I'm not married to the girl and doubt I ever will be. Aw, come on, Jim, let's celebrate my victory over 'the mountain' of labs, experiments, tough exams, and hard work. *I'm going to medical school*!

That was a glorious night. The movie was a tearjerker, and we both cried a little, then laughed to cover up. Afterward, we *did* split the coke and hamburger, and then we walked, slowly, back to the campus. Somewhere along the way we stopped and sat on a low brick wall.

"I have some good news to tell you, pretty girl."

"It must be good. I don't think I have ever seen you so happy. Tell me what it is."

"I hope you'll be happy about it, too. Today, I got that long-awaited letter from the University of Tennessee in Memphis, telling me that I had been accepted to medical school for the September class. Isn't that great?"

"Oh, yes, that's wonderful news. Congratulations! I'm so proud of you I could hug your neck, and she did (but no kisses to go with it).

"Thanks, honey. That is worth a zillion dollars to me. You'll never know how much it really means to hear you say that. Now my day is complete. We'd better get you back to the dorm, or you might lose your late leave."

We had one fourth mile to go, but it seemed to take only a minute to walk that distance and reluctantly say our good nights. I don't know what my date was thinking or doing, but I was walking on cloud nine and had conquered the world.

By the time I got back to the dorm, all of our friends had gathered in our room to congratulate me. We got so boisterous that the hall monitor came to our room to quiet us down. Somebody said, "Aw, come on, Jack, Doc has just been accepted to medical school. Don't you want to help him celebrate?"

"Well, congratulations, Doc, I'm proud of you, too, but you'll have to be a little quieter with the celebration, ok?"

"Sure, Jack, thanks."

It was very heartwarming to have so many friends that really seemed to care about their fellow man and which direction his life would lead him in future years. That night touched me deeply. That was the type of spontaneous action one would expect from college friends. It was also something one never forgets.

That quarter of college ended on a high note, and we were out for a two-week Christmas vacation. While at home I had a duty to perform. That "duty" was to see Marie and tell her that our relationship must end. That was a painful and dirty thing to do. After all, she had been good to me in every way, even to telling me she truly loved me and would do "anything" for me. That made it all the more painful. So I took the cowardly way out, telling her that I might not be able so see her again before having to return to school. That was December 30, 1938. On January 2, 1939, I knew that we had to go back the next day and I called Marie to tell her that. I heard crying on the other end. It hurt because I felt guilty that I had caused her pain and apparent sorrow.

"Please don't cry, Marie. I didn't intend to hurt you. You have meant a lot to me and have given so much time to me during the last three years that I don't want to keep on hurting you. Our relationship has to stop. Our directions in life are so different now that it wouldn't be fair to you to keep you from more freedom in life. You should see new people, make new friends, and leave us old ones behind. Don't think of me in a romantic way anymore. I have become involved with someone else, and I think you should too."

"I know you're right, but it hurts too much to talk about it. Good-bye." The phone was silent, and I hung up. This had to be the end of a romance that began innocently and got out of control along the way.

January 3, 1939: We were back on campus and gathering in the hallways to register for the upcoming quarter. It was like a family reunion when we saw old friends again. "Hey, Jim Baxter, how was your Christmas?" "Hello, Paul, ready for some more chemistry lab time?" "Hi, Margaret, you look great, good to see you." "Helloo, pretty girl, tell me about your holidays." This went on and on until we had all finished and cleared the halls.

That evening P'John and I discussed his college future, and he seemed very uncertain about what he wanted to do. I tried to encourage him to continue on in school. "You've made a good start this quarter, stay with it, and you'll like it much better. You're not wasting your time by getting an education. You never waste time when you're gaining knowledge. That is something nobody can take from you . . . think, P'John, you can be the boss of your division by getting a college degree. Besides, you'll have a position, not a job. You will also have a much better income."

"Ok, I'll stick it out for another three months—then decide."

The winter quarter was uneventful. I was happy with classes, fewer labs, more social life, and a bit more romancing. Now that my worries were behind, the world seemed to take on a more rosy hue. I liked everybody and everything. The classes were all interesting and enlightening. Life was wonderful and beautiful, and I wanted to live it to the fullest.

April, 1939: Spring quarter is in session. Trees are budding, flowers are blooming, romances are blossoming as lovesick couples stroll lazily around the campus, holding hands, stealing a furtive kiss and looking "moon-eyed" at each other. That was a dangerous time of the year for college students, a time when hearts ruled heads and wedding plans were made. I enjoyed the romancing part, but marriage was far distant in my mind. There were six more months of college to finish and then four years of medical school. No time for a serious courtship. That was not to say that I paid no attention to beautiful, sexy-looking co-eds. After all, all normal males will notice a female figure strolling by with a twist to her hips, a bounce to her bust, and a dreamy look on her face. Even if you were a fifty-year-old male with a normal testosterone output, that would attract one like nectar attracts bees. Thank God April is a short month or I couldn't have resisted the "thrust" of mother nature much longer.

Spring quarter, with all its glory and sensual side-effects of April finally ended. It was well worth all the pain, agony, daydreams, glory, and hopes that came and went like the mating of birds and the blossoms of flowers.

Now it is June, 1939, and time for graduating exercises. Although I would only get a "dummy" diploma, I would have the privilege of wearing the cap and gown. What a thrill to walk across the stage to get the false diploma and receive the handshake from Dean Beasley, then move the tassel from right to left across the mortar board, then walk across the stage, moving that tassel while gripping that "diploma." I was shivering by the time I sat down. While the last few are walking across the stage I am wondering, *Are any of my family here? I hope so because I am the first member to get a college degree since our father graduated from medical school in 1905.* As we are marching from the auditorium, I am looking in vain for a familiar Wilson face. None were in sight. God, was I disappointed! I ducked in the nearest bathroom to hide the disappointment. I wondered why no one was there and kept thinking, *Nobody cares what I've accomplished. It hurts, but if they don't care, then why should I? I'll show 'em. Now, I will really show 'em Ole Scrub from Bugtussle can amount to something.*

In spite of the disappointment, I knew that the family cared, so I swallowed my pride, hid my hurting, and went on home for the two-week break before going back to finish that last three months of college life.

June 23, 1939: I have completed registration, settled in Jones Hall with my roommate, James Armstrong, and am looking for my soulmate. There is a familiar voice: "Hey, are you lost?" Then I heard a throaty, teasing laugh. I jumped for joy!

"Where did you come from? You weren't here a second ago."

"Aren't you glad to see me?"

"What do you think? I'd like to give you a big bear hug and a "big red" kiss right here in front of God and everybody. That's how much I care."

"Aw, you—let's go to the cafeteria while you cool down."

"Have you girls registered yet?"

"Yes, have you?"

"Yes, we have—mostly crip courses like geography, home-ec, and entomology."

"Are you both taking home-ec?"

"Yeah, you girls said it was so tough we thought we would see for ourselves."

"I bet you both will regret taking that. It's really tough. Don't you think so, Lucille?"

"Yes, it's been tough for me."

"I don't see anything hard about cooking or decorating. Do you, Jim?"

These were our present girl friends, and we were actually taking the course to be around them as well as learning something, too. Everybody knew what the reasons were anyway. So all was well.

Lunch at the cafeteria was a great hour of teasing, holding hands, knowing looks, and light banter. By the time noon had passed, we went our separate ways, but not before all had agreed on getting together again for supper and a short visit afterwards. Everything went as planned through dinner, but shortly afterward, somehow we seemed to pair off into different directions (I'm sure that was not intentional).

In our wandering and talking, we wound up by the same bench under the same tree where we had our first tete-a-tete.

"Remember this place? How about stopping here for a minute?"

"I guess it's safe. I don't hear a mockingbird now."

There were deep shadows all around, no one else in sight, and she was irresistible in a pale-blue dress, hair falling around her shoulders, and her faint tantalizing aroma of perfume filling the air. My arms were around her in a flash, our lips met softly and then hungrily, but briefly. "God, I've missed you these three weeks."

"I've missed you, too. Let's walk some more."

The walk was slow and blissful with occasional questions about what the next ten weeks would be like and how we could handle the togetherness. We didn't see the girlfriends, except in class for another week or so. By then they were eager for male companionship. "Hi pretty girl, would you like to have a picnic?

"Oh, yes, that would be wonderful. Where are we going?"

"Just anywhere that there's a stream, a sand bar, and some shade."

"You don't want much, just a perfect spot."

Somehow we found all the things mentioned. The girls found baskets and food, somebody borrowed a car, and four couples piled in. We found the spot and spent the afternoon wading, walking, and exploring, and near sundown we were eating hot dogs and drinking cokes. It was old friends getting together again like a family. That day was a fun one, and by the time it was over we were tired and ready to go home.

Classes met daily from 8 o'clock to 4 o'clock p.m., but some of the group had only morning hours in class and were free to do other things in the afternoons. That meant more time would be spent with the opposite sex in whatever they wanted to do. That meant trouble sometimes, too. Our group was mostly campus-bound and had no problems, but some of us had a yen to have some off-campus action and looked for ways to make it possible. I happened to be the one that was lucky. My sister was teaching school, and she also had a car. Since her school was out for the summer, I asked if it would be possible to borrow the car for a month. "Think about it and I'll call back tomorrow," I asked. I called back the next night. While the phone was ringing I kept my fingers crossed for good luck. It did the trick.

"Hi, Sis, how are things?"

"Fine. Do you still want the car?"

"You bet I do. I'll take good care of it and keep it washed too."

"All right, you can have it for a month, but you'll have to come and get it."

"Thanks, Sis, I'll be in Lafayette on the 5 o'clock bus Saturday. Can you meet me then?"

"Yes, I'll be there," she promised.

We jumped for joy. "Hot dog, now we'll have some way to get off campus."

I spent six hours on the trip to Lafayette, stayed overnight, had three good meals, and then headed back to MTSC at 1 p.m. Sunday afternoon. I had no driver's license, no insurance, and about two dollars in my pocket. But I had a good-sized box of food packed by Mom that would last for three days. At the moment, I had no worries and very little sense, but I had a car.

That night James Armstrong and I had to inspect everything about it and take it by the dorm for all the girls to see. It passed inspection with flying colors, and I was in the driver's seat in more ways than one.

The car was a social asset, but from every other standpoint a definite liability. First of all, I did not have a driver's license and had to have that to drive legally. Two days after getting the car, my roommate and I (driving) went to the local Highway Patrol office to apply and take the test. I drove up, parked the car, and went in. We were greeted very politely by the patrolman.

"Come in, fellow. What can we do for you?"

"I want to apply for a driver's license."

"Oh, you do? I should arrest you."

"Why. I haven't done anything illegal."

"Oh, yes you have. You've been driving a car without a driver's license, and this is illegal in Tennessee."

"But, Sir, I wasn't aware of that law."

"That's no excuse. Where are you from?"

"Bugtussle." He didn't believe me. I could see it all over his face. "You don't believe me, I bet."

"No, I don't believe you. Where is Bugtussle *at*?"

I knew we had him then because he would have to admit that he was as ignorant of some things as I was.

"I thought everybody had heard of Bugtussle, particularly Tennessee Highway Patrol members. It is on the border of Tennessee and Kentucky, mostly in Macon County, Tennessee. It is pretty far back in the 'sticks'."

"It must be." He was pretty subdued by all of this explaining, and I could see that he was willing to concede. "Tell you what, Son. If you promise me that you will get a driver's license in your home county, we'll let you go. Now, how will you get back to where you are staying?"

My roommate spoke up, "I'll drive. Here's my driver's license."

"Ok, now get out of here."

"Yessir. Thank you, Sir."

James drove the car and I sat silent for a while. Finally he said, "If you were not going to medical school, you should be a lawyer or a preacher with all the BS you gave him."

"It worked. He couldn't admit he didn't know where Bugtussle was and fine me at the same time, so he saved face by scolding me and verbally throwing us out. I'm relieved he halfway believe my ignorant plea. I'll get a license Saturday." Four days later, Friday night, I drove home to Lafayette, sixty miles away, without a driver's license. The next day, my brother took me to the Highway Patrol office to make application for a permit to drive. I drove around the courthouse twice, parked and backed once, and was granted that license, a copy of which I have had since 1939.

About three weeks later, we same two went downtown on "business." Afterward, as I was pulling from the curbside parking, a car came from nowhere and, though the car was almost past, the corner of our left front bumper caught the end of his right rear bumper. He stopped, rushed over to me, saying, "What's the matter with you. Can't you see well?"

"I'm sorry, Sir. I didn't see how close you were."

"Let me see your driver's license." Boy, was I thankful to be able to show him my license.

"Yessir. I see. A new one, huh. What do you do?"

"I'm a student at MTSC."

"You are, huh. Can you pay for having these cars fixed?"

"Yessir." That was really stretching the truth. I had about fifteen dollars to my name. As he pulled away, I noted his license plate. He was a deputy sheriff! Then I began to sweat blood. We pulled into the garage, following the deputy, and I was relieved to see a familiar face. The fellow was the garage manager for the summer. He was also a friend and classmate at MTSC. Luck was on my side again.

"Hi, Wilson. What do you have against Deputy Ketchum? Let me see what we have. Oh, this won't be any trouble to fix. I can take care of both cars for twenty bucks. Is that fair enough?"

"Yes, it's fine with me. Okay, Mr. Ketchum?"

"So long as it's fixed, I don't care. But you had better be more careful with your driving from now on."

"Yessir, I will. Thank you." Both cars were soon repaired, and I was able to find the twenty dollars. I became a better driver due to that little accident. My sister never knew about the accident until years later.

Pretty soon everybody knew that "Doc" had a car, and there was many a request to borrow or share it. I refused to loan it to anyone except my roommate. The car was used a lot, but judiciously—usually for going to movies or just taking rides out in the country. Two or three couples usually went together. If we were out after dark, sometimes we changed drivers so we had equal "smooching" time. On one or two occasions we took trips to Nashville to sightsee or view a special movie. Those were the times when only two couples went. Since I was a senior, we had the privilege of occupying the back seat on the return to campus. That was when the "smooching" time tripled. Return trips were interspersed with periods of quiet, followed by excited conversation with driver and date. This was when the car was a definite asset to courtships and romances. The rest of the time it was a big liability requiring gas, washing, polishing, etc.

Classes were easy and pleasureful. We teased the girls, played up to the teacher, talked about how easy home-ec was and minimized the tougher courses. Before most realized it, summer school was over and exam time passed. This time I did not get a diploma either, just a promise one would be mailed to me in two weeks. I didn't care at that time. All I wanted was for the college to send a transcript of all my grades to the University of Tennessee Medical School so I could start the next chapter in my life.

The toughest part yet was still facing me. That was parting with long-time faithful friends and a beautiful woman I had begun to care for. Common sense told me this was just a romantic interlude that had run its course. But I could not leave at that and wouldn't leave without saying good-by in a romantic way. Packing my bags, I was thinking of how it should be done. Nothing seemed to be the right way, I just had to see *that* girl. I called and she answered the hall phone. That was very unusual. She had never done that before.

"Hi. What are you doing answering the phone?"

"Oh, I was hoping you would call, and I wanted to answer if you did."

"Thanks. Could I see you before we both leave here?"

"Sure, when?"

"In about five minutes. Meet me in front of the dorm, and we'll go for a coke."

I didn't wait two minutes. I couldn't.

She was waiting outside with that same pink dress on that she was wearing the first time we dated. It brought back fond memories and the hilarious "bird incident" also. "You look great in that pink dress. Do you want to sit on that favorite bench under the maple tree?"

"Yes, let's do." I parked the car, and we strolled and talked about that first time we sat there and got acquainted. We laughed nervously recalling that day, hoping there would not be a replay with birds. As we reached the bench and sat down we became silent, just looking into each other's eyes. She finally broke the silence.

"When are you leaving?"

"Whenever you have to go. When will that be?"

"My brother, Bill, will be here in half an hour."

"Let's walk up near the Science Hall to the spot where we had that first real meaningful kiss." She looked at me dreamily and with tears in her eyes, took my hand as we walked slowly to that "first-kiss hideout." During the next twenty minutes we relived and reenacted that day more than one time, making ourselves miserably happy as we did so. But neither of us would have been willing to go unless we had said good-bye in that way.

"I have to go. Bill will be here any minute."

"Just one more second of loving, then we'll leave." We were in each other's arms for a long embrace, then left in silence, afraid for the other to hear the tears in our voice. When we reached the car, she let go of my hand, and whispered—"Bye. Call me."

"I will, Sunday at 2 o'clock." At that minute I knew that we would see each other many more times before I left for medical school. That proved to be true, and it helped both of us to realize that we did not have a common interest that would hold us together for a lifetime. I hope she has as many fond memories of those years as I have.

My college friends have lasted for almost sixty years. I have had the opportunity to be the family physician of many that befriended me during those years. Without such friends as Edward Jennings, who helped me keep faith in God when it looked as though I had been forsaken. James Baxter who tutored me in math. Paul Stewart who worked with me in chemistry. Doyle ("Froggy") Smith who asked me to work for him so I could use his meal tickets when he was on road trips playing football, or James Armstrong, Raymond HIll, Hall Harris, Howard Lee, and Randy Wood. Last, but not least of these, Ralph Gwaltney, for helping me see the need of physical exercise and teaching me to play tennis—also, staying on the job with me when we waited tables at "Bock's Tea Room." I want to pay tribute to "Baker" who forced me to have an appendectomy just before it ruptured. If it had not been for "Baker," I might not have been here telling my story. Thanks, fellows, for helping me to be worth something to my fellow man. I will never forget those wonderful years.

Medical School

When I left home In September, 1939, it was for a cause and with a purpose. That cause was to become a physician, and the purpose was to work very hard to achieve that goal. Little did I realize what I was undertaking. Once again, I boarded a Greyhound bus for Memphis, Tennessee. The trip involved a 12-mile trip by car to Lafayette, a 70-mile bus ride to Nashville, and a 200-mile bus ride to Memphis, which consumed the better part of twelve hours.

We arrived in Memphis in late afternoon on September 18, 1939. Old friends from college, now medical students, met the bus and took me in tow. We went by the medical school where I saw the tall (three-story) buildings where we would be for the next three years. From there, I went to the Phi Rho Sigma Fraternity House where I would be living. I was made welcome by a friendly group of men, some I had known previously, and felt very comfortable there. The atmosphere was such that I felt at ease and a part of the group. The next morning at 8 o'clock they escorted me to the Medical School campus where we went through registration.

Then we were herded into a large room to meet the dean, Dr. O. W. Hyman. He was a small, intense man of about fifty years with thin red hair, a freckled face, small, piercing, gray eyes that seemed to bore through each student as he scanned the group as each one sat down. He was a no-nonsense type with no semblance of a sense of humor. As he stood before us, he leaned on his podium and said, "Good morning, ladies and gentlemen." You have now been enrolled into the School of Medicine, where each of you hope to become a physician. Let me tell you now that all of you will not do that. It is not that you can't but you just won't. Not because you are not capable, but because you will not apply yourselves. We are here to help you in any way we can, so long as it is honest and falls within the guidelines of this institution. My advice to you is to work hard, stay honest, and apply yourself to reaching that goal you have set for yourself. There will be a fifteen-minute break; then you return here for a personal interview in my office."

The class was interviewed in alphabetical order, which meant that I had to wait while forty-eight had their turn at being scrutinized, frightened, and at some time during the interview, even threatened. Sitting there waiting, each of us had become anxious and some had become angry. I, myself, was just plain scared. I knew that he would caution me because I had been through a small state college which he personally did not regard very highly. After about two hours of waiting, my time came. As I entered the room, Dr. Hyman looked up, nodded, and pointed to a chair. "Have a seat, Mr. Wilson."

"Thank you, Sir."

"I see you have no record of formal math courses during your college years."

"That's correct, Sir."

"How did you make it through those tough chemistry courses without the math?"

"A friend tutored me in the needed math courses."

"Did your friend come to medical school with you?"

I smiled. "No, he didn't, Mr. Hyman."

"Wilson, you are going to have a real hard time here. You will have to apply yourself 110 percent to make it."

"I am willing to do so, if it takes that to get through."

Dr. Hyman leaned forward over his desk, his small eyes boring into mine, and said, "I believe you will, Mr. Wilson. Good luck."

That interview haunted me for most of my first year in medical school and became very near to becoming my downfall.

The following morning we had an outline of the courses we would have. Then we toured the various classrooms, laboratories, dissecting rooms, and finally the basement area where they preserved the cadavers that the medical and dental students would dissect during study of gross anatomy. The place was dimly lighted, and as we proceeded along the hallways, a burning, sweetish odor engulfed the entire basement. It became stronger and stronger as we came to an oversized steel door, and I knew we had arrived at the "vat room." As the janitor unlocked this door, the stench multiplied tenfold; your eyes burned and watered profusely, your nostrils felt raw, and when you breathed, the rawness continued down the trachea into your bronchial area and into the entire lung fields. You felt like running out, but there was no place to go. Inside, the room was all concrete. First, a four-foot-wide apron surrounded the entire room. The central portion was partitioned off into many vats that were approximately two or three feet wide and two feet deep and eight feet long. Each vat had two bodies that were submerged in the foul-smelling formaldehyde solution. There must have been at least fifty to sixty vats in the room. It was eerie, but not scary. Each of us students had been used to the odors in smaller doses and had also had the experience of dissecting animal bodies before entering medical school. Even though we had done and seen all of these, it was far different when human bodies were to be the object of the scalpel, knife, scissor, bone saw, etc. I saw a few of the class members turn their heads and close their eyes. To me, this was an important part of the indoctrination into medical school.

The student assistant spoke: "Ladies and gentlemen, these are our preserving vats. We have other rooms similar to these with more cadavers. It is necessary for each specimen to be in the formalin solution for a number of months to be properly preserved for dissection. These bodies will not be used for another six weeks because they are not yet ready for dissecting. The ones you will 'operate' on are now in the dissection laboratory awaiting your 'introduction' tomorrow morning. Incidentally, each of you will need to have a dissecting partner selected by the time classes start tomorrow. You will also need to have a scalpel, strong dissecting scissors, skin hooks, strong cotton thread, a lab coat, and a strong stomach. Good luck. You are dismissed until 8 o'clock tomorrow.

The next day we were told to assemble in the chemistry lecture room at 8 o'clock to meet our professor. As we were seated, a fatherly 50-year-old entered the room. "Good morning, students. I am T. P. Nash. I will have the pleasure of being your caretaker and teacher for the next six months. To get acquainted, let's start by calling the roll. When I call your name please stand for a few seconds so I can recognize you the next time we meet." At the end of roll call he would call out a name then point to the right person, never missing. After that call work was outlined, and as we prepared to leave, Dr. Nash said, "Remember to be on time *every* time class meets. See you in the morning."

Next, we assembled in the hallway outside the anatomy dissecting lab. As we quieted down in anticipation of meeting the professor, a door to the dissecting lab opened and out he walked. You could hear a pin drop. His physical appearance and demeanor held us in awe. He was the epitome of my impression of "The Professor." He was a distinguished gentleman in his mid-60's who stood six feet tall, and was neatly dressed in a gray suit and navy-blue tie. He had closely cropped, iron-gray hair and a small mustache. His blue eyes twinkled, full of wit, wisdom, humor, and devilment. We were spellbound.

Cupping a hand to his ear he spoke, "Around here I am known as 'Dr. Witt,' your anatomy instructor. You may call me anything you wish, but only let me hear Dr. Wittenberg." That brought a laugh from the class and broke the spell he had cast upon us.

"Today we will start by having each team select a cadaver of their choice. Don't rush in and grab the first one you see. Act like gentlemen that you are supposed to be. All right, students, make your choices."

As the double doors swung wide open there was a rush of medical students that reminded me of women shoppers at an after-Christmas bargain sale or small children rushing everywhere searching for the many colored eggs at Easter time. I was thinking, *How foolish, one body would be as good as another for dissecting purposes.*

"Let's take this one, Wilson."

"That's ok with me."

"This one" was an 18-year-old black female with a perfect figure and not a blemish on her body. Then I noticed a small round hole in the center of her forehead.

"Looks like she got caught cheating, John."

"It sure does, but she should be a great body to work on."

How wrong we were! The next day was our first day of dissection. We started on the skin, studying every layer; the epidermis, dermis, subcutaneous tissue, etc. We quickly realized our mistake. We learned that curvaceous, young females have a lot of subcutaneous fat, which we had to deal with in order to study the other layers. This slowed and complicated our dissection as it masked other important structures, but we labored on.

"Dr. Witt" had an unorthodox teaching method, much like on-the-job training. He did not hold class in the designated classroom area, but in a corner of the dissecting lab or by the side of a cadaver where someone had demonstrated an anatomical structure in a superior way. He would call the class together and ask questions about the structure: "Name it. What is its blood and nerve supply? What is its function?" This way, each of us could picture this in our minds. He held some lectures each day with demonstrations of anatomical structures on students. Calling a name, he would say: "You come up here! Lecture about that particular structure." No matter what part of the anatomy, the demonstrating student had to expose that part. He was no respecter of students, but of the sex.

If the lecture involved the genitalia, the female class members were asked to leave the room. All of us cringed when he started a lecture concerning the "privates." Not one male could stand to be compared in "its" size to someone better "endowed" because he would be the butt of private jokes forever.

Concerning anatomical demonstrations, my roommate and dissecting partner had a dread (fear?) of being called before the class as a demonstrator. It happened one day, and I saw the fury in his face. He muttered, "That old S.O.B. I've a good mind to refuse."

"You go ahead, John, it's just your fingers."

Reluctantly, John walked slowly to the podium. "Let me see your hand, Professor," Dr. Witt said. John's face reddened as he stuck out his hand. "Thank you, Professor, now we can demonstrate the hand's functions. Now open and close your hand to make a fist. Now let us demonstrate some functions of the fingers, ok? Abduct your fingers (abduct means to separate). Good! Now adduct (close) your fingers. Good." Then "Dr. Witt" repeated in rapid-fire order; adduct, abduct, adduct, abduct, at least six times. John got so befuddled that he could not follow the correct orders. Then "Dr. Witt" added fuel to the fire by saying, in a sarcastic tone, "Thank you, Professor, you may be seated." After class, John was so angered that he hardly moved for a full five minutes and hardly realized what he was doing for the rest of that day. He couldn't let go of his anger for several days because he felt humiliated. Eventually, that incident would prove to be his downfall.

Dissection continued, day in and day out. Progress was slow on our cadaver, and I felt there was not enough time to complete each section of the body that had been allotted us. Under pressure we toiled on as "Dr. Witt" strolled up and down, observing each team as they labored, and discussed their work. All of this time, Dr. Witt was studying each student's attitude, sincerity, abilities, and reactions to the teaching methods. One of his habits was to suddenly stop by a student and start quizzing him about the area he was dissecting. If the student did not answer correctly, or was even hesitant with an answer, he would say: "You are not studying or working hard enough, Mister. *You* had better *get busy!*"

Dr. Witt's favorite thing was to have an appropriate nickname for each one in every class. My partner, an ex-teacher, was called "Professor," Lyon was called Lamb. A fine young man (Johnson) was called "Mama's Boy," as he came to class each day dressed in a suit, complete with white shirt and bow tie. He also lived with his mother. The female was called "Dahling," which she thoroughly disliked. A full six weeks went by, and I thought I had escaped the "Dubbing." The next day, he lectured on the esophagus. Suddenly, he stopped in the middle of a sentence, got everybody's attention, and blurted out: "You 'Voodrow,' *come up here.*" I felt weak all over. My knees trembled as I walked that "mile" (eight feet) to the podium. "Now, Voodrow, describe the swallowing mechanism, name the muscles involved, and the nerve and blood supply, plus the definite action of each. I did and I didn't. First, I gulped when I swallowed and then after a bit of choking, I was able to answer in detail. I was really lucky that we had spent a good two hours studying and dissecting the esophagus two days before that lecture. From that day until graduation and beyond, all my classmates called me "Voodrow."

Dr. Witt's teaching methods were so unusual that some students could never fully accept them. I thought they were the very best methods one could use to teach someone Gross Anatomy. Some of the students developed a thorough dislike for him, and my roommate, and dissecting partner actually had a hatred for him. This became an obsession with John.

"Woodrow, how can you like that man?"

"He has been good for, and to me, John. I also happen to think his method of teaching will instill anatomy into someone so well that he will never forget it."

"You may be right, but I can't stand the S.O.B. He's driving me insane. I am thinking of dropping out of school."

"Aw, come on John, you can't do that. Think what you have sacrificed to have this opportunity to study medicine. Don't quit now. At least think it over again before you make that decision."

"Ok, I'll think about it."

A couple of weeks passed, and I thought John was settling down and would stay in school, but again I was wrong! A night or two later, at about 2 a.m., I was awakened by shuffling sounds in the room. A dim light was on and John was fully dressed and filling his suitcase with his belongings. I was shocked!

"What are you doing, John? It's 2 o'clock in the morning."

"I'm leaving this damn place. That old S.O.B. is driving me crazy."

"Don't do this, John. He's a great teacher. Try to relax; you'll be all right."

"Hell no. I'm leaving! I'll go back to teaching school or join the Army—anything but this. I can't take anymore."

"Please, John, at least talk to Mackey (our senior student advisor) before you leave."

"No, my mind is made up. Just let me go."

"I'll miss you like the devil, John. Good luck. God be with you."

"Thanks, Wilson, you've been a good partner. You'll make a good doctor, too."

We both had tears in our eyes as we shook hands. John handed me an envelope. "Give this to Mackey before you go to class this morning." He picked up his suitcase, went down the stairs, and left. I thought, *What a pity that he didn't stay to fight the battle to win and realize the goal he had set years before.*

Getting back to sleep was almost impossible. I kept thinking: *but for the grace of God, there goes I.* Finally, I slept, but not soundly. The image of John carrying his suitcase haunted me, even as I slept.

My dissecting partner was one of the first to leave. Before the second quarter began, two more left. The attrition rate was high that first year. Some did not make the grade, some for lack of funds, others because of family illnesses and others realized that medicine was not their role in life. I stayed and fought on. After the other students dropped out, I moved to another table with a new dissecting partner and a much easier body to dissect. This one was old and thin, making everything easier to identify. In spite of that, time seemed to fly by, and we knew that we would have to ask for more time. I decided to ask Dr. Witt if we could dissect on Saturdays and Sunday afternoons.

"Yes, if you want to."

"My partner and I would really like to do that if it could be arranged."

"That will not be a problem. I'll take care of it today (Wednesday)."

The next day he let us know the arrangements, who to see, which route to take when we entered the building, etc. We spent many weekends in that dissecting lab, and it paid off. With fewer people around, less noise, and fewer distractions, we accomplished a lot more and caught up with the dissection. We almost lived in that lab. We ate there, we listened to football games, the news, and music. Eating was a problem since we had to arrange to get back in once we left. Instead of that, it was easier to bring a sandwich (peanut butter and jelly) than to waste time going out. We could eat and dissect at the same time. Never mind the stench—it was part of the learning we had to do. We had gotten used to the pickled bodies that had an indescribable odor. The strength of formaldehyde was so strong that it pervaded the whole body: your hair, your skin, the taste buds, and lungs. Washing your hands in strongly perfumed soaps did no good, for that certain odor was still there. We gave up trying to get rid of *that* odor and just carried the stench along wherever we went. When we met girls, particularly student nurses, they would ask, "Are you a medical student?"

"Yes, how can you tell?"

"By your hungry look and a certain odor all first-year med students have."

"I'm sorry if it's offensive."

"Oh, that's ok, we're used to it. It will leave by next year." The girls were right. It did take at least three months after we were through dissecting cadavers before the odors finally left our clothing and bodies. For me, it was well worth going through that demeaning period to achieve what we did.

About one week before the end of our first quarter of school, Dr. Wittenberg stopped by our table, watched a few minutes, bent down, and spoke softly to me. "Come into my office for a minute, Voodrow." Then he walked away. I watched him straight to the office. I knew I had to go right then. My knees were weak, and I could barely walk. It seemed to take five minutes to walk that thirty feet. I was imagining everything as I approached the door and gently knocked. "Come in, Voodrow. Have a seat." I just knew he was going to "ream" me out good. Instead, he talked in a kindly voice. "Relax, Voodrow. Let's just talk a minute. First, I think you are doing well enough, but not as good as you are capable of doing. You are not giving yourself a chance. I know you can do better. I've watched you work, and your dissection is *very* good. You know the anatomy well, but when it comes to examination time, you get so tense that you don't think logically. You try too hard, don't relax enough, and, right at this time, you are not believing in yourself. I want you to know that *I* believe in you, Voodrow, and know that you will be a very good doctor also. Let up on the work time, relax more, drink some wine, have a beer, and socialize more with a pretty female. This will probably help improve your grade level as well as your self-confidence. Think about what we have talked about, and come to see me anytime you feel I can be of help." I stood like a soldier at attention.

"Thank you, Dr. Wittenberg. I appreciate your advice more than you will ever know. I feel better already." Dr. Witt was right on the button with his prediction. I took his advice, within reason; my grades improved, my confidence was greater, and my outlook in general was much brighter.

Gross anatomy was not the only course we were taking. There was embryology, physiology, and last, but not least, chemistry. All of these combined to make a full work week. Chemistry was taught by Dr. T. P. Nash, and to him it was the most important course in medical school. That first day he impressed on us that he meant for everybody to be on time when class convened, and he emphasized it by pounding the floor with the butt end of his four-foot-long pointer. He certainly got our attention!

The first day in chemistry lasted a full hour, mostly outlining what we would cover that quarter with time scheduled for each section. At the end of the hour he said, "Tomorrow I want you to be able to recite the essential amino acids and what effect each has on our body functions." That really got our attention! You could tell that he was competing with Dr. Witt for teaching time. Having had three years of chemistry in college, I thought I had a good background for this course in physiological chemistry, but I soon found it was not quite as good as I thought. It was tough—a good, interesting, and stimulating tough. With lectures twice a week and a two-hour day in lab once a week, we stayed busy. I liked Dr. Nash. He had a tough exterior but a heart of gold, reminding me of my father. I knew that he liked for students to show an interest in his classes. I was interested, and it showed. For this, I was singled out more than expected. We had more than an average course had in exams, particularly "pop quizzes." That was to keep us on our toes. One such thing happened toward the end of the first quarter, and one of my classmates and I "flunked" the exam. It must have been bad because Dr. Nash asked us to report to him after class, and we did so with fear and trembling.

"Come in, gentlemen, and have a seat."

"Thank you, Doctor."

"Fellows, I won't say how bad you both did on this exam, but it is so poor that I don't know that a double X would be low enough. What happened, Wilson?"

"We just weren't prepared, Dr. Nash. I don't know about Burg, but I don't have any excuse. I just wasn't ready for the exam."

"Me either," Burg said.

"Ok, I'll give you another chance. The whole class did poor, but—he began to shake his head—you boys were by far the worst I have had in many a day. If you both get busy and try real hard maybe you will make it. Now, go home and think it over. Then get to work!"

"Thank you again, Dr. Nash." (We left with our tails between our legs like two whipped dogs).

We had to talk to somebody about it and went to our friend Mackey. He consoled us and then said try to forget it. "Come on, let's go down to Mike's Place (a small restaurant two blocks from the fraternity hours). We can have a beer and relax. That way it won't be so painful. This is not the end of the world anyway." Of course, his word was enough to convince us that it was the best course to follow and about 6:30 we walked the two blocks to the "beer joint." I had never had more than a few swallows of beer and didn't like the stuff.

"I may not be able to drink a whole bottle, Mackey."

"Let's give it a try and see."

The waiter came by for our order. "Hi, Doc Mackey. I see you have some new faces. What can I do for you?"

"Oh, just bring us three Budweisers." That was just the beginning of a long night. The first one I had to make myself drink. By the time it was finished my head felt light, my face was warm, and my tongue was loose.

"How about another one?"

Burg and I looked at each other and nodded. The second one tasted better, or it could be my taste buds were numb. Before we realized it, we had told Mackey all our problems, our life and family histories, and each of us was barely able to walk back and forth to the bathroom. We had also consumed four beers each.

"Mackey, I don't want another beer. Let's go back to the frat house."

"Can you make it ok, Wilson?"

"I may need a little help. Let's try and see. C'mon."

How the three of us were able to walk that three blocks is a miracle because none of us could walk independently. I barely remember our staggering along leaning on each other, never falling, as we made our way back. I also recall the crawling up the stairs and into bed. The worst thing of all was the nausea and vomiting that followed about two hours later and lasted until dawn. About 6:30, our "savior," Mackey, was shaking me awake. "Come on, Wilson, you need to take a cool shower and get ready for school. You have an 8 o'clock class. Remember!"

"I'm too sick to get up, Mackey, just let me die."

"You'll be ok. C'mon, get up!"

"I can't face Dr. Nash today. He has been too good to me."

"Yes, you can. I know how you feel because I have been there."

"Well, you'll have to help me, though. How's Burg?"

"He's ok. Thompson is helping him. You'll both make it."

We both made it to class, still nauseated and with awful headaches. The minutes seemed like hours as Dr. Nash lectured about parasites and their effects on our bodies' chemistry. Then he announced: "Now we will spend the next hour in the laboratory studying fresh stool specimens we have just received from the hospital wards. Miss James, our lab technician, will assist you in preparing any slides. We will demonstrate the proper method to prepare stools for mounting on slides."

When we arrived in the lab, we were met with a mixture of odors from fresh stool specimens. You can imagine what that did for my nausea. To complicate the problem, Dr. Nash chose to demonstrate his preparations at the sink next to mine. I was miserable. My head was splitting, my stomach churned as I fought nausea, and I felt dizzy and faint. Dr. Nash looked down his nose at me and muttered, "Are you not feeling well, student Wilson?"

"I'm very nauseated, Dr. Nash. May I be excused?"

"Yes, but come back as soon as you feel better."

I was very grateful to Dr. Nash. At the same time I was mad as hell at Mackey.

I made it to the bathroom, leaned over a sink, heaved three or four times, and spit up a small amount of bitter stomach acids and bile. I washed my face in cold water three times and felt a bit better. Then I made a mistake. I took two gulps of cold water which tasted sweet and wonderful—then immediately it came back up, followed by heaving again. Nobody came to see if I was ok and that made me worse. I felt abandoned, but knew this was all my fault. That helped as I was now remorseful for what I had done. Now, I was able to face the music. In spite of how I felt, I had to get back to class. The walk back was not so long, and I was able to make it through the day. That episode was a well-learned, bitter lesson for me. I didn't try any form of alcohol for the next eighteen months. To follow up on this, I apologized to Dr. Nash the next day. When he accepted, he said, "I'm sure you learned something from this. For what it is worth, don't let your social life interfere with your education too much."

"Thank you, Dr. Nash. I appreciate your understanding and I won't forget your advice."

From that time on I was more diligent with chemistry. It was enjoyable and fun most of the time. When we studied amino acids and their chemical effects on our everyday living, each of us had to eat a specified type of diet of our own choosing in the study. I chose a high protein diet which required me to eat "sweet breads" (pancreas). This required a daily trip to downtown Memphis to a certain meat packing company that had an agreement with the medical school to furnish the school at no cost. Our "house man" (Gus) did this every three months when a new class started.

Along with the special diet each had to collect all of his urine for a 5-day period. In order to do that we were issued a gallon-sized, brown, long-necked bottle with a cork to seal it. There was a large twine string around the bottle's neck that allowed us to carry it at all times so the student could collect his/her urine. I'm not sure they provided female students with funnels or not. Anyone passing the medical school knew we were freshman medical students when they saw a group of young men walking along with each one carrying textbooks in one hand and a large brown bottle with a string around its neck in the other one. If someone accidentally hit and broke the bottle, he would have to start all over with the procedure. This invariably happened with every class. Physiological chemistry became one of the most interesting courses in the pre-clinical years as we progressed to studying all the body functions. I was amazed how the instructors integrated each course with the other as we dissected certain anatomical regions of the body.

The other courses, embryology and physiology, we had in that first quarter seemed secondary to the chemistry and gross anatomy classes. They were interesting but not nearly so much as the latter two. The embryology lab was situated in a building across an alley from the Baptist Student Nurses dormitory. Buildings were of the same heights with nursing students occupying a floor of the same level as the embryo lab. Large windows of both buildings opened onto the alley, making a good view into each place. This was a boon to us medical students as the nursing students loved to tease us with their "striptease" acts. It was very deliberate with some. They would slowly remove each article of clothing as they moved about the room. When they were down to the underwear, most of them went no further, but some of the more "experienced" ones removed the "bra" too. Boy, did they get the attention. One of the fellows brought field glasses to share with the class so we could get a better view of the more titillating anatomical structures being exposed for our benefit. Of course, the instructor knew what was going on, so he would conveniently go into his office for a 15-minute period each day, timing it so we could enjoy the break. Some of the fellows found the identity of the "actress," and she was wined and dined constantly. She also managed to find a husband who greatly admired her acting abilities.

Physiology class was scheduled at 1 o'clock, about half an hour after lunch, when most of us had finished eating. That was an awful time to sit through lectures that were sometimes boring. Luckily, I had no problem with that, but a roommate did. He sat directly in front of me, and I could tell when he was getting sleepy as he would start wiggling his right knee in and out until he actually fell asleep. I would then "poke" him in the back to arouse him. If I did not watch him, the teacher would always ask him a question.

"Mr. Ryan! Define and illustrate the trace reflex."

Gene would stammer and try to answer, usually missing the question completely. "Mr. Ryan, if you can't stay awake in this class, perhaps you had best see your doctor or drop out of the class. I don't like students sleeping in class."

"Yes, sir, I'm sorry, Dr. Flanigan."

Dr. Flanigan was full of ego and did not like anyone to flaunt that. He developed a dislike for Gene, and it was obvious that he never gave him a second chance. Even though the sleeping stopped, Gene answered questions correctly, and he did well on his mid-term and final exams, the professor did not give him a passing grade. His ego had been injured too deeply. Because of that, Gene had to repeat the course. Thank God he drew a different instructor that time.

We witnessed that happening more than once in the pre-clinical years. All of us knew it was a great injustice, but were helpless to do anything about it. It was one of their ways of "weeding out" the classes since they had the reputation of doing so and told each incoming class that a fourth would never graduate from medical school.

We spent the first six quarters in the pre-clinical courses, adding microbiology, organology, pathology, pharmacology, etc., to the didactic portion of our curriculum. Those were the days we sweated through long hours in labs studying tissues of all kinds under the microscope. We looked at normal blood cells and abnormal blood from leukemia, anemia, and cancers of all types. Once we made it past those courses, we knew then we would be allowed to examine patients and do "hands-on" practice.

Gross anatomy and Dr. Witt were still a big hurdle. In spite of all the other courses, he never let up on us for one minute. By the time I was halfway through the second quarter, I was working with my third dissecting partner. One didn't make the grade, and two dropped out; then the fourth one joined me on Mr. Leukemia. We were studying the chest and its contents by that time. The abdominal cavity had been very, very interesting and intriguing to me. As we worked with the stomach, spleen, liver, gall bladder, small bowel, colon, urinary bladder, plus the pelvic structures (prostate in the male and uterus, tubes and ovaries in the female) my enthusiasm soared. I was *really* enjoying the dissection. What I learned then has stayed with me better than any part of the anatomy that we studied. With all of that the third partner left school because he was so discouraged. My fourth dissecting partner was enthusiastic also, and it helped both of us. He was a good student which helped a lot, but he lacked in personality and was not a disciple of Dr. Witt so much as I was.

"Good to have you with me, Blanton. You'll be able to help me a lot. Looks like we have both had bad luck with dissecting partners."

"Yes, we have. Mine decided he wanted to get a Ph.D. in pharmacology."

"Well, two of the three just quit, and you know what happened to Burg."

"Yeah, that's too bad. He would've been a good doctor."

"You're right. Shall we open this chest?"

"Guess that's the next step."

Each took our scalpel and made an incision beginning about two inches outside the suprasternal notch extending down to the lower rib cage just barely outside the nipple and then past the last rib. The incision was deep enough to reveal the fascia over each rib. We then took the bone cutters—a short-handled version of pruning "loppers" (shears) that had a hook and a sharp, wide, curved blade to divide each rib. Starting with the last rib, the hook was pushed under the rib, then the blade was closed and each rib cut through. The sternum (breast bone) was removed by dividing at the sternoclavicular junction. The ribs and sternum were laid aside to leave the chest cavity exposed for dissection and study of its contents—the heart, lungs, aorta, and its branches. The esophagus, trachea (wind pipe), bronchial tubes, and diaphragm were also exposed. Each of these was studied in detail as we removed them one by one, beginning with the lungs, trachea, and large bronchi into which the trachea divided so each lung could be inflated and deflated as we breathe. Attached to the lungs also were two large blood vessels, the pulmonary vein which oxygenated blood to the lungs and the pulmonary artery, which returned oxygen-poor blood back to the heart—for recycling and picking up oxygen, returning it to the left ventricle of the heart which pumps it to the entire body.

Looking at that "pump" I realized what a perfect engineering feat had been performed. We then studied the anatomical relationships of the heart with all of its great vessels and the lungs with their large vessels and bronchi. Realizing our early religious teachings of how God made man, then created woman in His image, I was awed and humbled as we tried to understand it all as we opened the heart and studied its valves, how they opened and closed in rhythm with each pulsation of the heart 72 times each minute, which supplied the oxygen-rich blood from our lungs as we breathe eighteen times per minute. What a wonderful, miraculous thing the human body is.

How fortunate we were to be able to study and try to understand its mechanisms. We spent ten days on the anatomy of the chest cavity and the external genitalia combined. From there we began the study of the skeletal parts, not as you seem them assembled, but each bone separately as it relates to the muscle, nerve, and blood supply. To do this we were allowed to sign out on each part as we wished, such as arm bones, leg bones, the skull, etc. As we walked that mile from school to the frat house, people would stare at us and ask questions such as, "Why are you carrying those bones?"

"Oh, these are a part of my grandpa. I keep them just so I won't forget him."

Or referring to a skull: "I have to count the holes Uncle John had in his head." They soon got used to our shenanigans and would refer to us as those crazy "doctor" boys.

At the fraternity house we would get together and study each in detail. Each was marked in vari-colored ink as to blood supply, nerve supply, plus muscle and tendon insertion. It was pure memory work. As we dissected, one would "out of the blue" ask: "Where do the biceps tendons insert?" Most of us could answer correctly in a flash . . . anyone who couldn't was almost ostracized from class.

The last thing to dissect was the head and neck. Reluctantly, we had to change professors. I dreaded that because the man we faced was hard-nosed and, in my opinion, narrow-minded. From day one there was a personality clash. Neither of us was happy and sensed it. I felt pressured the entire quarter and could not perform at my normal level. For that I got singled out in class many times. All of this made for poor grades during the quarter, and I almost knew that I faced repeating that three months. When final exam time came, the questions he asked happened to be ones I had prepared for and the grade I made was *very* good, but, in Dr. Mueller's estimation, not good enough, so I did have to repeat.

The next quarter we drew a different instructor whom I could relate with. Things went well and the first year ended on a good note. Boy! I was glad that first year had ended. Surely things would be better from here on.

The second year started off on a good note. We spent time in class and lab time in both pathology and pharmacology.

We also had class in orthopedic surgery and neuroanatomy. Some of the courses were tough, but we all made it through. At the end of the fifth quarter, we had our first taste when we were allowed to do clinical studies in psychiatry, which had become a new course in the school's curriculum. At the end of six weeks, the entire class knew no one would enter that field of practice.

Along with our lectures in pathology, we had to do a lot of microscopic study of tissue. We also observed and assisted in autopsies if our patient expired. The latter really put us into clinical medicine.

Some of the autopsies were gruesome. I recall one in particular that was the worst we ever witnessed. The student read the history, physical findings, and lab work. The treatment and hospital course was given, but the final diagnosis was not. The autopsy was being done to establish that. The autopsy was a total one, meaning it included the brain. Nobody flinched as the skull was opened and removed—no reaction to the chest contents being removed—but when it came time to open the abdomen, the "fun" began. The senior resident Surgeon made the usual, long abdominal incision beginning just below the xiphoid process down to the pubic bone. When he carefully opened the second layer, there was a sudden gush of greenish yellow, purulent material that had the worst, foul odor that could be imagined. The stench was unbearable. The student became ill and left the room. The secretary also got sick, covered her face, began to heave, and left. Within minutes, the resident was alone at the autopsy table. Then, one by one, students began leaving. The resident looked up to the empty seats. "What's the matter, MEN, can't you stand a little strong gangrenous intestine?" By the time he had finished, three of us were left, and all had been reared by physicians that did general practice. Two of us had been reared on the farm and had been used to cleaning out horse manure, cow barns, chicken houses, and outhouses. I guess the other thirty-nine students had never had those experiences.

In the sixth quarter we were allowed to wear our white coats, carry a stethoscope, a percussion hammer, and an oto/ophthalmoscope. Of course, we would let the instruments hang out of our pockets or wear the stethoscope around our necks. We had to be sure that people would notice that we were now "Doctors." We held clinics in various subjects which we were currently having lectures on. These classes were taught by practicing physicians in their respective specialties. For that reason, we saw the more practical side of medicine as how one would handle a problem in real practice. The physician monitored the clinics and graded us on our abilities to diagnose and treat. Cases were mostly easy ones, but some were hard to diagnose or treat, and sometimes we saw a rare case that required the attention of the entire class. One such case came to the urology clinic, and it so happened the clown of the class drew him. I saw the elderly, black male enter "Joe's" cubicle next to mine. Within minutes, Joe stuck his head in the door. There was an excited look on his face, his eyes sparkled with the excitement. I thought he had a case of leprosy he was so ecstatic.

"Come over here, Woodrow, I have something very unusual to show you."

"It must be something rate to get you so stirred up. What is it?"

"Come on. I'll show you. You may never see another case like this in your life."

As we entered the room, there was an elderly black male standing beside the table with his external genitalia exposed. Joe said, "Uncle John, this is Dr. Wilson. He wants to examine you."

"Yassa, that's ok."

"Hi, John, looks like you have a problem."

"I sho' has, Doctor, a bad'un too."

With gloved hands, his penis was examined. There was an ulcerating lesion one inch before the edge of the foreskin. It was ragged, firm to touch, and non-tender. "No doubt about your diagnosis, Dr. Lyon."

"I'll call Dr. Morgan." He came immediately and took one look at John, then called the class in and proceeded to lecture on carcinoma of the penis. He related the causes, diagnosis, treatment, and prognosis. Cause was uncleanliness for both sexual parties on a continuing basis. Diagnosis was obvious, and treatment was surgical, meaning amputation. Dr. Morgan turned to the patient, saying, "Uncle, you have a cancer on your 'organ,' and we need to do something about it right away." John's eyes widened, and in a trembling voice he asked, "What is you gonna do to me, Doctor?"

"We'll have to get rid of that cancer."

"Yassah, how you gonna do dat?"

"Well—we'll have to amputate, just cut the organ off."

Uncle John turned pale as he began to tremble all over, and with trembling hands he was replacing the penis back in his underwear, all the while saying, "No suh, you not gonna do dat, no suh you ain't."

"Why not, Uncle? If you don't let us operate, the cancer will eat the whole thing off. Why don't you want to have it removed?"

"Cause I've had this thing all my life, for 75 years, and I would feel so undressed without it." What that, he buttoned his trousers and walked out. The class broke out in laughter, but at the same time we all felt sorry for "Uncle John."

That is just one example of many cases we treated among the poor, indigent, and unlearned every day during the Depression years. It was a great experience for us to have for future successful practices.

Following the sixth quarter of class, we had a month of vacation to study for an oral exam to cover all the subjects we had studied through the entire two years. That involved more than one class, as the school admitted a new class every three months on an accelerated program, preparing for a possible war. After two weeks of vacation, most of us returned to school to start reviewing for the "practical" that meant so much for our future. The ruse was this: If you did not make a passing grade on a single subject, you would have to take the whole three month course in two weeks. If you failed in more than one subject, you were automatically dismissed from school. If you think that didn't make you sweat blood and shed a few tears—think again. The pressure became so great that I, personally, went into the exams with the attitude of, "What the heck? I'll just do the best I can. If it's not good enough, then I can always do something else for a living." Most everybody felt the same way, and only a few students had to repeat three months of one subject.

The next three quarters were devoted to Physical Diagnosis, Obstetrics and Gynecology, General Surgery, Orthopedics and Ophthalmology. Each of these had clinics that we attended once a week on a staggered basis. In addition, seventh-quarter students in "O.B." had to go on home deliveries with the senior student and a health nurse. That was the highlight of our seventh quarter for me. Before that three months was over, I had delivered five babies under the supervision of the senior student and his nurse. At that moment, I was an Obstetrician.

By the time we had finished that three months, all of us felt that the first two years of pre-clinical study had prepared us well for the real world of medicine and surgery. I was enjoying this more than anything I had done in my entire life. I was beginning to see an end to that goal I had set at age seventeen. If I kept on, it could be realized in another year.

I took a new job in the eighth quarter when I was named house manager of our Phi Rho Sigma Fraternity house. I got no salary, but free room and board and an awful lot of responsibility, plus a $2,500 grocery bill incurred over a 2-year period. How could I have been such a fool to have taken on all of this? Well, I had no money and didn't want to ask my father to support me completely, so I took the job. The first thing we did was to look at the areas where were spent the most money. First, we were eating good, expensive food, and large amounts of it. There was too much waste there. So I ordered smaller amounts.

Secondly, we ate better and less expensive foods, such as peanut butter and jelly sandwiches for lunch, and white bread instead of more expensive rolls and whole wheat. We also served dried beans and peas, cabbage, potatoes, and other soul foods that were actually good for us. For all of these changes, I took a lot of verbal abuse, for which I returned in equal amounts. Then I called a meeting to inform them of our financial status. Many of them were shocked. Someone suggested an immediate

20-dollar-per-month raise in room and board. That went over like a lead balloon. We finally compromised on a 10-dollar raise.

Then I mentioned a fact that shocked some members and humbled others. "Now that we have met and brought up everything in an open manner, some things have to be talked about frankly and openly. There are some of you that are too far behind in your room and board payments to be able to catch up if you don't start now. I want each of you to see me tonight so we can get your money in very soon. You know what the rules are as well as I do. Second, we have a huge food debt, and the grocer is threatening to cut us off. I have talked to both him and our sponsor-advisor, Dr. Lewis, and so far he won't refuse to deliver food. We have agreed to make a small payment on the back bill every week."

I waited for comments or questions, and none were forthcoming, so I continued. "There is one more thing that we need to discuss, and that is repairs and upkeep of the building. At the present, the gutters need cleaning, there are loose shingles on the roof, and some window frames are loose. Much of this we can do if enough volunteers will come forth. Remember, this is your house, too, not just the house man's." I wasn't too popular, but everything was done fairly soon. The large grocery bill was a problem that could be solved. The good fairy heard our plea for help, and it came in the form of the city water company. They asked for an easement through our back property which was not being used for anything. They were willing to pay us for the easement. Dr. Lewis advised to sign an agreement after we sought legal advice. "I'm sure you are right, Dr. Lewis, but we can't afford attorney's fees."

"Don't worry about that, Wilson, I'll ask my attorney to look into it, and it won't cost Phi Rho a penny. Be sure you ask and get enough to cover your debt with a little more for security."

The upshot of that was we made a deal through Dr. Lewis' attorney whereby they got the easement, we got $3,000 and paid our grocery bill, with some left over. The house man job lasted through the tenth quarter, and I was ready to give it up, and the members were ready to make a change. By then, my time was filled with classroom work, home deliveries, and a torrid courtship with a new love that was to be my wife. The ten months I had the job was helpful to me in two ways: I did not have to pay room and board, and I gained some business experience. I felt good about leaving because the fraternity was not so deep in debt and the building was in better repair.

During the time I served as house manager, I was also busy at school. We had six weeks on "outside O.B." where we attended lectures, went on calls as mentioned, then had six weeks with continued lectures, plus doing histories and physicals on hospitalized O.B. patients. We also learned to examine patients in active labor at different stages so we could recognize how a cervix changed with the progress of labor, particularly when it was fully dilated and thinned to allow passage of the fetus. It was interesting, and time passed too fast for me because I felt we were doing something worthwhile for people in need.

During that, and the ensuing eighth and ninth quarters, we attended classes in the subjects I mentioned earlier. They were all interesting but did not hold a fascination for me that O.B. did. Orthopedics was interesting and challenging, but I did not have the physical ability to be a good Orthopedic Surgeon. General surgery was very challenging, and I visited the emergency room to watch as the different types of cases came in. Sometimes they would recognize me as a med student and ask me to help in some small way.

A course that I thoroughly enjoyed was physical diagnosis. I guess my interest was at a higher level than most because I had observed my father doing the same things in his examination of patients over the years. The difference now was the fact that the instructor explained as he went along. For example: when he listened to a heart, he would mock the different sounds of a normal heart and an abnormal heart. Also, the difference between the sounds of an aortic stenosis and an aortic regurgitation. Or as he examined a chest and percusssed (thumped) it in different parts, he would note the different sounds such as dull or resonant, as over something hollow. He taught us how to palpate (feel) an abdomen for masses or an enlarged liver or spleen. He was so good that, as he described something, I could see or hear that particular thing. His teachings stayed with me throughout the ensuing forty years-plus that I actually practiced.

❖   ❖   ❖

One of the few times I was home long enough during my medical school years, I made calls and accompanied Dad on deliveries. This was at the end of my second year and just as we were starting clinic work. Being with him that summer was a big help to me as we began to study obstetrics in class and go on home deliveries shortly afterward.

That summer I spent three weeks "practicing" with Dad and really gained a wealth of experience, plus being able to understand what it was all about.

From the time I was about 12 years old until I was a college student, I used to go with my father as he would make house calls throughout the surrounding neighborhoods. This was mostly during the summer months or on Sundays. From Monday through Friday, we had to do farm work. In the wintertime, Dad made his house calls by horseback as roads were impassable for cars in much of the area where he practiced. I was glad when spring and summer came each year so I could "practice with Dad."

"Can I go with you today, Dad?"

"I guess so, if you really want to."

At that time I was looking for something to do that was exciting to tell my friends about.

"Where are we going today, Dad?"

"Three or four places. We will start at Punkin Town, then to Akersville, circle back to Bugtussle, then stop to see Kit Dyer in York Branch. Then we'll be through unless somebody else needs me."

"How will you know if someone else wants you to stop?"

"If they want me to stop, they'll have a white cloth on a pole beside the road in front of the house."

"That sounds interesting. Let's go."

We took off in a cloud of dust, at about 30 m.p.h., never slowing down for pot holes, ruts, mud holes, or flocks of chickens, and made our first call. At that age, 12, I usually stayed in the car while Dad was seeing the patients. By the time I was 16 or 17, I was allowed to go into the homes to observe. Soon after that, I quit going with Dad as often because the teenage girls suddenly became more attractive, interesting, exciting, and fun to be with. Besides, I was learning gross anatomy.

Through the college years, I again made more house call than in prior years. By that time I had a real interest in medicine and had decided to make that my career. By this time, I was able to visit patients, assist in some manner, and observe his practice skills. We saw cases of a type that I would never have seen in later years of private practice. Some of these were associated with malnourishment, superstition, poverty, illiteracy, and many with false pride. We saw typhoid, pellagra, scurvy, rickets, tuberculosis, and others that one would not expect to find in our country, the land of plenty.

On this particular day in 1935, we stopped to see a 16-year-old boy. "How long have you been sick, Hezekiah?" I asked.

"Aw, I ain't sick. I jist got this here breakin' out on my arms and my neck and face. I've had the runs fer 'bout ah week too."

"He jist lays 'round all the time too, Doc."

"I tole you I'm too weak to walk much, Mama."

"When Hezzie is well, what does he eat?"

"Mostly we'ns jist eat cornbread, white beans, and water gravy."

"Do you have turnip greens, squash, green beans, or sweet potatoes? Does he eat fresh or canned fruits?"

"Naw, I don't like that ole stuff."

"Let me see the rash on your hands and face. I could see the fine, red rash on the skin that looked rough and irritated. He had some peeling of the skin on his face also."

"Open your mouth and stick your tongue out." Both were slick and red, and there were red cracks in the corners of the mouth."

"I'm afraid you have pellagra, Hezekiah. You need to eat meat and eggs, fresh fruit and vegetables, and turnip greens. Be sure to drink milk also. I'll give you some vitamin capsules also. Take the vitamins three times a day and eat right or you'll get worse. I'll see you in a week." I missed seeing Hezzie again, but Dad reported that he was improved.

This was a hot dry, Sunday afternoon when we stopped at a small house beside the dusty road. An obese young woman was sitting in a rocking chair on the front porch. She held a small baby in her arms. As she gently rocked, she would wave her hand back and forth over the baby's face. As we walked onto the porch, we could very clearly see the problem. The baby she held was six to eight months old and appeared to be sleeping. There was a black ring surrounding his mouth, and as we got nearer I realized that black ring was house flies. As I watched, one would occasionally crawl in and out of the baby's mouth. The baby was not moving, his breathing was shallow and slow. He was limp and so pale that the skin seemed to be transparent.

"Hello, Dorothy, we stopped to see your baby. This is my son, Wendell. He says he wants to be a doctor." She barely nodded as she looked at the baby. There was terror on her face as she looked up at Dad, and her eyes were filled with tears.

"My baby is rail sick, Doc."

"How long has he been sick, Dorothy?"

"Four or five days. He wuz vomickin first, then he started runnon off at the bowels, then yestiddy, I seen some blood. He ain't been awake much today, and he cain't take nuthin' to eat or drink. I'm rail worried 'bout him, Doc."

Dad examined the baby, took the temp under the arm, and it was 101.8. He checked the eyes, mouth, nose and throat, chest and heart, then his abdomen. When he felt the abdomen there was a slight reaction as if it was painful. Dad shook his head.

"Dorothy, this baby is critically ill. I don't think he'll make it unless we can get some fluids into him and stop his diarrhea. Where is your husband?"

"I don't know where he's at . . . I tried to git him to stay home so's he could git medicine fer the baby." She began to cry. "I don't know what to do, Dr. Wilson."

"You'll have to get some help here, Dorothy, and we'll try to get this baby to the hospital before it's too late."

"Ain't no use in trying, Doc. My husband don't believe in hospitals—and not much in doctors neither. I wish he did—he's jist like his ole daddy!"

"I'm sorry about that Dorothy. I'll be back in the morning."

Next morning was too late. A neighbor came by home at about 7 a.m. to let Dad know the baby had died during the night.

Later that same day, in the same neighborhood, we had seen a baby with a high fever and vomiting.

"This baby is critical, Mr. Jakes. I'm afraid he has meningitis."

"He just got sick last night, Doctor. He can't have that stuff."

"Has he had a cold or the sniffles?"

"Yes, for a couple of days."

"That was probably the beginning of his problem. Give him this liquid for the fever, a lot of water, three drops of this every three hours for his vomiting—and do a lot of praying. Let me know if there is any change in his condition." This baby died also.

As we went into homes, we saw acutely ill patients in great numbers: typhoid was common, infectious diarrhea cases abounded, and malnutrition was rampant. The number of cases with tuberculosis was shocking to me. Dad was so used to seeing these types of ill people, with any of those mentioned he could almost instantly make a diagnosis. I was amazed. This man I knew as the avid squirrel hunter, the addicted fisherman, or a father who said, "No, Son, you have to do it this way." He would then demonstrate how to swing an ax, plow a straight furrow, or butcher a hog. I had a hard time realizing his medical skills. Had I not been allowed to go with him to make house calls, I may have never known how skillful he really was.

Not only was Dad able to easily make the mentioned diagnosis of diseases, he was also well-known for his ability to handle difficult deliveries and was often called to consult and do the actual delivery for his colleagues. He related some of the cases to me as we would discuss medical problems. Some had tragic endings, some were hilarious, but most of them turned out well and normal. With his fellow practitioners in difficult cases, sometimes he would recall some of these cases and discuss them with me.

Here is one of the hilarious ones, as he told it: "I was called to deliver Mrs. Woodside, a 38-year-old woman who had two children, 15 and 18 years of age. This one was an 'accident.' When I got there, she was alone and about ready to deliver. As I started to examine her there was a deep growl from under the bed. That scared me to death! I knew that she had a German Shepherd as a watchdog, and he would attack anyone at the hint of hurting this woman. I said, 'Irma, you will have to get this dog out of here and lock the door, or I won't deliver your baby.'"

"What happened then, Dad?"

"She got out of bed, and put him outside as I asked. Then she proceeded with her labor as if she had not been interrupted. The baby's head came down to the outlet—then I had to rotate and extract the head. This made if necessary to pull real hard. The membranes had ruptured earlier, and there was a lot of fluid on the floor. As I pulled on the head and rotated the shoulders, the baby suddenly popped out, my feet slipped, and I went under the bed, but I held onto the baby. There I was flat on my back, blood and amniotic fluid spilling on me, and I was still holding the baby. That was a mess!"

"How did you get out of that mess?"

"Irma sat up and took the baby. I crawled from under the bed and finished the job!"

As he told the story, he laughed so hard he cried. This was one of my favorite stories.

❖   ❖   ❖

We made six or eight deliveries during the three weeks I spent "practicing with Dad,", but two in particular made a lasting impression on me.

The first was a 16-year-old primipara. She was an average-sized girl with adequate pelvic measurements. Our first call there was at noon. When I stopped the car, we could hear the screams of agonizing pain as she labored. Going into the room, I recognized the couple as neighborhood children I had known. The expectant father seemed calm, but the expectant young mother had a look of fear and pain on her face.

"How long have you been in labor, Susie?"

"Since 8 this morning—Oh-h-h, give me something for this pain, Dr. Wilson."

"Let me examine you first. John, get me a pan of warm water. Son, put two tablets of bichloride of mercury in the water (this was a sterile solution he used to wash his hands after each exam). He washed his hands in soapy water, then without surgical gloves did a vaginal examination. As he washed his hands, he was saying she was not too small, but the baby's head was large and still high. She was dilating some, but labor would be slow. (I checked the baby's heart through the mother's abdomen, and it was 116, strong and regular). "We'll be back in three or four hours to see how she's doing."

As we pulled away from the house Dad looked glum. "That little girl will need a caesarean section, but I don't think he'll hear of it. You know that he has a large skull, and the baby does also. I don't believe she will ever push the head through the pelvic outlet, although it is normal."

"What makes you think he will not have the surgery?"

"Oh, they have some kind of foolish religious belief in that it would be an unnatural way and not what God intended to be done."

"Do you mean he would risk the baby and mother's life because of an ignorant religious belief?"

"Yes, Son, there are a lot of people like that in our neck of the woods. I have problems with many people because of superstitions, religious teachings, and old wives' tales.

We went back about 4 p.m. and she was still in active, hard labor. Again, Dad examined her. "John, your wife is not making any progress in having this baby. The head is too large for her to have this baby normally. She needs to be in the hospital where the Surgeon can do an operation and deliver the baby. If you don't agree to that, then you are risking both your wife and baby's life."

John shook his head vigorously. "No, Doctor, I don't believe in women having babies that way; that is not the way God intended it to be. I think you can deliver my baby."

"John, I have made many difficult deliveries, even you, but in my experience I don't think we will be able to save your baby unless she has the caesarean section."

John still shook his head "No!"

"I'll call Dr. Smith to see what he thinks, if that is all right with you?"

"Whatever you say, Doctor. I just don't want no surgery."

"But you want a live, healthy baby, don't you?"

"Whatever is the Lord's will, Doc."

I couldn't believe there were people like that in our world. I could tell by the look on Dad's face he wanted to let the fellow have it with an iron fist. He was trembling with anger as we left. "You drive son. I'm too upset!" In five minutes we arrived home, he called Dr. Smith, and they agreed to meet in an hour. By the time he was able to relax we returned to the Hix home. Dr. Smith came soon after. Both he and Dad examined the patient then went outside for a consultation. I went along to learn. Both agreed that something had to be done immediately. Since the father was so adamant in his beliefs to refuse surgery, the only thing to do was to attempt a mid-forceps delivery, which, at best, was a big risk to both mother and baby. Dad explained the whole situation again saying, "Dr. Smith agrees the only way to get a live baby is for your wife to have the surgery."

"No, Doctor, we have talked it over, and we don't want the surgery."

"Ok, if that is your final decision we will do the best we can. Wendell, give her Morphine 1/4 grain by injection and Nembutal, 50 mg. by mouth. Then we will wait twenty minutes and try to make the delivery.

Half an hour later, I checked the fetal heart. It was weaker and slower, 100/minute.

"Susie, we will try to deliver your baby now. Let's turn her across the bed and cover her with a sheet, but leave the bottom exposed." After that was accomplished, Dad took the forceps, lubricated the blades, which were gently curved with a metal bar, three to four inches wide, and bluntly curved on the pelvic end so they would encircle the baby's head. There was an open space four inches wide along the middle to allow tissue to expand into it. Those "blades" were inserted on either side of the baby's head, then grasped by closing the handles which interlocked smoothly if the forceps were applied correctly. If they did not fit and interlock, that means there was something wrong.

Dad slowly and smoothly inserted the left blade, then the right blade, and then interlocked them and began to pull, gently at first and then harder for twenty seconds. He separated the handles and resumed. "Dr. Smith, do you want to try now?" He was repeating what my Dad had done. Then they took turns and after the fourth try, Dad said, "Son, check the baby's heart." I listened and it was fainter and only 80/minute. "We have to get this baby out now!"

"John, get a pan of real warm and a pan of real cold water ready."

Now Dad was pulling real hard while Dr. Smith and I pushed on the uterus. With a last hard pull the baby was out. He was gray and limp. There were forceps marks on each side of the head, the neck looked too long, and he was not breathing. The umbilical cord was still pulsating with mother's blood. Dr. Smith was dipping him in first warm water, and then the cold water, but there was still no sign of life. "Dilate his rectum, Wendell." I did so, but there was no response. I spanked him—no response. I tried artificial respiration—still no response. Dr. Smith shook his head. At least ten minutes had passed, and all of us knew that there was no life in the infant.

The exhausted mother was barely aware of what was going on. We delivered the placenta (after birth), gave a shot of Pitocin to contract the uterus, which protects against heavy bleeding, checked her blood pressure again, and prepared to leave.

"I'm sorry we lost the baby, John."

"Wasn't your fault, Doctor. It was the Lord's will." I was thinking: *No, it was your ignorance and stubbornness that killed your own child.* I hope never to encounter such in future practice.

The second O.B. case I vividly recall was humorous and had a happy ending.

At about 7 a.m., "Rowdy" Morgan came galloping up on his mule. He was so excited he could hardly get words out as he said, "I need you at my house right now," and began to turn the mule around and head back home.

"Wait a minute, Rowdy, what's your problem?" Dad shouted. ("Rowdy" was deaf as a post.)

"Gerty is about to have that baby. Hurry, Doc." He took off, spurring the mule with both heels to hurry back to "Gerty's" side. He lived about a mile from our home, but we had to drive about eight miles to get there by car since there were two creeks to cross, and they both were too deep to ford. Dad didn't seem to be in a hurry to start the trip. I got a little anxious and asked if we shouldn't start.

"I don't think we need to rush. This is her first baby. She's 32 years old and will probably be in labor for 12 hours or more."

"Have you seen her on a regular basis?"

"Son, nobody is seen more than three to four times during a pregnancy unless they have some medical problem."

Then I recalled the many times that some man would ride up at 2 or 3 in the morning, yelling, "Hey, Doc!" I usually was the first to wake up. I raised the bedroom window and asked him, "Who are you and what is the problem?" The answer, "I'm Jim Jones, and my wife is a-granny-in" (meaning she was in labor). "I need yore daddy to come as quick as he can."

"Has be been seeing your wife for this baby?"

"Quit askin' foolish questions. Jist git Doc." I could tell he was irritated by the tone of his voice.

Some of those times Dad would still be sound asleep and often had not been in bed more than two hours. I felt sorry for him at times like that, but that was his duty. He would get out of bed, dress, go to the barn with his lantern, saddle his horse, and ride off with the expectant father as a guide. Reflecting on these situations, I understood why he wasn't rushing to start this time.

When we arrived an hour later at Rowdy's home, the patient's mother greeted us at the door. "I thought you got lost, Doc," Rowdy said.

"Is Gerty in trouble?"

"Naw, but she's havin' purty hard pains. This bein' her first-un, I knowd she'd have a hard time."

"Let me examine her. Gerty, this is my Son. He's in medical school."

"Yeah, I remember him. He don't seem to be old 'nough to be a doctor; he was jist a little boy when I seed him last."

"Well, he will soon be a real doctor."

"Hi, Gerty. Looks like you're going to be a mother. Is it ok if I help Dad bring your baby into the world?"

"Why, shore 'tis. We'uns are rail proud yore makin' ah' doctor. Be a good'un, like yore daddy is."

"I'll try."

Dad proceeded to examine her. "Everything is fine, Gerty. We're going to be here to watch your progress. I'll examine you some more so that we will know if the baby is all right, and if you will deliver normally. With your age it could be a bit slower in arriving than in a young girl. I'll need a pan of fresh water, Mabel" (the patient's mother). He dissolved two green tablets in the water to make a sterile solution.

Within two hours, she was having contractions about every fifteen minutes. As the pains came, Gerty began to cry out, "Caint you give me something fer these pains, Doctor?"

"Not yet, Gerty, it might stop the labor, and it wouldn't be good for the baby. Let's wait a little longer."

Dad kept examining Gerty from time-to-time. After each examination, he would wash his hands in the basin of water and let them air dry. Each time, after examining the patient, he would reassure that all was well, but the baby was just slow in being born. Before I realized it, the clock struck 12. Dad examined her once more. No progress.

The mother disappeared, then came back. "Dr. Wilson, we are cookin' somethin' t'eat. Will you eat with us?"

"I guess so. Gerty is ok, and it will be a while before this baby arrives."

Not long after that, Dad questioned Gerty, but did not examine her. At that minute, I thought nothing of his not examining her. In another five minutes, he disappeared and I heard him say, "I think we'll go home for lunch. Gerty is slow, and we'll be back in an hour." We prepared to leave. As we got in the car I was curious as to why there was a sudden change of plans.

"What made you suddenly decide not to have lunch with the family?"

"I missed the pan I had been washing my hands in (he didn't use gloves), went in the kitchen, and saw Mabel mixing corn meal for lunch in that same pan. I was afraid to say anything, but I knew I couldn't stomach any food she cooked."

I had a big laugh out of that and couldn't wait to tell Mom why we came home for lunch.

We went back to be with Gerty during the hours of labor and about 6 p.m. Dad delivered an eight pound, lively, healthy baby girl. (I suggested they name her "Clorine," but Dad didn't think that was a very good idea.)

I stayed around another week and had a great time "practicing with Dad. We continued to see patients up every road, hollow, and pig path at all times of day or night. Rain or shine we were on the go. It was an unforgettable three weeks. I realized what an advantage I would have over most of my classmates from having this 3-week "crash course" of general practice, but I had to return to the world of being a student and "embryo doctor."

❖ ❖ ❖

The third year of medical school passed much faster than the previous ones, and before we realized it we were registering for that last one as medical students. Coming out the door from registration, I bumped into my best friend, Joe Lyon.

"Hey, Joe, do you realize what we are now?"

"What are you talking about, Woodrow?"

"I'm talking about our status. We are seniors in medical school!"

"By golly, we *are*. I can't believe we made it."

"Well, it's true, and here is my registration to prove it."

As we began that last year, I never imagined what fate had in store for me. I felt good going into the quarter. Everything seemed to be falling into place during the last few months, and I knew that I had chosen the right type of field for my life's work.

The entire class felt that we had to prove ourselves ready for the acid test to become physicians. The upcoming quarter would be devoted to internal medicine, sprinkled with six lectures on business and legal aspects of practice. Internal medicine is the part that is the diagnosis and treatment of non-surgical diseases and/or acute illnesses. Members of the class were assigned to specific wards, which would be all males or all females. The patients were assigned in rotation as they were admitted. Whenever their patient was admitted, the student was notified to be there as soon as possible. The patient was in his hands to examine, write the history and physical, do the basic lab work, and give his diagnosis in writing. No only that, whenever rounds would be made, each student was expected to be there to present their case if called upon. That was the thing we needed to prepare us for future private practice. It was excellent training.

I was assigned to ward A, all female with acute illnesses, some terminal. My first patient was Mrs. Long. I was introduced by the head nurse. "Mrs. Long, this is your new student physician, Dr. Wilson."

"Hello, Dr. Wilson. I'm glad to meet you."

"Good morning, Mrs. Long. I'm happy to meet you, too. How are you feeling this morning?"

"Not too good, I'm afraid." I really looked at her for the first time. I noted the pale skin, blonde graying hair, and blue eyes. She was a bit plump and had a pleasant personality. I noted several small, shiny, black moles scattered on her neck and face: Then it hit me. *Mrs. Long must have melanomatosis*. Everything about her was typical to make her susceptible to that tumor. I turned the front cover of the chart to see the diagnosis: There it was! "Acute generalized melanomatosis." This meant that the patient had the tumors spread throughout her entire body. It also meant she had no chance of surviving. There was no specific treatment for her illness. I reviewed her chart, then I sat by her bedside to chat for a few minutes before leaving. Every morning as I made the rounds, I could see very small, pinhead-sized black spots everywhere. As I followed her along, I watched the pinheads grow rapidly into matchhead moles and become a deep, shiny black. I knew her time was short. I also felt helpless because all we could do for Mrs. Long was to relieve her pain and nausea. The third day, I decided to visit with her a bit longer and sat down by her bedside again. "Mrs. Long, I hope you don't mind if I ask you some more personal questions?"

"Not at all, Dr. Wilson."

"Where were you reared?"

"I was born in Mississippi. Then we moved to Memphis when I was six and have been here since."

"Were you active in sports like softball, swimming, and sunbathing when you were young?"

"Oh, yes. I loved the sun and stayed outside a lot. Every summer we would lie out in the sun to get a tan. But I sunburned easily and would get upset at my brunette friends because I was jealous of their beautiful tans."

"I know how you girls felt about that. Did anybody ever tell you that too much sun was harmful to your skin, and particularly to blondes with peaches-and-cream complexions, which you probably had?"

"Yes, my mother would say, 'You're blistering too easy. That will ruin your pretty, white skin.'"

"Your mother was right, but no one knew then that it might be a cause for developing tumors of the type you have."

"I know, Dr. Hall (her Dermatologist) told me to stay out of the sun. But by the time I saw him, it was too late. I know my condition Dr. Wilson, and at this point I just want to get it over."

"Thank you, Mrs. Long. Whatever you want or need in the way of medication, any one of us will be happy to help."

Daily visits for two weeks made me realize how bitter patients must get to know they can't get well, and the physician cannot legally, permanently ease the pain and mental anguish. "How much pain do you have today, Mrs. Long?"

"Not too much."

The next morning when the nurse and I made rounds, the patient was more cheerful and seemed stronger.

"Good morning, how are you feeling? You look chipper to me." The nurse said, "Yes, she sure does."

"Oh, I always feel better when my doctor comes."

"That's quire a compliment, Mrs. Long."

She smiled. "Do you have time to sit down for a minute."

"Sure! Excuse us, Mrs. Gray. Now what can I do for you?"

"I just wanted to thank you for taking such good care of me Doctor. Most of the other ones I have had seemed to be too busy or not to care. She held out her hands and as I held them briefly, Mrs. Long said, "I just wanted to tell you that you have made it easier for me to accept the inevitable. Good-bye Doctor."

"Bye, Mrs. Long." I turned away with tears in my eyes and hurried to the writing desk, hidden from the nurses. Men, particularly male doctors, are not supposed to cry—no matter what. That night Mrs. Long died, and the tears flowed again.

The second patient assigned to me on A Ward was a grossly obese, black female, about forty years of age, with multiple complaints. The most prominent was recurrent headaches and back pain. The nurse introduced us. "Florene, this is Dr. Wilson, your new student doctor. He needs to ask you some questions and examine you."

"That's fine. How is you, Doctor?"

"Hi, Florene. I'm fine. It's good to meet you. What's your problem?"

Florene then proceeded to tell me all of her ills, which took at least half and hour, as she had something wrong with every system of her entire body. That made me very suspicious.

"Are you married?"

"Naw, I ain't married. Why you ask that?"

"Oh, it's just the question. How many children do you have?"

"Three."

"Did you have a hard time having them?"

"I sho' did with that fust'un. Liked to ah killed my back."

"Oh, I see. Now let me check you and see if I can find anything wrong." I did it all even to a pelvic examination and neurological with all the hammers, needles, pinwheels, toe to heel walking, etc. I needed to impress this patient. Of course, it took the whole morning, but I knew the intern—he was a bastard! The writeup and lab work were yet to come. Together, they took another hour. Just as I was finishing, they paged me to report to Ward A immediately. I went on the double expecting a dire emergency. I approached the desk feeling anxious. "What is the emergency, Mrs. Gray?"

"No emergency, but Dr. James wants you to do a spinal tap on Florene, and you know how he is."

"I sure do! Ok, let's just do it now."

"We are ready. What size gloves do you wear?"

"Seven and a half."

"Florene, Dr. Wilson needs to do a spinal tap. You know what that is, I'm sure."

"I sho' do. I don't like them things."

"Maybe it won't be too bad. Turn on your side and curl up so the doctor can get to your spine."

As I put my gloves on, Mrs. Gray "prepped" the back. "This will be a little cold, Florene. I then draped her back. "We'll cover you with this sterile drape . . . the Novocaine is ready. Just a little pinprick to numb you. Is that numb?"

"Yassuh, it feels numb."

"Ok, now let's do the tap." I checked the intervertebral spaces again, took the long spinal needle, inserted it into the area marked, and slowly pushed it between the vertebrae a half-inch more, and I felt the needle pop through the tough dura, entering the spinal canal. I withdrew the stylet from the needle as I held my breath and as the stylet came out, it was followed by a steady flow of spinal fluid. Without realizing I did it, I yelled "Bingo!" We collected the three spinal fluid specimens, reinserted the stylet, and removed the needle. Then the nurse said, "Congratulations, you're the fourth one to try. One of the three failures was the intern."

I really felt that I had accomplished something great, but I hadn't. The intern had a dislike for me, and I never knew why. After that patient, he gave me every tough assignment possible, I thought, to see that I failed to do a job. I happened to luck out on every one he tried me on.

Ward A was a good beginning for me. I was challenged and met each challenge.

The terminally-ill patients taught me that I could empathize with a patient and not be criticized by showing my feelings. That was a real learning experience.

Not long after my experience on Ward A, I met my fate!

The next day or so we were sitting in a classroom before lectures. As we sat there, someone said, "Hey, look at all those pretty nurses going by." I noticed one in particular. She caught my eye because of her beautiful auburn hair surrounding a round face. Every step she took, that auburn hair bounced, as did her whole body. "Boy, look at that redhead. Who is she?" A classmate said, "That's my girl."

"What's her name, Keith?"

"You'll have to find out for yourself."

"I will. All's fair in love and war, you know?" During the day, I saw one of the members of that class and found that her name was Jessie Bess. She was working on C&D at the opposite end of the same floor that I had been assigned. So I found an excuse to go there and wandered by her desk. "Hi, are you Miss Bess?"

"Yes, I am. Why?"

"I saw you today and wanted to meet you. Is there anything I can do to help? You look awfully busy."

She looked at me with a mischievous twinkle in her eyes. "Yes, as a matter of fact you can, *student* Wilson. You can start an IV on a patient in bed two."

"Fine. Show me the patient." This would be only the third patient that I had to draw blood from. We went into the ward to bed two. The patient was a slender, young black who did not appear ill.

"Otis, this is Dr. Wilson. He's going to start your IV."

"He is?" He was looking at me with a question on his face which said, "I don't think you can do this."

"I'm going to *try*, Otis. Let me see this arm." The veins looked normal. I palpated the larger vein. It was pliable and did not roll. This impressed Otis. I applied the tourniquet. "Now, open and close your fingers and then make a tight fist." He was watching every move I made. I connected the needle to a 5. cc syringe, felt the vein again, applied the alcohol sponge, and stuck the vein very confidently in a swift motion, thinking, *I have to hit this vein to impress my nurse.* (She did not know how inexperienced I really was.) Luck was with me again. As the needle entered the vein, blood filled the syringe. Otis' eyes popped open, and he smiled.

"There you are, Otis. How was that?"

"That's fine. Thank you, Doctor."

"Good. Now let's start the fluids, Miss Bess." She looked at me with a disgusting expression and said, "Yes, Sir, *Doctor.*" Afterward, I found out that there had been three or four failed attempts, and she was going to put this little smart aleck student in his place.

I would hang around her ward each night, offering to help. She had little time for me and seemed to care less if I was there or not. That didn't bother me. I just wanted to be near her. She finally warmed up a little after she decided I wouldn't go away. "What night are you off, Miss Bess?"

"Thursday night. Why?"

"I thought we could go someplace for a coke and maybe dance a little, ok?"

"I'd like that. What time do you want to go?"

"How about 6:30? Is that too early?"

"Let's make it 7:00. That'll give me more time to get ready."

This was Tuesday, and I saw her on the ward Wednesday. I teased her a little, stayed until she got off, walked her to the dormitory, and said "Good night."

The first date went well. We talked about our high school and college years, our families, and things in general. Soon we were dating more often, and then on a regular basis. It wasn't long before things got serious. We had fallen in love. Although I had been in "love" many times since the age of fifteen, this time it was for real. I wanted to be with her all the time.

I'm sure that would have been disastrous. Nursing duties and class work kept us apart and away from each other, but we managed to work in a few dates. Sometimes it would last for only half an hour, but that was long enough to let each other know we cared. We would then prove it with embraces and long moments of sensual kissing. Those were stolen moments—therefore, the most powerful ones. Whenever she had a night off, dates began at 6 o'clock and lasted until her curfew at 11 o'clock. We usually made it back in plenty of time, but on one unforgettable occasion, we got into trouble. In those days, drive-ins offered curb service, and that meant anywhere in the parking lot. We chose a place away from the restaurant under an overhanging tree.

After having the burger and coke, we talked, held hands, and teased each other. Darkness came, and the "smooching" began. The radio was playing romantic music, and time meant nothing. Finally, Jessie asked what time it was. I checked, and she still had 10 minutes, and neither of us was worried. I turned the key, stepped on the starter, and nothing happened. "Oh, God, the battery is dead! We'll have to push the car out and down the hill to start it." We both got out and pushed it back—then she was back in the car and steered as I pushed. I jumped in as the car started rolling down the hill, put it in gear, and it started. I breathed a sigh of relief. "I'm sorry, Honey, I've made you late. I know that means two weeks without dates at night." Then she was silent.

Arriving at the dormitory, Jessie would not wait for me to escort her to the door because she was already three minutes late. Sure enough, Miss Huspeth stormed at her, threatened her, and said, "You have gotten yourself in a mess now, thanks to that no-good Wilson fellow. That means he won't be around here for the next two weeks anyway." At that moment Jessie was about as mad at me as Miss Huspeth was. I saw my beloved on the halls and had a little time with her as the two weeks went flying by. When she was able to get her late leave back, that first date was as though we hadn't seen one another for a month. We just had some freedom of expressing our pent-up emotions.

At the end of the tenth quarter, our grades came, and I was elated. Dr. Witt had been right. I needed to relax, have dates, and enjoy life. It reflected in my grades. Now we would have our day in pediatrics, as well as spending more time in O.B. At this stage of school, the senior students were the "attending physicians" on home deliveries. Half of the class had O.B. call on the ward, the other half was responsible for the home deliveries. After six weeks, we reversed our positions. This was done alphabetically with the last half being on home delivery first. My father was aware of our schedule and felt I needed a car. Again, the promissory note was used to enable me to get a car. I signed as primary payor. Dad and my brother, Barton, co-signed. This was no problem as my brother, Harold, had a car spotted for me already. Having a car while still in medical school was rare in 1942, but I was soon driving a blue 1940, 4-door sedan with a radio and heater. That was "high livin' " for sure.

In early September, we registered for the eleventh quarter of medical school. Classes began the next day: obstetrics and gynecology, pediatrics and public health. I was really looking forward to this three months. Our experience in O.B. had been very good and had kept my interest high. Pediatrics should be interesting, and we had to take public health to round out the curriculum.

That first day of class found two of our half of the class being called away from the lecture to make home deliveries. All of us knew this would become a routine for the entire quarter, and most looked forward to the calls. I was not on first call for delivery until the tenth day of class. That night we were called about 7 o'clock. Within ten minutes the county health nurse, the junior medical student, and I were on our way (in the nurse's car). When we arrived at the home of the patient, we could hear her screaming in pain. The nurse remarked, "She may be in trouble." "Gramma" met us at the door. "I sho' is glad you folks is heah. Lucy's hurtin' somethin' awful." The nurse knew "Gramma and Lucy since she had visited her for prenatal care. "What seems to be wrong, Sadie?"

"She's been in hard labor now for two hours, and nothing has happened."

"Maybe she's just hurting more this time. The doctor will check her to see how she's doing."

"Hi, Lucy. I'm Dr. Wilson, and this is Dr. James. Let's take a look." Before I could get the stethoscope to check the fetal heart, Lucy let out a scream that shook the rafters. I felt the abdomen. It was rock hard, and the contraction lasted for twenty seconds. "Let me check you now while you're not having a pain. How often are your pains, Lucy?"

"'Bout every three minutes, and they are getting worse. I had a glove on and checked her as instructed, by examining her through the rectal route. I could not identify any definite anatomical parts, just a soft "glob" of tissue. The nurse saw the look on my face, bent down, and asked if I would like for her to examine the patient. "Yes, please do. I don't recognize anything." Her glove was on in a flash. She examined the patient for five seconds and whispered to me, "We're in trouble. She has a frank breech and needs to be hospitalized immediately."

She called the ambulance, and within 10 to 15 minutes they had Lucy on the way to the city hospital. While we waited, the nurse and I had explained to Lucy that the baby was coming bottom first, and she had to be hospitalized for the delivery to be sure the baby was safe. We followed the ambulance. The junior student and I witnessed the delivery, which went well, and I learned a good lesson from my first "outside" O.B. call. The six weeks we spent on home deliveries was an education to me. Although I had seen my father deliver babies, some breech, I had not actually done a delivery until I was the junior on-call doctor in the seventh quarter. I found it a different ball game when I had the sole responsibility of two lives for a brief time during each delivery. By the time our inside rotation came, I had been responsible for more than twenty deliveries. You can imagine how busy we had been, as 14 of my classmates were delivering babies at the same time.

Just as the beginning of home deliveries and the first patient in particular was unusual, so was the last part of the outside O.B. deliveries. The rotation had me first up just at the same time the biggest school function of the year was scheduled. The annual dance was the time everybody came and brought their best girl/boy. It involved all schools: Medical, Dental, Nursing, Pharmacy, The Ph.D. candidates, and faculty. It was *the big blowout*. Jessie and I had made plans two weeks in advance, even though we knew there was a possibility I might be called to deliver a baby. I had no backup to see that she got to the dance, and I was prohibited from having someone else take my calls. It just so happened that I became first up on call two days before the dance.

We talked about it. "That won't be a problem. I'll get a delivery the night before and be home free," I reasoned. It didn't work out that way at all. During the 2-day period, I was up 10 times, and none of them counted. They were either false calls or BOAs (born on call). I was afraid to go to the dance and strand Jessie at one of the downtown hotels. At the last minute, a good friend of both of ours agreed to take Jessie to the big dance, and I was grateful because I had felt guilty since it looked as though she would not be going, and that would have been a heartbreaker to her. Sure enough, about 10 o'clock a call came. By the time the delivery was made and we got back to the hospital, the dance was breaking up. The next week ended our outside call time and I was glad. There was nothing good to recall about that six weeks except the great experience and the lesson learned by the first call when the "frank breech" gave me a scare.

After we made home deliveries, we were expected to make post-partum calls to check both mother and baby, which had to be done on the second and seventh days. I usually made them on days that my nurse girlfriend could go with me. Sometimes they required ten or more miles of driving, and sometimes we went by street car. I would make a late-afternoon date with Jessie and not tell her that we had to make the calls. Of course, after the first post-partum call, she knew to expect a trip to the slum or to a housing project. In 1942, it was perfectly safe to go into those areas. "Which housing projects are we going to today?" she asked.

"Oh, we're going to one close by the school in the 800 block of Poplar."

"That's in a better neighborhood than the one South of Peabody's 400 block. That visit was scary," Jessie noted.

"You'll like this one. Lucy was my first patient. Remember me telling you about the 'frank breech' that I didn't recognize?"

"Yes. So she's the one?"

"You'll be my nurse today, ok?"

"I guess so."

When we rang the doorbell, "Gramma came to the door. She greeted me with a big smile.

"Hello, Doctah, who you got with you today?"

"This is my nurse, Miss Bess."

"You sho' knows how to pick'um. She's pretty."

"She's a good nurse also."

"Hello, Lucy, how're you doing?"

"Fine as can be. Is this your nurse you tole me 'bout?"

"She sure is. This is Miss Bess. Doesn't she look like a nurse? Miss Bess, meet Lucy, my prize patient."

"Hello, Lucy. Dr. Wilson has told me about you giving him a scare. It's good to meet you."

"It's good to see you, too, Miss Bess. You sho' is pretty. I bet you is a good nurse, too."

"Thank you, Lucy. How's your baby? What's his name?" By that time she had him in her arms and was talking to him. I thought how natural she looked with a baby in her arms.

"Let's go ahead and check the baby since you have him in your arms." She deftly undressed him and cooed to him. My examination showed him to be normal in every way. "He's fine Lucy. Are you breast feeding him?"

"Yes, Doctah, and he sucks real good, too."

"What did you say his name is? I need to make a record on him, too."

"Theosis. You spell it jus' lak it sounds."

"Fine. Now let's examine you." We checked and recorded everything on her PP record—pulse, BP, heart, lungs, breasts and nipples, abdomen, uterus (size and consistency), etc. "You're doing real well, Lucy. Your womb is coming down fine, your blood pressure is normal, and I think you will do just fine. Have you been up any?"

"Yes. I've been going to the bathroom and sitting in a chair some. Mama don't want me to do anything much. She say it's too soon."

"Don't worry about that, Gramma, she needs to walk and be up more. She'll be a lot better if she moves about more. We'll be back to see you in five days Lucy, and I expect you to meet us at the door."

"Thank you, doctah, and you too, Miss Bess. I likes you. Be sure you come back with the doctah."

"Thank you, I hope I can. Bye."

As we got in the car, Jessie said, "What did you mean by saying we will see you?"

"Don't you want to come back with me?

"Well—I'd like to go to other places, too."

"Ok. We will—I promise."

We did go to other places. We even went dancing sometimes, but we also made post-partum calls several times again. It was a must for me, and she made it a much more enjoyable chore. Soon they were over with, and we rotated into the hospital part of the O.B. course.

The six weeks we spent on OB-GYN was interesting, tough, trying, and exhausting. These were clinic patients that had complications such as heart disease, high blood pressure, kidney failure, eclampsia, pulmonary emphysema, asthma, and the worst of all, psychiatric problems. When we were assigned a patient, it meant we had to be there immediately, if possible.

The lab work, general workup (history and physical), a diagnosis, and outline of treatment of her complication had to be on her chart within two hours of her admission. All of this was then checked and graded by the chief resident in the department. Our chief resident showed no mercy. You did it completely and correctly or found yourself answering to the head of the department. We never argued our case with Dr. Greene, the resident, at the time we spent that six weeks "in-house" O.B. training. The most severe complications were admitted that required constant, around-the-clock, bedside care.

"Student Wilson, report to OB stat!" That call meant real trouble. You didn't take time to call. You ran to get there—no elevators, stairways, same as level floors, you *got* there.

"I'm student Wilson, what's the problem?"

"You have a new patient in room 4. Looks like eclampsia."

Oh, no. How lucky can I get? Eclampsia meant constant, bedside vigil, taking pulse and blood pressure every 15 minutes, measuring urinary output every hour, urine analysis every 12 hours, and stat blood work with some elements, such as urea nitrogen, being checked twice daily. Monitoring the patient's state of consciousness was necessary since they were in a toxic state and could slip into unconsciousness without warning. These patients were also prone to having seizures, so there was no sleeping on the job. It did not matter if you had not slept for 18 hours and had not had any food for that same time. You were responsible for that patient's life, as well as her baby's life also. You *had* to be alert! Besides the 12-hour shifts at the bedside, we had to attend classes in three subjects, make rounds with instructors on the pediatric ward, plus do a workup on your patients on that floor. That six weeks was gruesome. It was the time that "tried men's souls." It also was a time that many, who would be obstetricians, decided to change to some other specialty. For some curious reason, I really liked that six weeks. You didn't eat or sleep much, you didn't spend much time with your beloved, but you were never bored either. I wanted to stay on for another six weeks, and let it be known. My "buddy," Joe, remarked: "I thought you were sane, Woodrow, but now I think you've lost your mind."

During the eleventh quarter, we spent six weeks on the pediatric wards seeing and treating babies and children that had the illnesses we heard about in the lecture room. They had multitudes of acute and chronic illnesses: feeding problems, pneumonia, malnutrition, allergies, appendicitis, strangulated hernias, orthopedic problems, meningitis, brain tumors, and on and on. I had never really thought of it, but I had the privilege of seeing many of the problems as I was making house calls with Dad during and after my teens. I had just not been astute enough to realize what I was experiencing at the time, but my recall worked well and helped me to recognize many of the ills.

Our class was unlucky enough to be taking pediatrics when a polio epidemic hit Memphis. Of course, we had to be involved with the diagnosis and treatment of the indigent infants and children. Because of this, we had a wealth of experience with poliomyelitis. It wasn't very pleasant. There was no specific treatment for the disease. A vaccine had not been discovered at that time, and the only thing to be done was to give them supportive treatment and some physiotherapy. The latter was in its infancy in 1942 and was scoffed at by many people in treating polio victims. It was discouraging to see small children become paralyzed or lose their life when everybody was doing their best to prevent that from happening. The one thing being done at that time was adopting the use of the "Iron Lung" to treat polio victims when the respiratory muscles would be involved. It saved many, many lives that would have been lost from respiratory failure without the device.

The University of Tennessee Medical units had an Isolation Hospital that was set apart from its other buildings. There we spent part of our training in caring for the infectious diseases that were isolated and life-threatening. This was where polio victims were housed for care. This included infants and children. They were the ones we had the responsibility for. It was heart-wrenching to see them fighting for their lives. The calls would come at all hours— "Student Wilson, you have a new patient in isolation. You need to come now." That made me angry, and I shivered to think this should happen to an infant that might end a life that was just beginning.

Poliomyelitis, like many other diseases, was no respecter of persons, but seemed to be more prevalent in children and young adults than the older generation. It also involved a higher percentage of the poor and indigent than any other groups.

Again, our class was fortunate. At the time of the polio epidemic we were visited by Sister Kinney, the Australian nurse Nun, who had developed a successful physiotherapy type of treatment. She came to Memphis and to our medical school, and her treatment was started very soon after onset of the illness. As soon as the patient had passed the highly acute stage, the hot packs, muscle massage, and passive exercises were begun. These were done two or three times daily and gradually increased to more active exercises, resulting in muscle activity returning more quickly and normally. What might have once been a useless limb would often be salvaged. After a month's stay in the University giving lectures and demonstrations, she won over many disbelievers that had been opposing her method of treatment.

The reason I said our class was lucky was the very fact that we, as medical students, became involved in and experienced a revolutionary change in the management of a dread disease that crippled or killed thousands and thousands yearly. To have had this experience was an immeasurable asset to me. Soon after, I began a private practice in Memphis where polio was endemic at that time. Again, when moving to Old Hickory, Tennessee, in 1951, we had a mild epidemic in the area, and diagnosing and treating those patients was made easier from the training and experience I had as a medical student.

Our active, interesting, highly involved, exhausting, and thrilling (for me) eleventh quarter of medical school came to an end, as did the year of 1942 at almost the same day. That year had been the most enlightening in medical school for me. The calendar year had also been the best to me for everything else in my life.

In early January of 1943, we registered for classes for the last time as students in the School of Medicine at the University of Tennessee. This was a day to remember. This last quarter was to be devoted to the surgical specialties. To me it was, what I thought, would be the most interesting of all the fields to be involved in. That was because it was more hands-on than most specialties, and it also involved gross anatomy, my first love, when I entered medical school. Also, my beloved was to be on duty in the operating room sometime during that quarter. The class work was interesting. We made ward rounds daily with demonstrations and questions that further stimulated students to be alert. The chief resident was the demonstrator and mentor in the wards. "Student Stevens, this is your patient. Tell us about his problem and how it was handled."

"This is Jim Matlock, age 22. He was admitted with lower abdominal pain, nausea, and vomiting for six hours. He noticed his abdomen swelling about one hour before admission. He felt the need to have a bowel movement shortly after his pain started, but has not defecated yet."

"Is this his first episode of this kind?"

"No, he had a similar one about one year ago. He got relief with a bowel movement after about four hours then. Since that time, he has had bouts of slight pain and loss of appetite that cleared spontaneously. He has lost six pounds of weight in the last three months, and his appetite is poor. What about his physical findings? His head and neck are normal, heart is regular with normal sounds, chest is clear to auscultation."

"What about his abdomen?"

"He has some problem there. It is moderately distended. There is generalized tenderness, which is most marked in the left lower quadrant. There are no masses felt on palpation, and the bowel sounds are hyperactive. On rectal exam, there is feces in the rectal pouch, which is negative for occult blood."

"Lab work showed an elevated WBC count to 15,000 with a shift to the left, polys being 75 percent. Red blood cells are normal in number, shape, and size. His urine analysis is normal. X-rays of the chest and abdomen have been done and interpreted by the Radiologist, which showed a few loops of distended small bowel on the left; otherwise, they are normal."

"Student Lyon, what is your diagnosis?"

"If he had right lower quadrant pain and tenderness, I would say he has acute appendicitis, but that can't be so because the appendix is located on the right side."

"What is your diagnosis, Mr. Miles?"

"I think he has an early intestinal obstruction."

"Tell us what you think he has, Mr. Tabb."

Tabb was an excellent student and number two in class, well-read, quiet, and very astute. "There are reports of left side appendicitis in cases where there is malrotation of the bowel which is congenital. I think that should be considered."

"Thank you, gentlemen. Those are very good observations and diagnoses. Now let's see what we find on the operating table."

Since we were not absolutely sure of our own diagnosis, we made a low, midline, incision in the abdomen, expecting to find most anything. What we really found was a surprise. He had an acutely inflamed appendix and nothing else, except it was on the left. "He was one of the 1 in 100,000 that you mentioned, Mr. Tabb. You are to be congratulated, Sir." Tabb just smiled and said nothing. The rest of us just shook our heads and said: "It's bound to happen to Tommy Stevens. Now he can brag some more about *his* cases."

We saw and discussed case after case on our rounds, which was usually preceded by an hour of lecture. That way the many things we encountered had been etched in our minds.

The class rotated through the OR and ER during that three months, so we had more free time than any previous quarter. That way we could review our work and be prepared for the final exams. We also had more time for recreation and to spend with our favorite girl; which in my case was my favorite recreation anyway. The last three months were wonderful. The classes were enjoyable and I looked forward to clinic hours and ward rounds. I was in love, seriously and hopelessly, as I walked on cloud nine. Everything just seemed to fall into place. The school work flowed freely and love was in full bloom. My beloved was working in the OR as the number one scrub nurse on the 11 to 7 night shift, the hours when gunshot wounds, accident victims, and dire emergencies of all types came to the emergency room and straight to the OR. She was usually totally exhausted by the time she got off duty. I would see her as she was on her way to the dormitory and I on the way to my class or clinic.

All of this was happening near the end of January and we realized that only a little more than two months of school was left. We both began to talk about what was going to happen. At the time our class would graduate, she would still have another year before finishing the course in nursing. At that stage in our love life, neither of us wanted to be separated, and we both avoided the word "marriage" because of financial circumstances. But we also knew I was facing active duty in the Navy as I had been in the V-12 program for a year. All of this haunted us, and the thought of it was more than I could stand. I thought of a way out, and we could be together while she finished nursing school.

"I know what we'll do, Honey."

"What?"

"I'll resign from the internship in Birmingham and take one at St. Joseph's here. I'll be off every other day and we'll have a lot of time together."

"That sounds good. Are you sure you can do that?"

"I haven't signed a contract with them yet, so I guess I can. I'll ask our law instructor tomorrow after class."

After class on Monday, I asked Mr. Skinner if he had time to talk to me. "Sure, I do. Stop by my office next door, and we'll talk there." After class, I waited a few minutes, rehearsed what I would say, and knocked on his door.

"Come in and have a seat, Mr. Wilson. Do you have a problem?"

"Yes, sir, I may have." I outlined the situation, telling him that I had not signed a contract with the Birmingham hospital and wanted to stay in Memphis and why. He assured me that it would be no problem, and he would send a letter to the hospital that would relieve me of any ties to them, and I would be free to apply anywhere else I wished.

"Thank you, Mr. Skinner. I appreciate your interest and your helping me out." We still had other decisions to make and I made one. I would propose marriage. Then she would be with me all the time. I knew the frustration of not knowing what was going to happen was really devastating to her as well. I didn't sleep much for two nights, and my roommates said, "You must have a problem, Woodrow. You have tossed, turned, talked, and carried on all night for three nights. Do you want to talk about it?"

"No, I'll be ok. I'll let you know when I do. I just need to think something out."

The next day after class, we went for a ride in one of the city parks. It was a warm, sunny day, and we enjoyed the quiet surroundings as we rode. We stopped and strolled a little while as we talked of our situation. We soon found a grassy spot under a large tree and sat down to ponder our problem. She was dreamy eyed and pensive. Sitting there with her auburn hair falling around her face, she was so irresistibly beautiful to me that I could not stand the thought of not being with her for the rest of my life. I sat down beside her, and the words automatically poured out. "I love you. Marry me and make me the happiest man in the world." She was so stunned that no words came as she looked at me in wonderment. Then the words came: "I want to more than anything in the world, but I can't say yes now. I need more time to think about it."

"I understand, but I can't wait for a long time."

"It may seem to be a long time, but maybe not. Now take me back to the dorm so I can think this through. Then I'll call."

We drove most of the way back to the dorm in silence, each with their own thoughts. I was thinking, *What will I do if she says "no" to my proposal?* At that moment, I couldn't bear the thought of that happening. I looked at her, and she was staring straight ahead, either deep in thought or dazed by what had happened. When we arrived at the dorm, she was out of the car by the time it stopped. I made a move to get out—"No, don't," and she hurried to the dormitory.

Two days went by. She didn't call. I stuck to my word; I didn't call and I knew better than to go by. It was agony not hearing her voice, not seeing or touching her, just wondering what was happening.

The third day the phone rang. Someone yelled, "Telephone, Woodrow." I knew that it was *her* and took a chance. "God, I've missed you. It seems like a million years since we were together."

"I told you I'd call, I've missed you, too. Can we go somewhere so we can talk?"

"Sure, Sweetheart, whenever and wherever you say. I'll be there."

"Come by the dorm in an hour. I'll be in the lobby."

Time dragged as I waited, then drove the two miles. When I started up the walk to the dorm, she came out the door. I had to control myself to keep from throwing my arms around her and smothering her with a longing embrace.

She smiled at me and said, "You look good. Let's go to Fortunes and have a coke while we sit in the car and talk."

"Don't you want to go inside where you'll be safe from me?"

"No, I'll take a chance with you."

"Ok, but I warn you, you'd better keep an eye on me."

"I will. Let's go." We made idle chatter on the way. I could see she was very tense and talked about school. "When do you go on duty again?"

"In two days. Why?"

"Oh, I just wondered if we might be able to spend some time together."

"I'll think about it and let you know. My calendar is pretty full."

"Ok, here we are." I pulled into the spot where we had parked the night the car's battery ran down. "Remember this spot?" The waiter came with a coke and chocolate shake for the lady.

"How did you know I wanted that?" she asked.

"Instinct, I guess." And before she could move I had her in my arms for a brief "smooch." "I love the taste of your lips. What do you have on?"

"It is called Longing Love." We were interrupted by the waiter. "That will be 75 cents, Sir."

"Here you are, waiter" (I gave him a dollar).

As we sat with our drinks, I had a hard time waiting to ask her that question again. She kept sipping her milkshake and smiling mischievously at me. I waited her out.

Finally, she asked, "Do you want to know my answer?"

"Yes, but let me ask you again so all the world can hear me. Will you marry me?"

She looked at me with a shy smile and spoke softly, "Yes, I will."

It was my turn not to be able to speak. I fought back tears of joy as we were locked in a long embrace. We pushed away from the embrace and looked at each other, drinking in the love we held for each other.

"Thank you, Honey. My heart is full of love for you and always will be."

"You know that I love you just as much in return. I'll be faithful forever."

The waiter came and took the tray. We hardly noticed what was going on around us as we drove slowly back to the dormitory as I held her close to me with our love overflowing into each other's life. At the dorm, leaving her again was agony. I wanted to hold her close again to show how I loved her, but had to settle for a whispered "Good-bye, I love you" as she went inside.

On my way back to the frat house, my sanity returned for a few minutes as I thought, *Oh, Lord, what have I done? Here I am a poor, penniless medical student asking an equally poor girl to marry me with nothing to offer but my love and devotion.* But we were in love—blind, deaf, and dumb love. Nothing else mattered at the moment. *We'll find a way to make it.* I had to tell somebody. I wanted someone that I knew would never tell until the time came. That person was Dr. Clyde Kirk, a former roommate, now an Intern at John Gaston Hospital. He couldn't afford to tell because he had been secretly married since he graduated from college. I was the only one in Memphis that he had every told about it. I called and asked to see him the next day. He was not surprised at all that we planned the wedding.

"What can I do to help you, Wendell?"

"First thing you can do is to do our premarital blood tests. The second thing I want you to do is to be the best man at our wedding. The third thing is to keep everything a secret until we have all our plans made."

"I'll do that, of course . . . I'll call you tomorrow to let you know where and when to have the blood drawn."

"Thanks, Kirk, you're a real friend."

The next day we planned to see "Gone with the Wind," then look for a ring. We did both. We looked in all the jewelry store windows on Main Street for six blocks in downtown Memphis. We walked oblivious to everything around us. We had but one thing in mind—find a ring that we could afford. (We should have shopped in pawn shops on Beale Street). Finally, we spotted one that we both liked, and it was reasonably priced. We had shopped as though my pockets were lined with gold. I had no money, but we shopped anyway. When we found "The Ring," it looked to us that it was pure platinum. "Do you like it, Honey?"

"Yes, it's beautiful. I love it!" We went inside and showed the clerk the ring we had chosen. Jessie tried it on and looked at me with shining eyes. "This one's perfect," she exulted. I made arrangements to buy it on time with a down payment of ten dollars. I gave him the date I would pick up the ring and we left.

On the street we both became sober. Finally, she said, "How are we going to pay for that ring?"

"We'll worry about that later. Let's get you back to the dorm before Miss Huspeth gets her shotgun and waits for me to show up so she can threaten my life for ruining the life of one of 'her girls.'"

The next day I called Dad with the good news. He was flabbergasted! "What do you mean you're getting married? Can't you wait until you graduate?"

"Well, I could, but I'd rather not. Do you think your bank would loan me 200 dollars? I'll sign a note if you can co-sign with me—I'll pay it back as soon as I start to work at 50 dollars a month."

"Yes, I guess so. I'll send the note and money tomorrow." I guess he couldn't say no. After all, he had done the same thing before he graduated from medical school.

The note and money arrived three days later, with an extra hundred dollars.

We had the lab work done. I told Kirk when we would be married and planned to get the marriage license on February 12 since we wanted to have the ceremony on her father's birthday, February 14. On the fourth, I met her as she came off duty from a *very* rough night in surgery. "You look exhausted," I commented.

"I am. We had cases continuously with one or two 15-minute breaks the whole night."

"Come on, I'll walk you to the dormitory."

"Wait, let's sit in the car a minute first so we can talk about our plans."

I though, *something is wrong or she would want to get some sleep.* We sat in the car. I couldn't wait. "Is there a problem, honey?"

"Not really. Why don't we get married this coming Sunday?"

"Suits me, but that's only three days away. Think we can get everything ready by that time."

"I think so. We already have the apartment. I've notified the school that I'm leaving after exams. Sure, we can make it."

"Sure we can. Now all I have to do is find a preacher, get the church, get your parent's consent, get a marriage license, buy furnishings for the apartment, and we'll be all set."

This was on Thursday. By Friday night, all arrangements had been made, and all we had to do was to get the license. Her sister and one of my roommates drove us to the courthouse. We found the County Court Clerk's office. A nice young lady greeted us with, "How can I help you?"

"We'd like to get a marriage license."

"Ok. Let me see your health certificates." She glanced at us and said, "I'm sorry, but I can't issue a marriage license."

I was indignant! "Why not?"

The young lady is not 21, and we'll need her parent's consent."

"We weren't aware of that. What else can we do?"

"Well, the young lady could swear she's pregnant—then they'll issue a license."

Jessie was furious and raised her voice, "I won't do that because it would be a lie."

"You could go before the Probate Judge and he might issue the license. He's three doors down the hall to your right."

I grabbed the paper and Jessie's arm and hurried down the hall. We found the room and stood just inside the door. The courtroom was packed. The Judge was trying a divorce case. The couple was "fighting" in loud voices while the Judge pounded his gavel to restore order, admonishing the couple to take a 10-minute break to cool off. By that time, we had gotten anxious and started inching out. The bailiff saw us and came up and asked if we wanted to see the Judge. "Yes, we want to get a marriage license."

"Wait right here for a minute and I'll ask the Judge now." He spoke to the Judge, then motioned for us to come down there. We walked meekly to face the Judge. I handed him the documents. "Thank you for seeing us, Your Honor." He looked the papers over, signed them, and handed them back to me as he smiled and said, "I'll give you these on one condition—that you'll promise me that you won't be back here in a few years like the couple that just left here."

"We won't, I promise. Thank you, Your Honor!" We took the papers and hurried out the door, happy as larks.

Late that afternoon we went shopping again, this time to buy cooking utensils, towels, etc., so we could "set up housekeeping." We had finished by 8 o'clock, and Jessie had to return to the dormitory. There we had a hasty good-bye, and I headed back to the fraternity house, not knowing what was in store for me.

As I walked into the darkened foyer, hands grabbed both arms and half-carried me down the winding stairs to the bar. Then I realized what was about to happen. One of my "buddies" was tending bar which was loaded with several, long-necked bottles of various alcoholic "beverages." They greeted me loudly, shaking my hand, slapping my back, congratulating me, and offering advice. "Come on Woodrow, you need a drink. What will you have?"

"Just a light bourbon and Seven-up."

The "bartender" didn't hear well and poured a stiff one. I almost strangled as I drank it. They watched me closely, and they weren't satisfied because I drank too slowly to suit them. "You're just sipping that, Woodrow. Drink up." Someone took the glass, refilled it, and handed it back. By this time, I was feeling the effects of the whiskey and joined the celebrating. We had a great time. The fellows told me what a great fellow I was and what a wonderful girl I was marrying and how I would be missed at the "house." Some of them talked about losing their girl back home and would never trust another woman because of that. Some shed tears as they talked of all their problems, and they all got drunk. During all of this time, I sipped my drinks very slowly and stayed a bit more sober. I knew that I would get sick and start vomiting if I continued drinking. Although I stopped taking any more, I felt the nausea creeping up on me.

By 2 a.m. I had persuaded two friends to go to bed and helped them get there. I wasn't doing too well myself, but kept busy so I would avoid the celebrants. It didn't quite work out that way as "Buck" Best cornered me, and I wound up in the bar again. I was doomed! Everybody gathered around and "sang" "For He's a Jolly Good Fellow," plus a half-dozen more before I could manage to get away. Somehow I found my bed and crawled in. When I lay down the bed started spinning and rolling so fast that I became nauseated and "tossed my cookies" two or three times. Now it was 3 a.m., and in 12 more hours I would be a married man. I had to get some sleep, then find some clothes by 8 o'clock. Then I had to meet the bride-to-be at our apartment so we could make it livable. I managed to sleep four hours, only to wake up with a bad headache. As I sat on the bedside, "Buck" came in, sober as a judge and smiling from ear to ear.

"What's the matter, Woodrow? You don't look so hot."

"I feel terrible and I need to leave here at 9. Right now, I don't think I can make it."

"Oh, sure you can. Come on, let's take a cool shower." He was very solicitous, helped me into the shower, then left me on my own." That was what I needed at the moment. Somehow I managed to get dressed, called Jessie, and drove to the dormitory, collected her belongings, and headed for the apartment six blocks away. By the time we arrived, the nausea struck again.

Carrying the bags upstairs was all I could manage. Within two minutes, I felt faint and fell across the bed. "Are you all right, Wendell?" (She seemed a mile away.)

"I'm sick, just let me lie here for a minute, then maybe I'll be ok." The next thing I knew someone was shaking me. "Wake up, Wendell. It's noon. We have only three more hours before the wedding. How do you feel now?"

"Much better, I think. Maybe I'll live. I'm sorry, honey, I just can't take the alcohol without getting sick. I had about two drinks too many last night."

"Are you able to drive me back to the dormitory now?" she asked.

"Sure, I can. Everything's clearing up now. I'll be in good shape before 3 o'clock. Trust me."

"I'm not too sure I *can*. Let's go." She glared at me, took my arm, and we went down the stairway to the car. Conversation was out! We drove in silence to the dormitory. She was out of the car in a flash. I wondered if she would go through with the wedding or leave me standing at the altar. At least her reactions served to clear my head, and I was cold sober by the time I got back.

My friend "Buck" accosted me again. "Hey, Woodrow, you look much better. How about some food? Maybe some cheese and crackers, huh?"

"Yeah, that sounds good. Bring me some while I take another cool shower." The clock struck 1, and I felt a cold chill over my whole body. Only two more hours to wait, wondering if my fiancee would be at the church. Now I was *really* sober. The shower and food helped a lot.

Everybody came to my rescue. I borrowed a suit from W. T. Mathis, a shirt from Tommy Stevens, and a tie from somebody else (I had my own socks and underwear). I was ready to meet the preacher, the best man, and go through the ceremony.

Arriving at the church, I was searching for the bride. My heart skipped a beat.

She wasn't there. "Have you seen Jessie, Gene?"

"No, but it's early. She'll be here. Quit worrying."

Soon the minister went in and motioned me in. My knees were so weak that I had to lean on Kirk, the best man, for support. Then the music began, and I knew *she* was ready to walk down that long aisle. By then my heart was pounding with anticipation of her walking *to* me. The wedding march sounded far away as I waited for my beloved. Then she was standing by my side as the minister was intoning, "Dearly beloved, we are gathered here today to ..." The next few words were a blur, then—"Jessie, do you take Wendell to be your lawful husband, to have and to hold until death do you part?" She looked into my eyes and whispered, "I do." "I now pronounce you husband and wife. You may kiss the bride." I did deeply and longingly.

After the wedding ceremony, we were driven around Memphis by a friend and Jessie's sister. We stopped for milkshakes and cokes. Following that we were honored guests at a dinner given by Dr. and Mrs. Kirk. That was a wonderful end to the most glorious day of my life.

By 8 o'clock we were anxious to leave. I gave my friend the "high sign," and we left for our "honeymoon cottage," a second-floor, efficiency apartment with a shared bathroom at the foot of our stairs. There we spent a wonderfully glorious, 4-day "honeymoon."

On the fifth day of our married life, I reluctantly returned to class to face some ridicule and to be the brunt of some poor jokes. Interestingly enough that was the same room where we had class that fateful day nine months earlier when I spied the beautiful, auburn-haired student nurse who was now my wife.

From that day my life wasn't quite the same. Everything was beautiful to me. Days went by swiftly and smoothly. Class work was enjoyable and more understandable than ever before, and before anyone realized it, our class faced the last final examination as medical students. They were practical and sensible, utilizing what we had covered for the last three months. Nobody worried about whether or not they passed because they felt that confident, and the professor felt the same way.

We had two weeks to wait for the results, during which time we continued to see the hospital patients and relax. That was a great ending to four years of hard work, frightening times, many frustrations, a lot of fun, and drastic changes in our lives. It was also the fulfillment of a dream come true for me. God was good to me. Not only did I realize the dream come true, but I found a mate that proved to be the perfect one for me. I was happy and grateful for all that I had been blessed with.

A week after exams were finished, and we had relaxed, our test results were announced earlier than we had expected. The class met with one of our sponsors. He passed out the grades, congratulated us on our accomplishments, and then announced the date and place for the brief graduation ceremonies.

That day finally came. A 7 p.m., on March 22, 1943, we assembled in the Student Center for the ceremony. There was a brief speech by the Dean, and then his secretary called the roll as each one walked to the podium to receive the diploma, a handshake, and "congratulations" by Dean Hyman. As I waited, it all seemed like a dream, and it was hard to believe what was really happening. As the Dean droned on and on—"Adams, Andrews, Tabb, Wilkening, Wilson . . ." *That's me, Wendell Wilson, M.D.!* I felt like jumping up and screaming to the world, "I did it, I did it, I did it!" Instead, I walked calmly to the stage and took my diploma, returned the handshake, and thanked Dean Hyman. Then I fought back the tears and sat down beside my wife of six weeks. When she whispered, "Congratulations, honey, I'm proud of you," the tears of joy and happiness flowed freely in spite of me, because I had finally reached that goal I had set some ten years before.

Inside me there was some pain and sadness. Pain because not one family member had attended this graduation ceremony, just as they also did not attend when I graduated from college in 1939 (a first for my ten siblings). Sadness that my parents were unable to attend to rejoice and celebrate with me and mine. The sadness was multiplied as I thought how they had sacrificed so this goal could be realized. This was the way they had proved their love and belief in me. Deep inside I knew that the entire family was proud of "Scrub." Life would go on, and the hurting would soon pass away.

Holding that diploma tightly in my hand as we left the Student Center, I made a statement that I had to retract: "I've been going to school for 20 years to be able to get this, and now I have it. I'm not going to crack a book for the next five years." We walked in silence for a few minutes. Then my sister-in-law asked, "Aren't you going to study for state boards?" Then it dawned on me that we had to face that chore to be eligible to do an internship. What a world!

At that moment, I was thinking of what all physicians had to endure to earn a degree and practice their profession. The "weeding out" began when you applied for admission to medical school. A certain grade level was required before you were even considered. Then one had to compete with 300 other applicants when the school would take only fifty each quarter in an accelerated program. As one progressed through the twelve quarters, many exams were given that you had to pass to be promoted. Then, if one survived the two pre-clinical years, an oral exam was given to include all subjects during that time, so the faculty could decide if you were "fit" to continue. At the end of the ninth quarter, the National Boards were given, a landmark for our class since it was the first time this had every been required before graduation at our school. Then there was another three quarters with several exams, and then the finals. If you passed this, you could get that M.D. degree. After that the last hurdle was "State Boards."

If you succeeded and made a passing grade, then you would be able to go out into the world and be responsible for people's lives.

The next two weeks, I was reviewing old exams, reading textbooks, calling and studying with classmates still in town, and, in general, ignoring my new wife. It must have been worth the time we spent, as everybody passed with flying colors. Now we could practice if we could find twenty dollars to pay for the license.

Internship

April 1, 1943, was a banner day in my life. That day I began my internship! A beginning of a busy, interesting, and often hectic life. New interns had gathered in the Hospital Administrator's office to become acquainted. In came the senior hospital resident physician, a quiet, no-nonsense type of man, very straightforward and helpful. He believed in hard work, honesty, punctuality, and accepting responsibility in all situations. The junior resident had the same attitude but was not as dependable or helpful. The administrator, a Catholic sister, was a kind, considerate, helpful lady who impressed me as an individual with a big heart, which was proven to me many times. I liked her immensely! I knew nothing of the Catholic faith, but she made me realize that we all worshiped the same God and that I was in good hands.

The senior resident then briefed us on our duties, responsibilities, hours of duty, and time off. The he informed us that there would be four interns and two residents to do the work that was usually done by twelve interns and six residents. "Because of this house-staff shortage, you may be asked to work extra hours on occasions, but as a rule you will be on for 24 hours and off 24 hours." It didn't work out that way very long. After the briefing we were introduced to everybody: then each of us were assigned to our service for that month. I was lucky and was assigned to the emergency room. We all left to begin our tour of duty the following day. On the way home, I took stock of where I stood. We (my wife and I) were in a financial bind. We lived in a 3-story attic apartment, with the bedroom opening out to an added outside stairway through a large, picture window, which could not be locked. This cost us rent of $55 per month. My salary was $50 per month, and my wife was unemployed. That was when I found out she was a jewel. We discussed the situation, and her answer was quick. "I'll go to work"—and she did—at Sears-Roebuck in the office. Her salary of $84 a month kept us afloat. That was $134 per month and was 100 percent more than our income had been since our marriage. We felt secure until she was forced to quit her job in the latter part of September, and we were back in the same spot again. My duty hours had proven to be two days on and then off when possible. She would be alone in the apartment much of the time, and I would be dead tired when off. Yet, we survived, and I feel our marriage was strengthened by that experience. Neither of us expected much and were happy just being together whenever possible.

April 2, 1943, was my first day on duty in the emergency room. I was busy with routine illnesses and minor accidents from 7 a.m. to 7 p.m., with short breaks for meals—a lull until midnight, and then the people that had been ill all day became frightened and came in with minor problems that kept me up the remainder of the night. This became a routine. I was glad to get the experience and see the variety of ills that came in for treatment. Since the hospital was only a few blocks from downtown it was always busy in the emergency room.

In addition to this, a very active ambulance company was nearby and brought most of their patients to our emergency room. Believe you me, they kept me busy. That first month of emergency experience was very valuable to me throughout my career. It was actually a triage center. I soon learned to make rapid diagnoses, to move patients to proper areas for treatment, learned the art of getting along with the staff physicians, gaining the confidence of most, learned how to empathize and talk with families during time of stress or loss of a loved one, and, most of all, how to use my God-given talents.

I treated a lot of trauma patients during my tour of duty in the ER. some were unforgettable. I'll describe a few of the most impressive cases I had the privilege to care for.

❖ ❖ ❖

It was Easter Sunday, my second week of ER duty, a beautiful spring day with clear, blue skies, and a light breeze from the south. Spring flowers were in bloom, and all was serene. This was a day meant for relaxing with families, and that was what most of the staff members were doing. The emergency room was quiet and peaceful.

My wife and her sister had lunch with me and had just left. As I walked into the ER, telephones were urgently ringing off the walls and the radio was on. I heard a program being interrupted with an emergency call for all hospitals and doctors to be alerted for action. There was a head-on collision of trains just outside the station downtown. Three people were reported killed and scores injured. By the time the nurse could hang up the phone we could see an ambulance in the distance with its siren wailing, horns blaring, and red lights flashing. We thought we would be ready, but not for what came in. The assistant resident and I were the only house staffers on duty at that moment. Most active staff members were out with families. We had 32 injured patients arrive in a short period, with a myriad of types from very critical ones to minor ones—head injuries, a variety of fractures, mangled limbs, profusely bleeding, open wounds, all degrees of burns, and shock from blood loss. It was bedlam! People were screaming for help, and some were crying out, "Oh, God, let me die!" It would be etched in my memory forever. We were working frantically to save the critical ones. We stopped the profuse bleeding wounds, started IV fluids, gave transfusions when we could, bound wounds, and gave pain shots. Some went to x-ray, and we sent the most dire surgical patients to the operating room, and then prayed for help. Thank God no one panicked. We were too busy doing those things we had been trained to do in emergency situations. In less than 30 minutes, staff physicians came pouring in to take care of the patients, and by nightfall all was back to normal. What a day!

From that experience I had made friends with several families and one in particular. A 32-year-old railroad employee came in in deep shock from a mangled leg. He was conscious, but near death. By the grace of God we saved him with quick work by the entire emergency room staff, IV fluids, transfusions, and other supportive measures. I had the duty of telling his young wife the situation—that he would probably lose a leg, but he would live. Shortly after talking with her, he went to surgery, had his leg amputated, and recovered quickly.

As soon as he regained consciousness, I was called from his floor and asked to come up. I rushed there not knowing what to expect. "Mr. Johnson wants to see you, Doctor." He was amazingly alert, and again I was relieved. He looked like a million dollars to me.

"I want to thank you for saving my life, Doctor, and if you ever have a practice in this town, I will be your first patient."

That really touched me. "Thank you for the compliment, Hal. I'll hold you to that promise." Fighting back the tears, I left the room. Of course, I visited as often as possible during his 6-week hospital stay. He went back to work with a prosthesis a few months later. I finished my internship, went to active duty in the Navy, and didn't see or hear from him for three years. I returned to the city for a residency at the same hospital and got in touch with them. We renewed our friendship, and a year later I was in private practice there. He kept his word and came to see me the first day of practice. His entire family became my patients. I saw them through many trying times of various illnesses. They were loyal and understanding patients, referred their friends to me, and when I left practice there, they hosted a going-away party for us. In later years they visited our home in Old Hickory, Tennessee, to renew friendships.

❖   ❖   ❖

Many exciting, comical, happy, and tragic events occur in a hospital emergency room. Most of them you don't recall, but some you can never forget. I can recall some very vividly.

An ambulance came "blaring" in, the attendants poured out, hurriedly removed a stretcher from inside, and came running in with it, and then a second stretcher was rushed in. Each one had a young man of about 20 to 25 years of age lying on it; each had burns over their entire body. Their eyelids were seared together as though they had been welded that way. Removing the sheet from each one, I saw that everything was burned away except the seams of underwear and collars. the eyes were sightless, ears burned to a crisp, palms and soles were solid blisters. Yet, they were still conscious, asking for a cigarette, able to give their names, calling for water, and walking about.

"What happened, Joe?"

"They didn't make the sharp curve going west over the Mississippi River bridge in a gasoline tanker truck and it exploded and caught fire as they 'bailed out.' "

"What is your name?" I asked.

"I'm Jim Kowalski."

"Where do you live?"

"110 Oak Street, Little Rock, Arkansas. Could I please have a cigarette, Doctor?"

I couldn't believe this was happening. We gave morphine, called the attending physician, finally found a vein, started IV fluids, wrapped each like a mummy and sent them to the floor. Within two hours one expired, and not long after, the second one also died. That was a moving event and kept the entire staff sober and silent for many hours.

❖   ❖   ❖

"How old is your son?"

"He's eight."

"When did he get sick?"

"Oh, two or three days ago."

"Tell me what happened."

"He got sore in his muscles and said he was hurting all over. This morning he was 'jumpy' and his face twitched some. He just kept getting worse all day, Doc. Now he can't open his mouth."

"Has he been hurt, stepped on a nail, or stuck a splinter in his hand or foot?"

"Yeah, he did stick a splinter in his hand five or six days ago, but he pulled it out."

"Where was he when this happened?"

"At the barn."

"Where do you live?"

"On a farm near Batesville, Arkansas."

"Has he been sick before?"

"He's had measles, mumps, and colds, but nothin' like this."

"Has he had DPT shots?"

"Naw, we ain't never give our kids them shots."

"Why, Mr. Ward?"

"Didn't think they needed them."

"Well, they did." I shook my head and examined the boy. He was very spastic. Just touching him would throw him into a severe spastic state; his back would arch and he would become rigid all over.

"Open your mouth, Dennis." He would roll his eyes and become spastic all over again. His abdomen was rigid, and his leg muscles twitched. This was a classic case of tetanus. I had an empty feeling in the pit of my stomach. I had never seen a case before. When they had progressed to this stage it was usually fatal. I turned to Mr. Ward and said, "Sir, your son has lockjaw." I could see the terror in his eyes.

"He has?" He shook his head as tears came to his eyes. He implored, "What are we gonna do, Doc?"

"We will do everything in our power to make him better, but he will have to be moved to another hospital where he can be quarantined because we don't have the facilities here for that. Now, you had better start praying (I didn't use the word isolate purposely because he wouldn't understand). I called the hospital. We gave the boy something to relax as they instructed and sent him to the other hospital. I could not get that boy off my mind day or night. I called the attending physician daily or watched for him when he arrived to follow the case.

After a few days he came in with a smile on his face. "Your tetanus case is going to make it, good Doctor." I felt like hugging him.

"Thank you, Sir, that's the best news I've had in a week." Then I relaxed.

❖   ❖   ❖

Soon thereafter, I rotated off ER service and through all other services, except psychiatry, since we did not have that department. Internal medicine was next. I had some interesting cases on that service, also, but not as exciting as my stint in the ER. Luckily, I had a sharp attending physician who was an excellent teacher with a lot of practical common sense. "Doctors, when you see a case, remember two things. when you take a history, take time to listen to that patient, give him your undivided attention, make him (or her) think they are the only patient you have in that hospital." I tried to remember that advice as long as I practiced. I was busy day and night on that service. Heart attacks, heart failure, pneumonia, high blood pressure, bronchitis, bronchiectasis, hepatitis, pancreatitis, ad infinitum. These were the days we were treating patients with sulfa drugs, cough expectorants, supportive measures, and prayer when all else failed.

"Doctor, come to 208 quickly, Mr. Smith is having a hard time breathing. It's 2 a.m." I jumped out of bed half-asleep and ran up the stairs from my first-floor quarters. By then I was awake but not thinking too clearly.

"What's wrong, Mr. Smith?"

"I can't get my breath, Doctor."

He was wheezing and trying to cough. "Just try to relax and let me see what is wrong," I urged. His pulse was rapid, his breathing labored; he was in a cold sweat, and his color was getting ashen. "Get the oxygen, Nurse." I examined him with the stethoscope and heard many rales (abnormal breath sounds) all through his upper chest. The breath sounds were distant to absent in his lower chest. Then I "percussed" (tapped with my fingers) in his chest and found dullness all over.

"Nurse, this man is in congestive heart failure." I checked his abdomen and found his liver edge was down about two fingers below the costal margin, his lower legs were edematous and pits on pressure. "Put him in the oxygen tent, Nurse. give him 50 Mg. of Diuretin by IV route and 1 Mg. of Digoxin IM while I call Dr. Brown."

"Doctor, I hate to call you so late, but Mr. Smith in Room 208 is in congestive failure. I have started oxygen by tent at 4 liters per minute."

"That's good, Dr. Wilson. Give another milligram of Digoxin in two hours and eight hours from that time, stop his fluid intake, repeat his diuretic in six hours, stay with him, and call me if he gets any worse."

"Thank you, Dr. Brown." I stayed with him for four hours.

"He's looking better now. Why don't you get some sleep," said the nurse. "I'll call you if he gets worse." Thank God for a capable, conscientious nurse!

During the six weeks I spent in internal medicine service there were many interesting cases that kept me busy. Some I still recall, such as the 200-pound man admitted with "hiccups."

"Hi, Mr. Parker. I'm Dr. Wilson. What can I do for you?"

"You can (hic) stop these (hic) damned (hic) hic (hic) cup (hic) sss (hic)."

"How long have you had them?"

"Three (hic) ddd (hic) days (hic), and they (hic) (hic) are k-k-killing mmme."

I had never seen a patient with such a severe case of hiccoughs. Talking to his wife, I learned they had started after a sneezing attach that lasted longer than usual. After they didn't stop with all the usual home remedies—such as holding your breath as long as possible, drinking a glass of water slowly, or eating a spoonful of sugar—they called the family doctor. After two or three days he was hospitalized. When he proved normal for all possible causes for this problem, he was given large doses of sedatives, but he continued to hiccup in his sleep. Gastroscoping did no good. Antispasmodics were tried to no avail. Withholding oral intake did not help. We were "stumped." During this 2-week period, he was fed by IV route. In spite of all measures, he continued to hiccup. Finally, the attending physician started gagging him repeatedly, and that seemed to help. It was then my duty to keep this treatment up every 15 to 30 minutes until we got results. Finally, after two weeks of this, plus sedatives and IV fluids, he stopped. He had lost thirty pounds from the day of onset, suffered physical and psychic trauma, and almost lost faith in all doctors.

One more case I recall vividly. Tom had a severe urinary tract infection for ten days and was getting worse. He was admitted for treatment with a new drug, sulfathiazole, which had proven to be very effective for this problem. He was given the prescribed dosage, his infection began to clear—then something happened. He couldn't urinate! I was called that night to find him in great distress. We inserted a Foley catheter—no urine, then only a few drops. Then we remembered that some people would have complications of the drug, forming crystals that would block the renal tubules and prevent normal flow of urine. This was the problem we faced. It was a life-threatening situation.

I called the Urologist to report the complication. "Dr. Allen, this is Dr. Wilson at St. Joseph's. Tom Judkins in 324 has a problem. He has severe pain in the kidney area bilaterally and is unable to void. He is a little tender over both kidneys. The bladder is not distended nor tender. We inserted a Foley catheter and got less and a c.c. of urine. He has been on sulfathiazole and I'm thinking this may be his problem. The renal tubules may be clogged with crystals."

"You're probably right. Let's leave the Foley in and check his output hourly. Stop the sulfathiazole now. Keep his I.V. going at 75 c.c.s per hour, give Diuretin 50 mg. by mouth every 12 hours, apply hot packs to the kidney areas, and give phenobarbital every eight hours. I'll ask Dr. Black to see him early in the morning."

All of this was done and within another 12 hours there was some output of urine, I.V. fluids were increased, and within three days, this had returned to normal. His infection cleared within the week, and he was dismissed home. We all learned a valuable lesson—with a new drug always watch for warnings of the possible reactions and complications.

Soon after this episode I rotated off of urology to pediatrics for six weeks. It was quite an experience; so much so that I decided then that I could never specialize in that field. I did learn the art of examining infants and small children, thanks to some older men who took the time to give advice to us interns. We were also taught how to insert needles and catheters into scalp veins on infants and small children. Here again we were aided by experienced nurses who knew how to wrap the patients so they were immobile while we performed/learned the technique. I did not like to see and treat sick, suffering children, and I was relieved that no severe complications or tragedies happened while on that service.

Following the six weeks on "peds," I then rotated through OB-GYN and surgical reviews. These were the fields I was looking forward to being involved more in. My first rotation was on OB. By that time, we were expecting our first child. As it happened, I had an active part on this service, examining and watching patients during labor, delivering some when the attending physician was not able to get there on time, and caring for newborns on many occasions. Unfortunately, we had some newborns with congenital abnormalities along the way, and I naturally would worry that our baby would have one of the several things that I saw happen to parents at those times. As a medical student I had delivered more than 30 babies, and some of our teachers were staff members at this hospital. They naturally thought one of their students would be capable of caring for his patient. For that reason I was given more leeway than some fellow interns.

"Would you like to deliver this patient, Dr. Wilson?"

"Yes, I would Dr. Rich. Thank you for standing beside me."

"You're doing ok, or rotate a little more, deliver that shoulder now, fine, that's it. Good job."

Boy! I felt like a real obstetrician then. Delivering a "frank breech" (bottom first) baby was a challenge, but I did some without any real problems. We had one event occur that was so unusual I will relate it since I played a major role at the time. A call came from the emergency room. "Dr. Wilson, you have an OB patient here that you need to see right now."

Arriving in the ER quickly, I saw a real problem. A large 200-pound plus woman was in hard labor. The fetal head was in the birth canal and the scalp presenting. The nurse gave me a rundown of the problem: fourth pregnancy, no prenatal MD visits, in active labor for eight hours, blood pressure 170/100, pulse 110, no fetal heart sounds. She had been seen by the county health nurse with quick evaluation and sent immediately to our hospital. My examination confirmed everything the nurse had related to me. I now had the task of telling both husband and wife that we suspected the fetus was dead in the uterus and that the mother was in trouble with high blood pressure, and the baby was "stuck" in the birth canal with the possibility we might not be able to remove it from below. I called Dr. Rich. "Doctor, we have a critical problem with an indigent patient." Then I outlined the case.

"Take her to the delivery room. I'll be there in 20 minutes."

She was on the table, the I.V. was going, and blood was being typed and cross-matched, just in case it was needed. We had the blood pressure down by that time, and I felt a bit better concerning her condition. Dr. Rich came in and looked things over, shook his head, and said, "Boy, you *do* have a problem."

"No, Dr. Rich, *we* have a problem."

"It's your patient. What have you planned?"

"Give her a general anesthetic, as much as we dare give, try to apply forceps, and attempt a delivery from below."

"That is good, Wilson, go ahead. I'll stand by."

What a burden! Applying the forceps was a tough job. That accomplished, we all began to pull and push at the same time; finally the head advanced a little. I was able to get two fingers in the baby's armpit, which helped to improve my grasping the baby. We were then able to rotate the shoulders, and with all the strength I had, plus two nurses pushing on the abdomen with all their might, out came the shoulders, the body, and lower extremities delivered easily. The baby had no sign of life. It was a huge boy, weighing 14 lbs. 8 ozs. The mother survived the tragic ordeal and was dismissed thereafter. She never returned as we requested.

My OB rotation time was enriching, as well as rewarding. I had a wealth of experience, developed my skills more, saw a variety of complications, met many fine people that were lasting friends, and most of all, learned the art of private practice. It was a wonderful, unforgettable, and happy experience.

After that time, I spent the next period in gynecology. I worked with many of the same staff physicians as before in OB. General Surgeons also did much of the OB-GYN surgery. The chief of service game me a resume of duties while on his service. "You will take all histories and physicals when patients are admitted. This will be done within 12 hours of admission. You will assist in surgery at all times as first or second assistant. On all house cases, you will follow the same routine except you will be responsible for her entire care, from the day of admission until discharged. You will also be responsible for follow-up care in the clinic." We were busy, and I found myself asking for advice quite often.

"Dr. Long, I have a patient in distress with pelvic pain and fever. She has a tender mass in the left adnexal region that is rather hard to touch."

"What do you think she might have, Wilson?"

"I think she either has a cystic ovary that is bleeding or a true tumor."

"Is she in the child-bearing age?"

"Yes, but there is no history of a missed cycle, so I feel she does not have an ectopic pregnancy."

"Very good. Get a chest X-ray, the lab work, give her morphine, 1/4 grain, and get her scheduled for surgery."

"Dr. Long, do I need to call the resident physician?"

"No, we can handle it without him."

I sweated, thinking he might expect me to do the surgery. Thank God he didn't. A few minutes later he was there and examined the patient.

Dr. Long said, "I agree with your diagnosis. Let's take her to surgery."

In surgery he took charge. After we prepped and draped the patient, Dr. Long made an incision from pelvic bone to the navel. When the abdomen was opened and pelvic structures exposed, we could see the problem.

Doctor From Bugtussle

"There you are, Doctor. I see what you were feeling on the pelvic exam."

"Yes, sir, it is a cyst and there's blood in the sac."

"We're pretty good diagnosticians! You did real good this time, Doctor," Dr. Long noted.

Inside I was ecstatic at being correct, but I just said, "Thank you, Sir." Since she was my first case, the lady got a lot of attention post-operative. The remainder of the time I was on that service, things were "popping" every day. I saw cases of advanced endometriosis that involved all of the pelvic structures, endometrial implants on the colon and omentum, plus practically destroying the ovaries.

Two or three cases of ectopic (tubal) pregnancy came in. One was in shock from blood loss. When we opened the abdomen it was amazing the amount of blood throughout her abdomen. This had all come from one small artery the size of a corsage pin. Each of those young women suffered the loss of a fallopian tube and the severe case, an ovary as well. I was unfortunate enough to find cases of cancer of the cervix and the ovary. It depressed me when I discovered the latter because almost every case of it was fatal. Today, that diagnosis is a death knell 95 percent of the time.

Again, I was sorry to leave that service. It too had been interesting, helpful for my future in practice, educational, depressing in some instances, but overall, rewarding and a pleasure.

❖   ❖   ❖

The next service I had was general surgery. This I was really looking forward to with great anticipation. I had fantasized many times of the cases I would be doing, when in reality I knew that I would be fortunate to do more than close incisions, remove a toenail, or incise and drain abscesses. After about three weeks of holding retractors for four to eight hours, tying sutures (after hours of practice at home), of dressing the surgical incisions post-operatively, I was unexpectedly rewarded.

One more call came from the emergency room. "Dr. Wilson, you have a surgical case here."

"I'll be right down. I was there before they hung up the phone. There the case was—a thin 12-year-old with a tummy ache.

"Hi, Jake, I'm Dr. Wilson."

"Hi. Are you going to hurt me?"

"No, I hope not. Let's see your tummy."

"How long have you had this stomachache?"
"Two days."
"Have you been throwing up?"
"Yeah, a couple of times."
"Where did the pain start?"
"Right here," pointing to his navel.
"Where is it now?"
"Right here," pointing to his right lower side.

I checked his abdomen all over. He was very tender over the anatomical site of the appendix, contracting the muscle when touched.

"Does this hurt much?" I asked, as I quickly let up finger pressure from over the appendix. He almost came off the table. This was a classic case of acute appendicitis. His lab work showed a high WBC count with a shift to the left, typical of an infection. I called Dr. Jordan, the staff M.D., gave him all the facts and waited. "Admit him, start an IV, call OR, and I'll come over. He made a cursory exam on arrival. "Let's put him to sleep, Nurse, and we'll scrub. We had already talked to the family and had the operative permit signed. As we scrubbed, he shocked and delighted me.

"You will do this case, Doctor." This would be my first experience. I was really proud to be the Operating Surgeon.

"Thank you, Dr. Jordan."

At the operating table, after draping, I assumed the correct position to do the surgery.

"Are you ready Miss Mullinax? (the anesthetist).
"Yes, Doctor.
"Scalpel."

The nurse deftly put the knife handle in my palm. I was making the incision, and my hand was shaking so that I wondered if I could make it. I looked at Dr. Jordan. He nodded and said, "You're doing fine."

I went through each layer as I had done before. All went well until the last layer. The assistant (Dr. J.) and I each grasped a bit of peritoneum (last layer) with a hemostat. That was the crucial second. I nicked the peritoneum with the scalpel and pus came pouring out through the small slit. I was not panicky and opened the incision more. "Suction, please," I requested. It was already there. I suctioned out all of the pus, then looked at my mentor—"Go ahead, Doctor. Look for the Appendix. Everything will be ok. You can't stop now." My hand was steady now. He had given me confidence I desperately needed. Inserting my finger in the incision, I located the appendix. With good retraction and packing we delivered the swollen, discolored organ that was covered with shaggy, purulent material. It was not perforated. We proceeded with the surgery, removed the appendix, irrigated the peritoneal cavity with large amounts of saline, inserted two Penrose rubber drains in the area of the appendix, closed the abdomen, supplied a copious dressing, kept his IV fluids going, and hoped he would soon recover. I visited often and observed closely as he recovered.

In those days we didn't get patients up so soon as we do now. This patient taught me something: he got out of bed the second day, and it seemed to speed his recovery. I continued to get him up each day, and he was walking before going home a week later. I learned by that case to get them up sooner. After that I was given more leeway and had the good fortune to gain needed experience as an Operating Surgeon. I did six appendectomies, several D&Cs, salpingectomies, oophorectomies and a gallbladder operation, all with the attending physician "holding my hand." Of course, that was not a wealth of surgical experience, but more than most interns would get. It also prepared me better for military service which I was facing at the end of the year. I had not finished eight months of internship, with one more to go before the call to active duty. Then the senior resident called me to his office. I didn't know what to expect. "Come in, Wilson. Have a seat."

"What's the problem, Dr. Sid?

"No problem. I heard that we will be losing you to the Navy."

"I know. I wish I could stay around, but I'm obligated to do my part."

"I need a favor of you, Wilson."

"I'll be happy to do what I can. What is it?"

"I would like for you to take over the ER for the rest of your time here."

"That's great. Just what I wanted. Thank you, Dr. Sid."

Right back where I started. I felt relaxed and comfortable in what I was doing again. I had many interesting cases to see and was happy there until I was called to active duty by the Navy Medical Corps. Leaving St. Joseph's was sad and tearful. I visited all the floors, hugged and got hugged and kissed by the nurses, embraced by the sisters, and I cried along with each of them.

Then I went to say good-bye to the administrator, and that is where I "lost" it. "Good morning, Sister. I just came to thank you for all the wonderful things you've done for me and my family. They will never be forgotten."

"Dr. Wilson, you've done a wonderful job here. We'll miss you terribly. We hate to see you go, but also know that our country needs good doctors like you."

When she held out both hands to me, saying, "I wish you well, and God be with you," that's when the tears flowed freely while I "blubbered," "Good-by, Sister." It was like leaving family. But I had no choice—duty called, and I left to serve my country, ending a year of wonderful experiences that would help me do my duty far better for my country and fellow man.

The Navy Medical Corps

They came, on December 29, 1943, my call to active duty orders. "To Lt. (jg) Wendell W. Wilson, MCUSNR, you are to report to active duty on January 2, 1944, etc. to Capt. John Jones, MCUSN, Commandant of Naval Hospital, Millington, TN @ 0800 hrs." How lucky could I get? Duty only 15 miles from the house. "Jessie, I got the orders. Guess where I will be going?"

"Where?"

"Millington Naval Hospital! Can you believe that?" We jumped for joy, for we could still be together.

At the hospital on January 2, 1944: "May I help you, Sir?"

"Yes. I have orders to report to Capt. Jones for active duty."

"Just a moment, Sir."

I sat and waited for five minutes.

"This way, Sir."

I walked into the Captain's office and stood at attention. "Lt. J.G. Wilson, Sir."

I was greeted by: "Where the hell is your uniform, Lieutenant?"

"Sorry, Sir. I don't have a uniform and am not able to buy one."

"What is your problem, Doctor?"

"Sir, I just finished my internship three days ago, and I haven't enough money to get a uniform."

"We'll fix that. Miss Enoch, get the uniform stores for me."

On the phone: "'Scissors,' I'm sending Lt. (jg) Wilson by for a dress blue uniform. Get him ready for duty by 0200 today. Get up there now, get fitted, and be back in this office at 0400. Dismissed."

"Aye, Sir. Thank you, Sir." I saluted and left. Somehow I got that uniform, complete with socks, shirt, tie, and hat, without paying any cash. I went home long enough to change into the proper dress and reported back *early* to Capt. Commander Jones for assignment. "Dr. Wilson reporting for duty, Sir."

"That's better. Have a seat."

"Thank you, Sir."

"You will report to Dr. Skelly on Dermatology Ward D1 immediately for duty assignment."

"Aye, Sir." With a sailor leading the way across the grounds, all the while I was thinking: *Dermatology! God, I know nothing about that dull skin stuff.*

"Here you are, Doctor. This way, Sir."

"God, why did I get into this?" (to myself)

"Dr. Wilson, I'm Dr. Skelly. Welcome aboard. I have just finished rounds and we will make out a duty roster for O.D. (Officer of the Day). Let's see, you will be on duty on Friday, January 5, from 0400 to 0600 January 6. The nurse will direct you to that duty station. I'll see you here at 0800 tomorrow."

"Thank you, Sir." We saw forty different cases of skin disorders the next three days. Half of them I had never seen before and probably would not recognize again when I saw them. To me they were all dermatitis, not diseases.

❖ ❖ ❖

I was OD January 5th, a Friday. For the first few hours all was quiet—then I got a call from the corpsman.

"Doctor, we have a real sick sailor on our hands. Can you come as soon as possible?"

I went immediately to the emergency room. He was right. *This was a very sick man.* "Seaman Cockrill, I'm Dr. Wilson." Very little response—a very low voice replied: "I'm real sick, Doctor. I have a terrible headache, and I'm throwing up."

"How long have you been sick?"

The corpsman answered, "About 10 hours, Sir. It started with a sore throat and a stuffy nose, then fever, headache, nausea, and vomiting for the past three or four hours." Temperature is now 103, pulse 120, BP 106/65.

He was very drowsy but responded appropriately. Examination revealed a fiery red throat that was edematous; ear canals and drums were normal; chest was clear and heart was normal. Neurological exam showed the patient to have a very stiff neck and exaggerated reflexes of his extremities.

With history and physical findings, I suspected meningitis. We obtained permission for a spinal tap. Other lab work was being done at this time, and I explained everything to him. As we began the procedure, he was very tense in spite of his drowsiness. I anesthetized the skin and inserted the spinal needle between the vertebral bodies, felt it enter the spinal canal, and slowly removed the stylet from the hollow needle. As I did so pus literally shot out of the needle into the test tube being held by the corpsman.

My heart sank! With spinal fluid being purulent and under such pressure, he probably had streptococcal or staphylococcal meningitis. In 1943, we had very few drugs to fight an acute fulminating infection of this magnitude. A specimen of the purulent spinal fluid was rushed to the lab for examination and culture. We soon had a report: staphylococcus! I called the Chief of Medicine with a complete report. The 18-year-old was admitted into the isolation ward where very intensive treatment was begun. We checked on him every two hours, but in spite of heroic efforts he died in less than 24 hours. I wondered then how it would feel as a parent to learn that a son had died under these circumstances, far away from home and family, in perfect health until two days before his death, then not to know of his illness until it was too late to be with him when the end came. We, the medical personnel, who were used to seeing patients die, were shocked at the suddenness and swiftness of this case.

❖ ❖ ❖

My stint at the Naval Station was very brief (19 days). On January 21, 1944, I received orders to transfer to Nashville for further duty. We had seven days for travel and to relocate. I did not have to report to headquarters until the sixth day. We proceeded to find an apartment in Nashville, thinking I would have duty in the city. Jessie was in her seventh month of her first pregnancy and had to find someone who would take her and deliver the baby. We were fortunate there. A sister-in-law was in the same state, and her attending physician agreed to care for my wife. On January 27, I reported to the Nashville headquarters office to find that I would be on duty at an Army post (Camp Forrest) near Tullahoma, Tennessee, some 65 miles away, and there was no housing on post for married officers. Of course, I had to stay on post except for times when the commanding officer would grant me a few hours leave. I requested as many overnight leaves as possible, and everything was fine. My wife had excellent care, the elderly couple where she lived treated her as a grandchild, and some of my family members helped out. I was busy at an Induction Station where we were examining 300 to 400 new recruits each day. The chief medical officer at the induction station was an Army major with an ego complex, plus being a "damn" Yankee.

Doctor From Bugtussle

I saw a few people from time to time that I had known prior to this duty, even examining one brother that came through. For some reason the chief medical officer didn't particularly like me, so he soon assigned me to the dirtiest part of the physical examination, that of checking for hernias, hemorrhoids, lesions, or problems with the genitalia and rectum. I have always wondered why the "asshole" gave me that "crappy" assignment. I had observed the procedure by my predecessor and continued his routine. I examined six men at a time. They stood in a semi-circle facing me. As would a tobacco auctioneer, I instructed each one to place his hands on his hips. Starting from left to right I would check each man for possible problems in the anatomical regions (groin) aforementioned. As I check the last man to my right, I was saying turn around, bend over, and hold your ankles.

As they did this they were checked one by one in the anal region, usually with the same glove. All the time I was doing the exams I could see the major out of the corner of my eye as he timed me for the procedure. I must say one had to become very proficient to do this 65 times a day. Soon he stopped timing me after the captain, my predecessor, told him I was faster than he had been. That didn't make the major like me any better. Soon after that things came to a head. The OB man called me to say we had a problem in that the baby was large and in a frank breech position. Since she was a primipara, he felt he should do a caesarian section because of the risk to the baby, and he would like for me to come, if at all possible. Instead of going to my senior Navy medical officer, I went directly to the "Chief" and asked permission. I explained the situation to him and asked for a 2-day leave on these grounds. He refused. We had words.

He threatened to have me court martialed. I retaliated by saying that the whole damn Army could go to hell, that I was going to see about my wife. My senior Navy medical officer appeared and interceded for me. I went to Nashville and reported to the Naval Commandant of the district, who gave me a dressing down that I have never forgotten, as I stood at attention for 10 minutes. Then he said, "At ease, Sailor." I was shocked as he then offered his hand, saying, "I've been wanting to do what you just did to that SOB for the past two years."

"Thank you, Sir. I'm sorry for what happened."

"How much leave do you think you will need, Doctor?"

"Four days, Sir."

"Granted, but don't ever take that chance again!"

I thanked him profusely, left the station, and went to Jessie's bedside.

Doctor From Bugtussle

❖ ❖ ❖

During the time I was on leave we sought consultation, had X-rays, and various measurements. Then, after this was done, the decision was to go ahead with the C-section. A definite day was set, and I was granted an emergency leave by the Navy Commandant in Nashville. The day arrived. Jessie was in the community hospital, and I was walking the floor as an expectant father should. I met with Dr. J. and the consultant that would be doing the actual surgery. The date was March 8, 1944, the time was 8 a.m. and the weather was cold and snowy. The hospital was a 1-story structure with porches connecting the wings.

As my wife left the room for the operating room, it was windy and cold with snow blowing. On the stretcher she was completely covered, but by the time she arrived at the OR, her blankets were covered with snow. This made me very anxious, and I'm sure Jessie was scared stiff. My sister-in-law, an RN, was with me. I had mixed emotion about the procedure, as well as the hospital and staff (later I found them to be capable and caring people). The surgery went smoothly, and the beautiful daughter was shown to me. As they were cleaning her and attempting to suction her, I noted a change in her color, and her breathing was obstructed. I rushed into the room. I hollered, "Give me that baby. You're going to let her die." I grabbed her feet, suspended her in the air, stuck a finger in her mouth to remove a large mucous plug, slapped her sharply on the buttocks, and she cried sharply and then strongly. her color changed to a beautiful pink, then red, and I knew she would be all right. I held her close (and tried to hold back the tears as I smiled, and then handed her back to the nurse). I apologized for "taking over" and went to report to the family that all was well. Mother and daughter did well and two days later I was back at my post with the "Major" standing watch over me. After about a month we were able to find housing in a nearby town, Winchester, Tennessee, and we were together as a family.

We had some feeding problems with our baby (Rachel), but finally this was solved, and we enjoyed our stay there, visited my family some, and made lasting good friends with many fine people. That duty lasted until mid-October when I received orders for change of duty. I was ordered to Newport, Rhode Island Naval Station to join the group that had been selected to form a ship's company for a new vessel that was to be put into service in early January 1945 at Baltimore, Maryland. There was to be a 10-day leave for travel time and family visits. Taking my orders, I reported to Nashville, thanked the commander and bade him good-bye. We packed our entire belongings in our Ford car (they consisted of a baby bed, a radio, baby clothes, other necessities, and our clothes). We drove to my parents' home 70 miles away for a 2-day visit, and then to Indiana to visit her family before I left for "foreign soil."

I had orders to obtain my own transportation. We went to nearby Terre Haute, got my tickets for travel to Chicago, from there to New York, and then to Newport. That was to be my maiden voyage on a train! I was to report for duty on November 1 at the Navy installation. At the ticket office in Terre Haute, we were assured that I could leave on the morning of October 30 and have plenty of time to make it to Newport long before the deadline. Jessie and I spent the night in the city, saying our good-byes, and I left for parts unknown the next morning. The hardest part of that was saying good-bye to our baby, not knowing whether I would ever see her again. The tears flowed freely, and as I cried, so did she and her mother. Leaving was a bitter pill to swallow.

❖   ❖   ❖

That first train ride was quite an experience. As we left the station a porter came through the car to see that everybody was comfortable. Then the conductor came by to check our tickets and help us relax. I guess he could see that I was a bit jittery, and he noticed the insignia of the Navy medical Corps on my uniform, and he engaged me in conversation.

"I have a son in the Navy also."

"Oh, is he at sea?" I inquired.

"I'm afraid so."

"Do you know what part of the world he's in?"

"Not for sure, but I think he's in the Pacific Fleet and headed for Japan."

"I hope not, Sir."

"Well, we can only hope he'll be ok."

He walked away, and I was left to my thoughts about what I was facing. The train rattled on as I watched the countryside fly by. Pretty soon we were in Chicago where I had to transfer to a train bound for New York. With a 2-hour layover time dragged, and I walked outside for a while. The place was depressing to me, but I saw enough of Chicago to know that I didn't like it. The train was delayed an hour. That didn't help any. I kept thinking about meeting the deadline to report in Newport. After endless hours, we arrived in New York. The conductor came back through to wish me luck. He called out the station, as they used to. I remembered the time the train was departing for the Navy base in Newport. It was scheduled to leave in 10 minutes! "god, I hope I make it." Almost on a dead run, I saw a conductor at the head of a stairway and slowed down long enough to ask where the train was to Newport. I was lucky once more.

"Right there at the foot of these stairs (he must have read the terror in my eyes), and you had better run like hell if you want to get aboard." I took off with my coattails flying, my orders and ticket in my hands, and just like in the movies, I jumped aboard as the train moved slowly out of the station. I saw the conductor and asked, "Sir, where is the car to Newport?"

"Next car to your left." Opening the door, I finally found one vacant seat. Sitting in that seat was a Navy enlisted man, a black fellow as scared as I was. Without hesitation, I took that seat. As it so happened, I was lucky again. He was headed for the same base as I, but he was already stationed there and knew how to get around the base. we were 10 to 15 minutes late, but they knew the train was late leaving so I had no problem except I was not billeted with the rest of my ship's company as I was told. It did not matter to me any way since I knew none of them. Although I was an officer, they directed me to eat at a mess hall with enlisted men, which was fine too. The day after arrival, I reported to the senior medical officer and was assigned to Psychiatry, Ward A. I was there for two weeks and then assigned to an internal medicine ward. I had some good experiences on the "Psychic" Ward. I had an unforgettable experience—it was a "once-in-a-lifetime case." A "pregnant" sailor (male). The Chief said, "Today we will present an unusual case—a 25-year-old male with the following history." He then proceeded to recite a history typical of a pregnancy of five month's duration.

"Any questions?"

"Sir, did you say this is a male patient you are referring to?"

"Yes."

Of course, we were all astounded. The patient came into the room, and he *did* have the physical appearance of a pregnant woman with an enlarged abdomen, shaped like a pregnancy. The breasts were bare, and they were enlarged; his feet and ankles were also swollen.

"Why is your abdomen swollen, John?"

"I'm going to have a baby, Sir."

"When?"

"In about four months."

"Is this your first child?"

"Yes, Sir."

"You're married?"

"Yes."

"Has your wife been married before?"

"No, Sir."

"How long have you been married?"

"Three years, Sir."

"Have you been on sea duty?"

"No."

"Have you been worried that you would?"

"Yes, Sir."

"I see—that's all, sailor."

"Thank you, gentlemen. This is a classic case of 'mind over matter.' This man feared that he would never have a child, and if he should be assigned to sea duty that he would be killed in action. This became an obsession with him, and since his wife could not conceive, he assumed the role of an expectant mother, even to the point that he took on the physical appearance of being pregnant." After seeing that, I could believe anything. I then knew for sure that this was not a branch of medicine I could be comfortable with. I never saw him again, but wondered about the outcome of his care. I suspect he had electro-shock treatment.

I survived the two months tour of duty there without any problems and on or about December 16, 1944, orders came to report to Baltimore, Maryland, Naval Headquarters, to be attached to the *USS Queens* for training for overseas duty and to commission the ship on a stated date. I was glad to leave the dismal place in Newport. The ship's company arrived in Baltimore on December 16, 1944, and boarded the *USS Queens* en masse. We were shown our quarters and got acquainted with our state roommates-to-be for the next several months. The next day we were assigned duties other than those of our regular ones. I was lucky. The Captain appointed me mess officer. That meant I would sit at the head of the table in the Officer's Mess Hall and be served first at each meal, according to Navy protocol. I certainly had to brush up on my etiquette after being put in that position. The next day I noticed a bit of nausea after breakfast, and by lunchtime it had gotten worse. I had a hard time choking my food down, as I was seasick, embarrassed, and took a lot of ribbing from my new friends because of that. It took two or three days to settle down to where I could eat.

After that we had to take "at-sea" training, which was a mockup of a ship that was anchored out in the bay a mile or so from shore. Going out in a small boat, we took our "gear" with us. When we boarded ship we put the "gear" on our backs and climbed a large rope net to get aboard. We also "went overboard" in the same way. Aboard, we were assigned to quarters and moved about on the "ship," going up and down "ladders" (stairways) through hatches, passageways, and to quarters as alarms were sounded. All of this was done with the ship's motion being simulated as if at sea. Of course, I got seasick along with most of the other "landlubbers." The Navy knew this would happen as they provided three times as many "heads" as were normal aboard a ship. We were "piped" to and from quarters, to different stations as if aboard ship—also when announcements would be made and at "chow time." All of this was done to get us used to life at sea before we actually did set sail.

"Now hear this, this ship's company will be prepared to go ashore at 0200."

This was good news, since it meant that would end the training cruise. Promptly, at the designated time, we were ordered to "go ashore." Going down that large rope net was twice as easy as climbing aboard, and three times as fast. Now we cold be considered true sailors.

On the trip back to the ship, I was jubilant as I realized my wife would be arriving the next day. Man, how I had missed her! It would be our honeymoon. All arrangements had been made as soon as our orders came in Newport. We were fortunate to find a room in a hotel near port since Baltimore rolled out the "Red Carpet" for our ship's crew. The day arrived and time dragged as the hour neared. By the time I made it to the train station, *she* was already waiting for me. I stood still as I saw her standing at the top of a stairway. What a beautiful woman she was with her beautiful auburn hair blowing in the breeze, a smile on her lips, and her eyes shining. My heart skipped a beat as I ran up the steps to hold her close. To me, she was the most beautiful woman in the world. We had our "honeymoon" with shipmates and their wives. We painted the town red. There was a ship party during that time, and Jessie was treated royally. "What a beautiful wife you have, Doc," they exulted. My chest swelled with pride every time. Time flew by and near Christmas the ship was christened. After the ceremony, lunch was served to the ship's company and special guests. The most special guest of all was my wife. Since I had the title of "Mess Officer" we sat at the head table in the officer's dining room (mess).

"Honey, look at this," I urged. We both were stunned at the site of the dining area. Everybody took their usual place in order of rank and with their guests, except us. We had to sit at the head table and be the first ones served to honor my position. They had brought out the silver, china, and crystal for the occasion.

Alongside the plates, there was an array of silverware that I had never seen. I glanced at Jessie and saw a scared little girl. At the same time, I was shaking inside. The black "mess boys" were in dress blues and wore white gloves. As we had a blessing by the chaplain and sat down, the waiters were by her side and seating her first of all the 50 to 60 officers and guests. We somehow did very well—two country bumpkins that had never been in this predicament before. I was so proud of her that it was hard to contain myself. What a sendoff that was for everybody, and for us in particular. Neither of us have ever forgotten that event. Those were 10 glorious days! But those days together came to an abrupt halt the night of December 25, 1944, as we had to stay aboard ship to ready for sailing the next day.

At 6 a.m. on December 26, the boatswain's pipe shrilled again, "Now, hear this. Be prepared to sail at 0700." This was "The Shakedown Cruise." We got underway promptly, setting sail for Norfolk. With a brand-new ship, we did not expect to have any mechanical problems. but we had been forewarned of probable rough seas as we had to pass Cape Hatteras. We were not disappointed! As we entered the area, the seas took on a different look; huge waves rolled in, striking the ship with all their mighty forces, striking first at the prow, then the port side, followed by a greater wave on the starboard side. As the waves struck, the ship rolled and pitched to the tune of the sea. As it did so, the prow would lift, then dip, as the fantail would rise to keep the ship on an even keel. It would roll with the awesome force of the 10- to 15-foot waves as it did everything, and all hands aboard would have to struggle to stay upright. As the angry sea continued its ships assault, the skies became more overcast. The wind velocity picked up, and visibility was zero. A fog rolled in, making everything worse. As time dragged by most of we "landlubbers" were seasick and miserable. The nausea seemed to start at my toes and then engulf my whole body. Each time the nausea started I rushed to the nearest head or to the side of the ship and emptied my stomach's contents. When the stomach was empty, the dry heaves started and continued until I was too weak to move. At that stage, I didn't care whether or not I moved again. That was one of the most miserable feelings I had ever experienced. Momentarily, I didn't care whether I lived or died.

"Now hear this—mess will be served at 0600 hours."

God! How could anyone think of food at a time like this? Then reality struck me. I had to go so those fellows that wanted to eat could begin because I was the "Mess Officer" and had to start the motion of eating.

Somehow, I made it to the mess hall, took some food on my plate, then it hit me again. I made it back to my bunk and stayed there until morning. During the night, I could hear the fog horns, like giant bullfrogs, as they blared their positions to other ships to avoid a collision, which meant we were in a dense fog. I slept, and as daylight came, the sea seemed to calm to welcome the new day. Like magic, that awful nausea was gone, and I was left weak and "hungover," with an awful taste in my mouth. I took a cool shower, and I could face the mess hall and my "friends" that started ribbing me about having "morning sickness." Routines of the day went on. I held sick call to treat sailors that had not fared so well. We all survived the "shakedown," and at sometime that afternoon we pulled into port in Norfolk, Virginia. All we "new" sailors could say that we had a full indoctrination into life at sea. From our "home port" (Norfolk), we had more sea experience (and seasickness) as we maneuvered about the Atlantic to get our sea legs.

After that we set sail for the Panama Canal. Two weeks later, January 24, 1945, we arrived at our destination. As we came into sight I couldn't believe what I saw. We were sailing uphill! I'm sure it was an optical illusion, but the horizon seemed to be upgrade from our anchor point.

"Look Jones, the locks are higher than we are."

"That's impossible, Doc."

I was right. As we got underway the next morning, the locks came into full view, and as we approached them and entered our slot, water rose to accommodate the ship. We barely had room to squeeze through, and it was an all-day affair. We were now on the Pacific Ocean. During this time all decks were filled to capacity as all sailors could leave their posts for short periods to see the ship slowly move through the docks into the Pacific Ocean.

The night after we had shore leave for five hours in the port city of Colon, Panama. What I saw and heard was unbelievable — whores walking the streets advertising their wares, quoting prices and procedures. There were houses of "assignation" throughout the city with heavy traffic through their doors. As the ship's doctor, my job was to inspect their quarters, check health department reports, and interview the "madam." An armed member of the Shore Patrol was on each side of me as we made rounds. Wherever we went all was in order, but we did not examine each girl that worked in the houses. As we left each place, sailors, soldiers, and marines would be waiting their "turn." Fully 90 percent of personnel ashore were intoxicated. Because of the state of sobriety, or lack of it, they were careless, fool-hardy, and ignorant of the consequences. A few of ship's company unfortunately paid a high price for a few hours of "freedom," getting V.D. (syphilis and gonorrhea).

We set sail for Pearl Harbor on January 26, 1945. It was gorgeous. the sea was smooth and calm, a perfect blue-green color that seemed to stretch on forever. Nights were usually beautiful with starlit skies, full moons, and soft breezes blowing over a phosphorescent sea as dolphins played in the moonlight.

Needless to say, homesickness was plentiful, and romantic letters filled the mail sacks as young boys and new husbands dreamed of home and loved ones. This peaceful voyage lasted for 13 days. During that time, we had further "at-sea" training, the most memorable of which was the "abandon-ship" drill. Fully clothed we had to jump from heights of 15 to 25 feet into a large, 20-foot deep pool; then as we would "go under" we would undress as we came to the surface, removing shoes, pants, and shirt. Then we had to swim to "shore."

I panicked! "Chief, I can't jump. I'll drown."

"No, you'll be ok, Doc. Just jump."

I shook my head, "No, I can't."

"Jump, Doc, damn you, or I'll throw you in."

It was a "mile" to the water—I said a prayer and jumped! To my surprise I did the procedure as we had been instructed to do, didn't drown, and got a pat on the back from the "Chief." After that I felt like an "old salt."

We arrived in Pearl Harbor on February 7, 1945, our second wedding anniversary. Nostalgia hit me when I thought of that, but soon left as we came into port and saw the awful devastation that still remained from the infamous Japanese attack. Parts of ships showed above water, docks were still only rubble. Areas were roped off and constantly patrolled. As we saw more of this, my anger rose to the point that it became hatred for all Japanese. For a long time after that the desire to kill (the Japs) stayed with me. I still mistrusted the race and am intolerant of their actions, but have many fine Japanese friends. After my experience, I doubt it will ever change.

We left there for further training in the area and 17 days later arrived in the port at beautiful Honolulu. What a sight this was; beautiful white beaches that were clean and peaceful. Palm trees lined the port areas, swaying in the breeze just as pictured. It looked like heaven to me. We remained there for nine days, getting to enjoy the relaxing atmosphere and tropical magic. We then set sail for the South Sea Islands, leaving Honolulu on March 2, 1945, and arriving March 10, 1945, at Eniwetok, one of the

Marshall Islands where we stayed until March 19, 1945. While there all was quiet. We were able to go ashore to an officer's club, which was mostly a bar, to keep in touch with people from other new ships, and to hear news from "home" as we relaxed and enjoyed our mixed drinks.

We got underway in the early morning of March 19, 1945, and six days later wound up offshore of Iwo Jima. during the voyage to Iwo, we had two or three alerts that never materialized but did make us accustomed to rushing to our battle stations faster and with more readiness. We discharged a contingent of marines onto Iwo Jima the day of arrival. The island was in "secured status" before arrival, and we felt "our Marines" would be safe. In the early morning hours of the fourth day, a radio message came for all medical personnel to stand-by to receive wounded from the island. At 4 a.m. small boats arrived with 36 wounded that varied from modest lacerations to serious, open chest wounds. As we treated the wounded, acting as a triage station, hospital ships were contacted, and the more seriously wounded were transferred to their care. All 36 survived, and all hands relaxed once again. the history of how the wounds occurred was sickening, and once again stirred my severe anger toward the Japanese. The victims were all attacked and bayonetted while they were sleeping, and after the guards were all killed by slashing their throats. That further strengthened my feeling of the treacherous nature of the Japanese.

After Iwo Jima, we touched Guam to take weary troops aboard for rest and recreation after duty on the islands for several months. Then we set sail for the U.S.A., stopping along the way to pick up more weary troops. Our home port was San Francisco, where we arrived on May 30, 1945, and stayed until June 13, 1945. Leaving there, we sailed to Everett and Seattle, Washington, for repairs and stayed for two weeks. Two memorable events happened while there: first, my beloved wife came to visit, and we were together for the last week of that stay. We had a wonderful visit.

The last night in port she visited aboard, and an incident occurred that was unforgettable and a bit scary. All was quiet when I was paged to report to sick bay on the double, which meant an emergency. A corpsman met me: "Hurry, Doctor, the man is about dead." He was right! A cyanotic sailor lay on the floor, unconscious, struggling to breathe. His pulse was weak, his heart sounds were faint and slow, and we had to act quickly. "Pump his chest, Smith." I gave him mouth-to-mouth resuscitation, the oxygen arrived, an airway was established, and the mask was applied.

"He's getting pink now, Doctor." Soon he was fighting, tearing the mask off, and had to be restrained. After he was stable, I heard the story. He had been ashore and had several drinks, disturbed the peace, was picked up by the shore Patrol, and taken to his ship where he landed in the brig. He then attempted to hang himself with the bunk chain and by the time he was discovered it was almost too late. I contacted the senior officer aboard and transferred the sailor ashore to a Navy hospital. All of this required about two hours and caused a lot of stress for that last night. There were repercussions the next day when the "Exec," still not entirely sober from his shore leave, jumped me at breakfast, threatening to "put me on report for doing my duty." I stood at attention: "Sir, I was only doing my duty as a doctor and would do the same thing again. Come on, let's go to the Captain right now." We were both out of line — he for questioning my medical judgment, and me for talking back to a superior officer. I was right, but a hothead, and didn't care at the moment.

Forty-eight hours later, we had orders to prepare for departure that night. At about 2 a.m., we got underway. A storm was brewing, and I couldn't sleep. An hour at sea, the boatswain's pipe sounded: "All hands secure your gear, batten the hatches, and clear the decks." I was already in the sick bay area with the duty corpsman when we got the first blast of wind, rain, and hail. The ship was tossed about like a bottle cork as it would pitch, then roll. As it creaked and groaned, the engines struggled, the fan-tail kicked upward, the screw came out of the water as the ship nosedived, and the entire ship shook like in the throes of a mighty chill. Then came the dreaded word "man overboard!" I felt a chill up my spine and into my body as a picture of a fellow man, struggling in that awful heaving, swirling mass of waves 10 to 20 feet high, flashed before me. The Sick Bay door opened and three people were there, all soaking wet and two of them bleeding.

"Mr. Bailey! Mr. Moss! Corpsman, bring the gurneys," I shouted. As I examined them I asked, "What happened out there?"

"We almost got washed overboard and were slammed against the bulkhead. I was knocked down by a huge wave and injured my leg."

"Were you unconscious?"

"No, I wasn't, but Moss bumped his head and has been groggy since then. Lucky that seaman came along just as it happened or we may have been washed overboard for sure."

"Let me take a look at your leg, Mr. Bailey. Uhhuh, that's not too bad, but we'll have to patch it up."

I then turned my attention to Moss. "How do you feel, Mr. Moss?"

He answered in a slow voice, "My head's killing me, but I'm all right." I checked him closely to find his vital signs were normal and his neurological exam negative. However, he did have a fairly large laceration of the scalp that was bleeding freely and needed suturing.

"Break out the suture tray, Corpsman, and I'll need #3-0 catgut and silk as well. Prep the scalp so we can close this wound and stop the bleeding."

"Aye, aye, Sir."

Within minutes the sutures were in place, the bleeding was controlled, and Mr. Moss was feeling much better. "How about a 'shot' of Brandy, Doc," Moss asked.

"Ok, I guess both of you deserve one, but we'll have to keep you here for a few hours to be on the safe side," I replied.

I made a full report to the senior medical officer, gave each a shot of brandy, and put both to bed for observation. When I sat down for a few minutes I realized that I wasn't seasick and hadn't been during the entire storm. Thank God I was never seasick again as we ran into rough seas during the last months of my Navy career.

After that episode we spent two weeks at sea, had two or three threats of air strikes, which always sent us scurrying to our battle stations when general quarters was sounded. None of them materialized, but each one scared the daylights out of us. When the alarm sounded the adrenalin began to flow, and the flight or fight syndrome went into effect as everybody acted on impulse, doing what he had been trained to do. Although nothing did happen, the GQ alarms served the purpose to keep us ever alert and mindful as to what *could* happen at any time.

We soon arrived at Eniwetok again where we spent two days "recuperating" from our sea experiences of three "near misses" by the Japs, then we moved on to Saipan for a 5-day stint. On the second day of that stay we had an interesting incident happen. After lunch four senior officers went ashore for R&R at the officer's club. One of these officers was our senior M.O., my "boss." Two or three hours later a radio message came for all medical personnel to stand by to receive an emergency from the officer's club. Somehow our chief petty officer and corpsman knew who the patient would be and had a wire-basket stretcher attached to a boom and lowered to the water's edge ready to accept the patient.

Within minutes from this finding, a horn sounded and the captain's gig appeared about 300 yards off the port side, running at top speed straight for the ship another 100 yards, and he slowed and came on in gradually, coming to a full stop alongside. Then the patient was transferred quickly to the wire-basket stretcher where guy-ropes had been attached and the unit was rapidly hoisted 40 feet up to the main deck and gently deposited there. In that "basket" was my senior medical officer who was quickly and expertly removed to a gurney and swiftly examined to ascertain his status. All vital signs were normal, his face was flushed and warm, an odor of alcohol came from each breath of air he expelled, and he snored deeply as he slept the sleep of the inebriated. I winked at the corpsmen that had been standing by, and they instantly knew what the situation was.

"Corpsman Sharp, will you take Dr. Bryan to his stateroom, have him undressed, and I'll be there shortly. Corpsman Swain, bring a liter of 5 percent dextrose to the stateroom and a Foley with bag attached, on the double! Ok, everybody, the Doctor is going to be fine. You can report back to your stations now, and thank you for standing by."

Corpsman Sharp and I stayed with Dr. Bryan, gave him the IV of dextrose, inserted a Foley catheter, checked his vital signs every half-hour, and waited. Within another three to four hours he began to arouse as the alcohol was being excreted from his system. He became combative and loud. In trying to get out of bed he bumped his head on the bulkhead (wall) and I felt we had to quiet him down. We gave him a light sedative intravenously, and he slept another three hours. By the time the sedative had worn off, when he awoke this time he was calmer, gradually became fully awake, and began to ask questions.

"What happened Dr. Wilson?"

"Oh, I think the two or three quick, deliciously cool, mixed drinks you had, along with the heat, overpowered you to the point of intoxication and you 'passed out!' The officers with you panicked and sent you back as an emergency. We had to handle you as such, gave you intravenous dextrose, inserted a Foley catheter, and flushed the alcohol from your system. When you first began to wake up, you hit your head on the bulkhead, and it will be sore. So you will have two sources for a big headache. You're ok now, so we can remove the catheter and finish the IV and let you get some rest."

Dr. Bryan stayed in his cabin another 24 hours. I visited him three times, and assured everybody that he would be fine. He thanked me profusely, treated me royally, and stayed sober the remainder of his time on shipboard.

From there we sailed to Oakland, California, stayed eight days, took on supplies, checked out the ship, and visited old friends ashore in "Frisco." We then picked up fresh troops and set sail once again for Pearl Harbor. We were there for two weeks as we had war maneuvers and learned all about the area. This was a great two weeks.

❖   ❖   ❖

September 1, 1945, we set sail again for Saipan, dropped off troops there and at Iwo Jima, then back to Sasebo, Japan, for four days where we participated in the surrender of that harbor to the U.S.A. This took place aboard our ship as the Captain was the senior Commanding Officer in the harbor. I have never seen hatred like that in the eyes of the Japanese naval officers when the ceremony took place.

From Sasebo harbor we sailed to the Philippines. We first went to the island of Luzon to Manila Harbor, then to Linguyan Gulf where we took aboard a hospital complement that had been on duty in that area for several months. We then began our return trip to Sasebo. Once again, my dislike for the Japanese increased three-fold as I saw the severely emaciated group. Some required IV fluids and supplementary vitamins before they could function again. Luckily we had the needed medications and all recovered.

During the return from the Philippines, a tragedy occurred aboard ship. A young officer took his own life because he was unable to tolerate pressures from superior officers. Because of our location and lack of embalming facilities, he was buried at sea. The ceremony was conducted at night with no prior notice of the time or location and in the presence of a few of us officers and six enlisted men. It was very depressing, something I have not wanted to remember but couldn't forget. The entire ship's company was saddened by the event.

❖ ❖ ❖

We returned to Sasebo Harbor on October 14th until the 27th. By this time Dr. Bryan had been rotated back to shore duty. I had been promoted and was the senior Medical Officer aboard., with private quarters and my own "cabin boy" at my beck and call, living the life of luxury. One evening my "luxury" was interrupted as the cabin boy knocked on the door.

"The Captain wishes to see you in his quarters, Sir."

"I'm on my way."

As I walked I was wondering what I had done to deserve this. As I arrived his cabin boy saluted sharply. I returned the salute and stated my mission.

"Aye, Sir. This way, Sir."

As we arrived the salutes were repeated. I knocked and stated, "Dr. Wilson reporting, Sir."

"Come in, Doc. At ease. Have a seat. How would you like to take a trip to Nagasaki?"

"I don't know, Sir. For what reason?" I vaguely recalled that was the city where the last atomic bomb had been dropped in late September.

"The Chief Engineer needs a piece of equipment for the ship's engine from there, and I want you, as Chief Medical Officer, to go with him."

I was astounded! "Thank you, Sir, but I won't be of much help."

Captain Mourning leaned forward and looked at me sharply. "I'm ordering you to go, Doctor!"

"Aye, aye. Sir!" I stood and held salute until he stood and returned it.

"Dismissed, *Doctor*!"

"Thank you, sir." I turned on my heel and left — a bit unhappy.

At 0700 the next morning, in mid-October, 1945, the Chief Engineer, his lieutenant, myself, and a seaman/driver loaded in a jeep and took off to Nagasaki, Japan, just as if we were going into downtown in Nashville, Tennessee. We had no idea of what to expect when we arrived at our destination. We soon found out as we arrived in "jig" time. What a shock! There was utter destruction and desolation! No sign of life any way we looked. We searched, wild-eyed and open-mouthed, with disbelief, as we looked at each other shaking our heads!

"Look, Commander, did you ever see such devastation?"

"No, never in my life have I seen anything like this."

The destruction was almost indescribable. Twisted steel was everywhere, in all shapes and sizes. Some reminded me of a wet dish rag that one would twist to dry, others looked as though it had been in a molten state. As we drove along we could see a huge crater in the center of the destruction. It looked as though a giant crane had been excavating for a 50-story building that would cover a square block. This crater dwarfed any excavated area we had ever imagined. From the center of this monstrous crater everything was utterly destroyed, or pushed uphill from its center as if one had stood dominoes on end and pushed them down and they all fell in the same direction in a gigantic circle around and away from the center of the crater. We saw scattered walls of buildings on the periphery of the crater which seemed to stretch almost to the horizon. The sun was shining through a haze that seemed to engulf the entire visible area. As we drove away from this area we could see no sign of life anywhere. We finally saw walls of a building with no roof, windows or doors. We drove toward it and decided it had been a school.

As we approached, we spotted someone near the building. It was a middle-aged Japanese man who smiled at us as we greeted him with "Good morning." To our surprise, he returned the greeting in perfect English, saying "Welcome to Americans." The Chief Engineer informed him of our purpose there, and he gave us directions to find the needed part. We thanked him and asked many questions.

"Can you tell us about the bomb dropping?"

"Yes, I can."

"Go ahead and describe it for us, please."

"It was just before noon, a bright, sunshiny day. We could hear the plane but could not see it. From the sound of the motor, I knew it was an American plane and felt we would be bombed, so I moved all the children to safe places in a building."

"What happened when the bomb fell?"

"All windows and doors fall out (gesturing in one direction), then roof blow away, but wall stay here."

"How many of the children were killed?"

"Two—not from bomb—they hit in head by something else."

"Did you go to school in America?"

"Yes, to college, so to teach English. I'm glad war is over."

"Are there many people around?"

"No, only a few."

"Were very many killed from the bomb?"

"YES! Many killed."

He didn't want to talk anymore about that. Then we wandered around in the area, ignorant of what the consequences might be by staying in the area because of what the central nuclear area could do to us. I, myself, picked up an egg-cup, a rice bowl, and a small vase as souvenirs—and still have two of them. Had I known then what we have learned since, I would have never agreed to obey the ship Captain's order to go into Nagasaki. I must have not have received much radiation, as we had three normal children afterwards. Now that I look back, I realize what fools we were to take that trip. But the "Chief" got his parts for the ship, and we left after our "shopping" was over, ignorant and oblivious of what we had done.

❖   ❖   ❖

On October 27, 1945, we set sail for Manila once more before returning home.

Prior to our first visit to Sasebo, Japan, we had received orders to join with the fleet designated to invade and take Japan by sea and air. The fleet was joining forces from several areas, and we had been fortunate enough to be in Hawaii at the time our orders came. After the second atomic bomb was dropped, the Japanese decided to call it quits, but the fleet still sailed as planned, and our wing went into Sasebo as originally planned. Boy! Am I glad they surrendered. When we entered the harbor area it was through

Doctor From Bugtussle

a narrow channel surrounded on both sides by sheer walls of granite, with gun emplacements pockmarking the walls. We would have been "sitting ducks" for them to pick off. The water ended gently into a sloping hill on which the city of Sasebo sat. Our stay there was peaceful except for the aforementioned events. We were happy to know that we would soon return home to join families and friends.

Following that, my Navy career was one of travel back and forth across the Pacific Ocean, putting into port in several cities and sometimes staying there weeks on end. In the latter part of 1945, I received my promotion (the senior medical officer was discharged from active duty). I was made Chief Medial Officer aboard, making all the medical decisions concerning ship's company and was leading "the life of Riley." This was not what I wanted, and I became restless with no medical challenges. I decided then that would not be the life for me.

After traversing the ocean for several months, I was called to the Captain's cabin and told to start taking inventory and to get rid of all surplus material that we possibly could. We went to work as we set course once more for home shores.

Time flew by. We inventoried, threw good stuff overboard, gave away what we could, and were ready for inspection and approval long before the deadline. My conscience bothered me because of the new and good usable materials and durable goods that disappeared, which are probably rusting away on the floor of the Pacific Ocean today.

On or about May 5, 1946, we docked in Norfolk, Virginia. After a visit to the Captain's cabin with two long socks full of bottles of "medical alcohol," the ship's Captain said, "Doc, you have done a good job. Your department is in excellent shape; it has been approved for closing. The ship is to be 'mothballed,' and I see no reason for you to hang around any longer. We will expedite your discharge tomorrow." That was music to my ears.

"Thank you, Sir. I appreciate your help. I have enjoyed my experience aboard, but will be glad to become a civilian again."

"Good-bye, Sir, and happy sailing."

I took off (almost at a run) and contacted the railroad, called my wife, packed my personal gear, and checked with the chief petty officer in transportation, who assured me that my foot lockers would be on the way in two days. Next, I visited the Naval headquarters office to receive my final discharge papers and was met with a pleasant surprise. The commander in charge of that office was a first cousin to my wife. He was a pleasant fellow, whom I had never met, and had everything ready in short order. At 4 p.m. that day I was aboard a train headed for Terre Haute,

Indiana. It was an all-night ride on a hard, wooden seat, but at that time I would have been glad to stand all the way just to be with my family. So ended my Navy career.

❖ ❖ ❖

On May 7, 1946, I was honorably discharged from the United States Navy at Norfolk, Virginia. I was now a civilian again—also unemployed. Now my immediate problem was to find my way to the depot and locate the train I was to board for an all-night ride to Indiana to my wife and child. At 4 p.m., we boarded and pulled out, heading west, northwest to our destination. All seats were bare wood, as were benches scattered through the train. There was no food service aboard, but there was a restroom. Most of the passengers were servicemen and, like me, were headed home after being discharged from the military. None of us cared whether or not we had plush seats. We just wanted to get home. After a 16-hour ride, we finally arrived at Terre Haute, weary and tired, but feeling like a million dollars.

As we got off the train there were at least 600 people waiting to meet us, but I had no trouble spotting my beloved, who was waiting with open arms. That thrilled me to my toes. We spent a blissful week there before we came back to earth again.

"Honey, do you realize that I am unemployed and we have no income?" I inquired.

"Yes, of course I do, but we can live on love a few more days."

"I'll have to do something fast. What do you think of my getting a residency?"

"Where are you thinking of going?"

"Back to Memphis, I guess."

"What will you be able to find?"

"Let's go back and see."

I made a few telephone calls to find if anything was available. They were not too encouraging, but St. Joseph's Hospital, where I had interned, promised to find a place for me on a rotating basis for a year, when a residency in OB-GYN was to become available. I took it! That did not start for another six weeks. We sat down to figure what to do, and I came up with an idea.

"Hey, Honey, why don't we go to my folks' place for the next five weeks, and I can practice with Dad."

"That's fine with me. I'd like to visit with your mother for a while anyway." The next day we settled things in Indiana and prepared to migrate to Tennessee. The following day we threw our belongings (a baby bed, a few pillows, our clothes, and a radio) in the car and headed South.

We surprised my folks by arriving unannounced at about 4 p.m., but they were glad to see us anyway. I had been home only once in over three years, and they thought this would be another short visit. The next morning we surprised them and asked if they could put up with us for a month or more. Then we explained our plight. I saw Dad's eyes light up as he said, "That'll be fine, Son."

Mama added, "We'll be glad to have you. We can all get acquainted again." We looked at each other and breathed a sigh of relief. I had a job, but no income and no expenses. We had a roof over our heads and free meals, and I was looking forward to getting back into general practice again.

The following day I began making house calls with Dad once again, only now I was a bonafide M.D. with a license to practice. It was a relaxing, informative, rewarding, and enjoyable five weeks. We again saw many interesting cases that I might never see again. We did minor surgery, delivered babies in the homes, treated major illnesses without benefits of hospitalization, consulted with each other with some differing on diagnosis and treatment of patients. Before the month was up, I had realized what a wonderful job Dad had been doing in his rural practice throughout the years. We had some interesting experiences in that short period of time. I was regarded as Dr. Wilson's "little boy" by some, at first, as they remembered me as a plowboy or a kid shooting marbles with their sons in the backyard. However, some people saw me in a different light and accepted me as a doctor. I still had to prove myself in all cases. Rural Tennessee folks did not readily accept change, especially with their doctor. Being a genuine rural Tennessee hillbilly myself, I understood their feelings and acted accordingly. Sometimes their attitudes caused problems. One case Jessie (my wife) and I had is a prime example.

About two weeks into the practice, two calls came within three minutes. Both were OB cases in active labor. One of the patients I had visited with Dad. I remembered her as being a primipara (first baby) with some medical problems and hoped Dad would take her. No such luck!

"Son, you know Mrs. Long and where she lives. You take care of her, and I'll deliver the other one."

"Ok, Dad, we'll do our best. Jessie, how about you being my nurse?"

Her eyes lit up. "Sure, let's go, but first we'll have to make up a sterile delivery tray."

Miss Dee said, "You don't need a delivery tray. You'll scare those people to death with all of that stuff." She didn't know my stubborn, red-headed, Irish wife. We made the pack!

"How do you plan to sterilize it, Jessie?"

"In the oven of course, just like they taught us in nursing school." In went the pack, perfectly prepared and neatly wrapped in a freshly laundered sheet.

Again, Mom spoke up. "Don't you foolish kids know it'll burn up?"

"No, it won't, Miss Dee." But she immediately saw smoke coming from the oven. I jerked the oven door open and put out the small blaze. "It's well sterilized now, Honey. Let's go deliver that baby."

Mom shook her head. "I told you it'd burn up. Go ahead. I'll take care of Rachel."

We were soon on our way through unpaved country roads, around sharp curves, up hills, through mud holes, and across small streams. Pretty soon Jessie looked at me and asked, "How do you know where you're going? There are no road signs anywhere."

"Oh, I've been here twice with Dad. Besides, we hillbillies drive by instinct in this environment."

A half-hour later we arrived at our destination—a small 3-room house with a front porch, sitting in a grove of trees on a hillside. As we got out the husband came to meet us. We introduced ourselves, and I explained the problem about Dad. "It's ok, Doc, I trust you. Come on in."

As we stepped onto the porch, I could see a room full of people As we went into the room, I saw the patient in bed and in no pain at the moment. She was an obese woman about 30 years of age at full term. Standing by her bedside was a woman of 50 years. She stood about five feet nine inches and weighed about 200 pounds. There was a scowl on her face. She spoke up. "I called for Dr. Wilson, not you." I introduced myself and Jessie, giving our credentials and explaining that Dad had another case he was delivering and asked me to deliver Mrs. Long.

"Well! I hope you know what you're doing."

"Thank you, Mrs. Snively. I'll do my best."

I looked around the room and noted five or six men sitting in straight chairs tilted back against the wall. I thought to myself, *I'd better take control of this situation before things get out of hand.* I also needed to gain their respect. "I would like for all of you folks to move outside while we take care of Mrs. Long." They slowly got up from their chairs and, with sullen faces and threatening looks, looked at me, took their chairs, and went outside. Right then I knew that we were on the "spot." If something should happen to the mother or baby they would not hesitate to do me bodily harm.

Turning our attention to the patient we took her blood pressure, which was 175/110. Pulse was 110. Her heart was strong and regular with no murmurs. We checked the fetal heart. It was strong at 120/minute.

"Let's examine her, Nurse, so we can see what station she's in."

Her mother said, "What's station, Doctor?"

I explained that it was how far the head had come down into the pelvic outlet and how much the cervix had dilated and thinned out. She seemed to be satisfied, but not very impressed.

"Let's give her something for the pain, Nurse, then you can 'prep' her."

Mama again asked, "What do you mean 'prep' her?" I again explained this procedure also.

"This time, Mama hit the ceiling. "What air you shavin her fer?"

Now it was my turn to speak out. "Mrs. Snivley, I came here to take care of your daughter and to deliver her baby, your grandchild, and I intend to do just that, whether you like it or not. If you really want to help, go out to the kitchen and boil two pans of water, which we will need pretty soon."

"Well, I never," and she stormed out. She came back in to say something, but her daughter spoke up: "You hush up, Mama, the Doctor knows what he's doing, and I like the way they're taking care of me." Mama hushed, but if looks could kill, both Jessie and I would have died instantly.

The patient progressed well. her pains came at 2- to 3-minute intervals. She dozed between pains, and pretty soon she had fully dilated, and it was soon time to deliver the baby. We placed the newspapers on the bedside, placed the sterile sheet over them, and had the patient across the bed, draped and ready. I had the Novocaine drawn up in the syringe with needle poised, ready to inject the perineum, when Mama came back in the room. "What air you doin that fer, Doc?"

"To numb her bottom so we can do an episiotomy to keep her from tearing open when the baby comes."

"Well I never seed that did afore."

I held my temper as Grandma watched and grumbled. When I did the episiotomy, I was sure she would "bust a gut," or attack me. She just gasped and whispered, "Good Lord, Doc, you have 'ruint' her. She will never be any good for Josh again." Soon the baby came, we suctioned his nose and mouth, wiped his face and head with a towel, then fully delivered him. He came out with a lusty cry as I held him up and spanked his feet.

"You have a healthy baby boy, Mrs. Long. Here, take a look at him." As she looked at him, she was laughing and crying at the same time. Grandma beamed, and all was well until she noticed the incision I had made to protect her daughter. She opened her mouth to speak, but words wouldn't come. She was too dumbfounded! I carefully closed the incision in three layers, using a subcuticular stitch on the last layer so there would be no suture ends to annoy her. Then I called Grandma in to show her everything was ok. I wanted to prove to her that her daughter was safe from her delivery. She made no comment, and I knew she was satisfied. We checked the baby, and he was perfect. We asked the patient to call if she had any problems, gave her a sedative, and promised to see her the next day. Just to aggravate her, I looked at Grandma and grinned. "Is everything all right now, Mrs. Snively?" I asked.

"Well, I guess you knowed what you wuz doin', but I'd still druther had yore Daddy."

I heard Jessie snicker as I was congratulating the new father. As we were driving away she said: "You didn't get the last word this time"—and laughed at me.

As we made calls, I observed how Dad cared for and handled each case when we went from home to home. Most all of the people were poor, many were illiterate, and disease went hand in glove with their living conditions. Telephones were few and far between, and some still had no electricity. For these reasons, they had developed an innovative way to let the doctor know he was needed. They would put a white rag on a long stick in the ground beside the road as a signal for him to stop. As we drove along, we watched for these signals. Driving along country roads at 40 m.p.h. there were a lot of rough stops with screeching tires and clouds of dust.

One day we made such a stop, and Dad was driving. It was so sudden he had to back up and was a bit irritated. In his rough voice he asked, "Who's sick here?"

"Senny is, Doc. She's rail puny. Been sick 'might nigh' a week now, and she's gittin' worse."

We went in to see Senny. She *was* a sick woman. She was lying in bed, dressed in three layers of clothing, wrapped in a quilt, and sweating profusely.

"What's wrong, Senny?" Between coughs, she answered: "I caint hardly breathe, Doc."

"Does your chest hurt?"

"Yes, sir, hit does when I take a big breath."

I took her temperature, 102 degrees. Pulse was 120. Respiration 28 (normal is 18). Dad listened to her chest, through her clothes, and then asked me to examine her chest. I tried to get the stethoscope on her skin, but it was impossible with all her clothing. I made a pretense of listening and in doing so, got too close, and the body odor was so strong I had to hold my breath. When we finished, Dad said, "You have a bad case of pneumonia, Senny." You need penicillin, but I can't get any for a few days, so we'll give you sulfa drugs, cough syrup, and aspirin. Take these sulfa pills one every four hours with a full glass of water and watch your kidneys. I'll be back in a couple of days to check on you."

As we were getting into the car, I couldn't wait any longer to ask Dad, "How did you know that Senny had pneumonia? I couldn't hear anything through all of those clothes she had on. Besides, she smelled so bad I had to hold my breath."

"You'll just have to get used to the odors, learn to listen through clothing, and learn to *listen to the patient's history.* I have seen so many cases of pneumonia through the years that I can diagnose some of them by their appearance and body odors."

I took that with a grain of salt, but remembered his words during my 40+ years of practice. My reply at that time was, "I bet you had to hold your breath too." He just laughed and never bothered to reply. Two days later we saw Senny again, and her condition was much better. Her temperature was down, she was no longer sweating, and she could breathe without pain. I thought, *this is almost a miracle.*

One other unusual case we saw before we had to leave for Memphis was a pregnant 43-year-old woman Dad was taking care of. Everything was normal until about the fifth month of pregnancy when she had vaginal bleeding for two days. On bed rest for a week all seemed to be normal again. However, the baby did not move, the mother-to-be had no further noticeable abdominal enlargement, and her breasts did not enlarge as with a normal pregnancy. Dad related the history to me one day and before we left, I recalled the patient and suggested we see her again before I had to leave.

Dad called to ask how she was and added that his doctor son was in and we wanted to come by so we both could examine her. With her consent, we did go to the home. As we arrived, the husband came out and introductions were made all around. Afterward, I talked to Mrs. Pardee to get a more detailed history. Then we got a consent from both she and her husband to do a pelvic examination, which was done while both Dad and I were present. After the exams, we went back to the car for a consultation, compared notes on both history and physical findings. Our findings on pelvic examination were identical. The uterus was enlarged to the size of a 5-month pregnancy. It was smooth and symmetrical but *very hard*, much more so than a normal pregnancy. To me it was typical of a missed abortion with a calcified fetus still undelivered.

"Well, what is your diagnosis, Son?"

"I think she has a missed abortion with a calcified fetus. I have never seen one *in situ*, only a specimen in a jar, but the history is like reading the textbook. What do you think?"

"I agree. Now what do I do?"

"Well, Dad, I would watch her, and maybe she'll go into spontaneous labor and deliver the fetus intact. If she does, everything should be ok. If she doesn't, she may get an infection, and there will be the devil to pay. Just pray she does go into labor. In the meantime, I would give her some penicillin as a precautionary measure."

"I have thought of all those things. Now, let's tell them what the problem is, then tell them what they can do and expect. Nothing happened before we left, but I called about two weeks later, and when I talked to Dad the first patient he mentioned was Mrs. Pardee.

"You remember the woman we saw with the possible calcified fetus?"

"Yes, I do. What has happened?"

"Well, about a week ago she went into labor and within four hours she delivered. And guess what it was?—a calcified fetus. Weren't we smart—or just lucky?"

"Did you preserve the specimen?"

"No, they refused. They wanted to bury it in the family plot. I guess that was best for everybody concerned."

"I understand, but it's so rare that I just thought it would be good for teaching purposes. Is everything ok with you now, Dad?"

"Everything is going along fine. I kind of miss you making calls with me, though."

"I miss it, too, but I feel like this was the wise thing for me to do."

"*Oh, yes*, staying here would be the last thing I would advise. Hope everything is going well with you, Jessie, and the baby."

"Yes, we're fine. Just wanted to let you know our address and phone number, and to find out how you and Mom are doing. Take care of yourselves, and we'll be in touch."

That six weeks had flown by so fast it seemed like only six days, but we had to move on. Deep inside I knew that I was sorely needed by the people in this backward, down-trodden, uneducated, and diseased rural community—much more than I would be in a city. I also knew that I had to have further training before I had the knowledge and maturity to start a private practice anywhere. I also felt it would not be fair to patients under my care if I didn't further my education at this time. At the same time, I realized it would not be fair to my wife and family if I chose to practice in this rural area where there were few opportunities for proper education and social life. We packed our meager belongings and headed back to Memphis, where we had met and married and where we would remain for the next five years.

Residency

We returned to Memphis in late June of 1946, found a place to stay—a bedroom, kitchen, and bath—in a private home. We felt fortunate to find anything at that time. It was five miles from the hospital, but we took it. Jessie was treated like a daughter; the landlady fell in love with our baby, and we were happy.

I began my residency one week later, and we soon found that we needed more room, if possible, and could find any. Soon after going back to the hospital I saw one of the staff members and told him of our needs: we were in luck! He had a duplex near the hospital, and one of the furnished apartments would be available in a month. I asked him the cost, and he said, "It is usually $150 a month, but I'll let you have it for $90 if you will help my mother who lives in the other apartment." I jumped at the chance. It was within two blocks of the hospital. I could walk to work. It was by a city bus stop, an ideal location for us. We moved at the end of a month and spent the next year there.

I had agreed to a rotating type of residency while waiting for an OB or surgery position to become available. My first rotation was on Internal Medicine, which was interesting and allowed me to have more time with my wife and child. I was on duty 24 hours and off 24 hours, which meant I had to be at the hospital half of the time or more. The pediatric resident and I roomed together and became good friends. Again, I was lucky. My second service was in Peds and with him being the senior resident. I was given preferential treatment. He was a good teacher, and I enjoyed the service. One case was of particular interest to both of us. A 14-month-old baby was admitted with pneumonia and malnutrition. We had a difficult time with the mother understanding the gravity of the illness or in cooperating with us. We concluded she was psychotic and proceeded to talk to the staff physician about her problem. "Dr. Bluestein, the mother is not capable of caring for this baby, and she might do it bodily harm."

"I don't have time to do anything about that. The baby is well enough to be sent home, so we will dismiss it in a day or so." His word was law and the baby was dismissed.

Doctor From Bugtussle

My third rotating service was the emergency room again. I was back home; this was the area where it was more like private practice because of the variety and number of cases we saw each day. That service lasted six weeks. As we saw patients, there were some that I have always remembered.

❖   ❖   ❖

My first week on duty at about 11 a.m., a familiar face came in the door holding his right hand that was wrapped in a bloody towel.

"I asked, "Dr. Pharr, what as happened to your hand?"

"I'm ashamed to tell you. I was in my shop with my bench saw and got careless."

"Let's take a look, Doctor." I took the towel off very gingerly. The blood was pumping from two fingers. He had amputated the distal parts of his right, middle and index fingers! "You have really played hops, Dr. Pharr." During my internship I had assisted him in surgery many times, and I remembered he was right-handed. I also recalled that he had lost the tip of the left index finger previously in a similar accident.

"Guess I won't be operating for a while now, Dr. Wilson. Well, I'm old enough to let you young fellows have it anyway." We, of course, called his surgeon and sent him to surgery immediately.

❖   ❖   ❖

A second dramatic case I recall vividly. A 45-year-old executive came to the emergency room about 4 p.m. with chest pain, shortness of breath, and profuse sweating.

"When did you pain start, Mr. Josephs?"

"About an hour ago. I need something for this pain."

"Where is the pain?"

"Right here," putting his fist in his sternum. "I had some in my neck and left wrist also."

His color was ashy, he was a bit short of breath,a nd he was sweaty. Examination revealed pulse of 110, blood pressure of 172/110, and his heart sounds were distant with a faint murmur. There were rales in both lung bases. *This man is in the throes of an acute myocardial infarction*!

"Nurse, give this man Morphine, 1/4 grain, oxygen by mask, and Seconal 25 mgs. STAT. Who is your doctor, Mr. Josephs?"

Doctor From Bugtussle

"Dr. Black, said Josephs.

I called his doctor, gave him the findings, and was told to admit him to the heart ward (we did not have coronary care units in those days), and he would see him as soon as possible. After the medications and oxygen, he was relieved of the severe pain and was sitting in a wheelchair.

"Can I have a cigarette, Doctor?"

"No, sir. It might be the end for you."

The resident M.D. came by at that moment, smoking a cigarette.

The patient asked me a second time to give him just one or two draws. "Absolutely *not*! It might be your last one."

The resident spoke up. "Aw, give him a cigarette; it'll be all right."

"You'll be responsible if anything happens. I won't." The resident gave the patient a lighted cigarette, the man took two or three "drags," and almost immediately he stared, went limp, grunted, convulsed, stopped breathing, became cyanotic, and was dead!

I was furious. "I hope to hell you're happy now. Dr. Swann. You can also call Dr. Black and tell him what happened to his patient." The resident was almost in shock as he realized what he had done. He went pale, his mouth fell open, and he left. The patient's family had not yet arrived at the hospital, and I was left to tell them we had lost him with a myocardial infarction. That was a tough assignment.

❖   ❖   ❖

The third dramatic case shook me to my toes. It was about 8:30 a.m., my last week on the emergency room service. An ambulance came in without the siren and lights on.

"We have a good one for you this time, Doctor."

"What is it?"

"Take a look. You won't believe it if I tell you."

He opened the rear door. I saw three "bundles" covered with two sheets. I drew the sheet back and was shocked and horrified at what I saw. It was the most gruesome sight I had ever seen. Three children, ages eighteen months, 7, and 10 years old, had been brutally slain by blows to the head that crushed their skulls. They had multiple stab wounds to the chest, neck, and abdomen, and large open wounds to the bodies. I recognized the baby. It was the same child that we treated for pneumonia, whose mother was psychotic. "Who did this?"

"The mother."

"How do you know it was the mother?"

"The father came home from work to find this and a bloody ax standing in the corner of a blood-spattered room. His wife was gone. By the time we were ready to leave, the police radioed in to say that they had found the mother wandering along the street. She was bloody from head to toe and babbling incoherently."

How could anyone ever forget such a sight? The incident left the entire emergency room staff in shock.

Next came OB service. It was great. I was back among old friends who had confidence in me and allowed me to do many deliveries of their private patients, and also to do the follow-up while in the hospital. That experience was invaluable to me as I went into private practice later. The staff members in practice were overworked and when a patient came in at night they would ask me to evaluate them and call them when needed. I was awake all night, 90 percent of the time, as I cared for the patients, wrote histories and performed physicals, saw obstetric patients in the emergency room, and made follow-up visits on the floor. I had far more than average experience as a resident would have in a private hospital.

This was immediately post-World War II, and the baby boom was just starting. In those days, patients were treated far differently than are present-day obstetric patients. They were usually given small doses of analgesics, along with a hypnotic, to relieve the severe labor pains in the later stages. The hypnotic drug most used was Scopolamine, which some patients reacted to adversely. They would become wild instead of getting drowsy. They would be unmanageable, sometimes getting out of bed, screaming for the family members (usually their mothers), and then fall asleep. The drug was also an amnesic, and they would not be able to recall their reactions. The drug fell into disrepute and is no longer used in that manner. In my estimation that was an intelligent decision.

❖   ❖   ❖

After I had been on the service about two weeks, I received a call to report to the Administrator's office. I was puzzled about the call and reported quickly. The visit turned out to be a pleasant surprise. The secretary greeted me in a friendly manner, not brusque as usual. "Come in, Doctor, how are you this morning?"

"Fine, thank you (in a questionable way). Sister Margaret called for me to come down."

"Sister will see you now, Doctor—right this way."

I was still puzzled at the attention I was getting.

"Good morning, Doctor, come in."

"Good morning, Sister, and how are you?"

"Have a seat, Doctor."

I sat down, expecting to get the "ax." Instead she said, "A position as Chief Resident in OB will be available on July 1, and you have been recommended for the position." I was totally unprepared for that. Sister picked up on my reaction and helped by saying, "You don't have to make a decision this moment, but think it over and let me know within a month."

"Thank you, Sister. I'll have to think it over. I do feel honored to have been recommended by the committee to fill that position. Thank you again, Sister. I'll make a decision soon and discuss it with you." I offered my hand and bade her good-bye, as if I were headed for outer space, and almost was.

There were several problems facing me now. Did I want to do just OB for the next 40 years? Could I ask my wife to keep sacrificing her life while I took another three years of training at $100 a month, and incur a big debt she would also be responsible for? Would I prefer to go into practice as a General Practitioner and find a residency in a specialty of choice later? I had about decided to do the latter when several things happened.

We ran out of money! I was being paid $100 per month salary. The rent was $90 a month, and $10 a month was just not enough to buy milk for a baby. The Navy had not sent the mustering-out pay I was to get. They had not started the $100 a month for further training as promised, so that left us in a bind. By this time, we were down to $11 in cash, and payday was a week away. Something had to be done. A few days later we found out that another baby was "on the way," and there had to be clothing for our child. I had no choice but to sell the car. We sold it in two days. That $1,400 was enough to keep the wolf from the door for about three months. About a week later we had a windfall. We received a check from the Navy for four months' training, another for travel pay, and a third one for mustering-out pay. That same day we received a box of food and two live chickens from Jessie's mother (by parcel post). You never saw two such happy people. Some tears of joy were shed. "Honey, let's celebrate!" We killed and dressed the chickens, and while Jessie was cooking, I called my buddy, Joe, who was still in Memphis, to come to dinner. I walked three blocks to the liquor store, bought two bottles of champagne, and we really lived it up that night. The next day I told my landlord, a General Practitioner with an office nearby, what had happened. That night he stopped by the house with a proposal that was one I had been praying for.

"Dr. Wilson, how would you like to work in my office on my day off each week?"

"That would be great, Dr. Sam, but I'll have to discuss it with the hospital and Chief Resident."

"I'm sure it will be ok because I have already talked to Dr. Seagraves and Sister Margaret."

"Thanks Dr. Sam, I do appreciate your offer, and I will talk to Sister and Dr. Seagraves tomorrow."

That was the first thing I did the next morning. What a pleasant surprise I got! They had already worked out a schedule for me to be off the same day each week so I could be in Dr. Sam's office. That Thursday, I was in the office, saw 10 or 12 patients, and kept that up until I finished my training. After I had been in that office for several days, another General Practitioner approached me to "fill in" for him on occasions when he was out. I was paid $25 for each day I worked (that was big dollars then). These two offices helped us meet our obligations, kept us from worrying or borrowing money, and at the same time, I learned how to conduct an office practice. I was one of the first "moonlighters" in Memphis.

After that, I made my decision to forego the obstetric residency and look for a place to practice in Memphis. By this time I was on the surgical service and liked every minute of it. The chief of surgery was asking for me to assist on a lot of his cases. That, of course, bolstered my ego, and I worked harder because I wanted to improve my surgical ability. I dreaded to see that service end, but it didn't! Dr. Grobmyer asked to see me one day. As I went in I was asked to "have a seat."

"Thank you, Dr. Grobmyer. Is something wrong?"

"No. I just want to know if you would like to stay on my service another month."

My heart came up into my mouth. As it raced, I tried to be calm. "That would be quite an honor. Doctor! Thank you.

"You have worked hard, improved your surgical skills, and are very dependable. I think you have a lot of potential in the surgical field."

"Thank you again, Doctor. I hope I can prove your confidence in me." The next month was hard work, long hours at the operating table, loss of sleep as I had to keep up my routine duties of history and physicals, doing follow-ups on the patients on the service, and finding a little time to spend with my wife and child, plus doing office work that my friends who were generous enough to allow me to do. While on that service, I learned more than just surgical techniques. I learned much about the various people that did surgery. The real person came out when under stress in the operating room. Some would lose the ability to continue on, some would take their frustrations out on the scrub nurse, some would rave at the MDs assistant, and some would hit the assistant on the hand with hemostats or retractors when under pressure. Nothing made me so mad as the fellows who did that. I considered them second-class people. It happened to me only one time. The attacker was not much older than I and I let him know immediately, in no uncertain terms, that I would not stand for that treatment. Using some of the language I had acquired in the Navy I let him have it with both barrels, telling him what would happen if he tried that again.

❖ ❖ ❖

While on surgical service we had to take shifts in the emergency room where a lot of action occurred. As I took my turn one day, I had another gruesome case come in. This happened near noontime. An elderly lady had been attacked by a pack of dogs as she walked to her mailbox, which was 100 yards from her house. Not long after the attack, a passerby heard weak cries, saw a commotion, and investigated. He was horrified at what he found. Several dogs were eating away on the woman's arms and legs while she was struggling and crying weakly for help. "I had a hard time getting them off her. They almost attacked me too," said her rescuer.

"How many dogs were there?" I asked.

"I would say six or eight," he replied.

He flagged down a motorist to call an ambulance. By the time she arrived in the emergency room she was in deep shock from trauma and blood loss. I examined her and was shocked at how she was still living. Both arms and legs had been eaten and gnawed from the hands to well-above the elbows and from the toes to above the knees. Muscle had been utterly destroyed in most places. The tendons were left intact for the greater part of both. There were some bites to her body that were minor. She had no blood pressure, the pulse was thready, her skin was cold with a grayish tint, and she was unresponsive. She was transfused as fast as possible, and I.V. fluids were given.

I called the Chief of Surgery to inform him of our problem. "Get her to surgery immediately, and we'll get some more surgeons to help us, and maybe we can save her," he advised. We did as he instructed, and for the next four hours four teams of surgeons and six or eight nurses worked rapidly to repair tendons, lacerated muscle, torn skin, and injured nerves. Thank God she had enough blood supply left so the tissues would be viable.

By the time the teams finished the patient was beginning to react. She had a blood pressure of 100/60, and was breathing on her own. With the copious amount of dressings on her extremities, she looked like someone from a horror movie. With all of the surgeons doing their part in salvaging her, you know that she was well cared for. She lived and did remarkably well with very little loss of function from her injuries.

This was near the end of my time on surgical service, and I don't recall any shocking events taking place during that time. The long hours, missing meals, not having time to shave, losing sleep, and not having time with my family continued on. These were the worst things about being on that service. It was the exciting, dramatic, and sometimes tragic part of practice. It was the specialty that could make you a hero one minute and a criminal the next. I reveled in that service.

❖ ❖ ❖

My next service was on urology which was very interesting, but not as dramatic as was general surgery. I learned the technique of examining prostate glands and how to differentiate between a malignant and a benign, diseased prostate. This early teaching was extremely valuable to me later on. I also learned that there are more people born with congenital deformities of the gento-urinary tract than any other system of the body. Many people live for most of their lives before they would find that they had only one kidney or had four instead of two. There were many with deformities, such as a horseshoe-shaped kidney or a double ureter (the tube from the kidney to the bladder), two instead of one. A small percentage of girl babies are born with an extra ureter that opened into the vagina instead of in the bladder. In the days I was in training, the latter problem was not discovered in early childhood as it is today. Male infants are born with some of the kidney deformities, as are females. They are often born with undescended testicles or hypospadias, neither of which are discovered until they are older. I was also surprised at the percentage of tumors of the kidney in both adults and children. Malignant tumors of these systems are not uncommon either. That month was well spent and enlightening.

❖ ❖ ❖

Neurology and neurosurgery service were only fairly active, and I was not too busy during that time. We had some interesting cases such as brain tumors, subdural hematomas, and skull fractures that required surgery to remove a blood clot from between the brain and its covering, the dura mater, which is the thick covering around the brain itself. Sometimes the fracture would cause pressure, and it would only need to be lifted off the brain to relieve the pressure symptoms. I was fortunate enough to assist in some of these cases and was amazed at the changes wrought by appropriate surgery. Some cases of brain tumors were inoperable, and most were soon fatal since we did not have the tools to treat them at that time. Again, I was fortunate because of previous association with some of the Neurosurgeons and felt more at ease in asking questions and assisting. It was an interesting month.

❖   ❖   ❖

Orthopedics was one specialty in which I could not drum up much interest. I spent my time and did my job, but was never enthusiastic. I saw the fractures and deformities, helped to treat them, to reduce simple fracture, how to properly apply a plaster cast and what to watch for afterward, plus all the many things required to pass the test. I did not enjoy assisting in surgery when the fractured hips had to be reduced and "pinned" into the normal anatomical position again. The time dragged on, and the month felt like three to me. I was relieved when it was over.

❖   ❖   ❖

My last month of residency were spent on gynecology and emergency room. I was happy in those areas and enjoyed them to the fullest. I was also relaxed and looking forward to finishing because I knew what I would be doing. This fact I will relate first. A few days before I was to start on GYN I talked with Dr. Grobmyer about whether or not he might need a third man in his office since his new associate was unhappy and was planning to move. "Dr. Grobmyer, I would like to have the opportunity to be associated with you and Dr. Pearce. I could assist you in all your cases, do my own with your help when needed, do office work, and make home calls when necessary."

"That sounds good, Dr. Wilson. I'll talk to my partner and get back with you in a day or two." The next morning while making rounds, I was paged. It was a phone call from Dr. Pearce. He was never one to mince words. "Wilson, can we get together for a few minutes?" he inquired.

"Yes, Sir. When and where?"

"In 15 minutes in the third floor waiting room. I'm here now, and it's empty."

"Thank you Dr. Pearce, I'll be there." We met at exactly the appointed minute, and I could tell he was pleased.

"Boy, you are prompt. Are you always this way?"

"I try to be, Dr. Pearce."

"Dr. Grobmyer tells me that you're ready to start a practice."

"That's right. If I can find somewhere to work."

"How would you like to join us? We have plenty of space and could use a third man for our overflow patients."

"That would be great, Dr. Pearce, but I still have some time before finishing my residency."

"How soon could you start after you finish your training?"

"Within a week."

"Then let's say you'll have an office and that you can start about July. We'll work out the details before you start."

"Thank you, Dr. Pearce. I consider it an honor and privilege to be associated with the both of you. I promise to work hard and hope I can be an asset to the practice." I couldn't wait to tell Jessie and phoned her immediately. She was overjoyed that we were staying in Memphis and more so that two men of such high caliber would ask me to join them.

The remaining time flew by, and nothing earth-shaking happened. A week before my residency was to end, Sister Margaret called me to her office.

"Dr. Wilson, you have worked hard and also have done a good job while in training. You are also very fortunate to soon be associated with Drs. Pearce and Grobmyer. They are two of the finest members of our staff. They are most capable in their respective fields and highly respected by the entire staff."

"Thank you, Sister. I feel honored by your trust in me and the work I have done while a member of the house staff. I hope that my work as an active member of the hospital staff will be satisfactory."

"I'm sure it will, Doctor. Now I have some good news for you. Since you have applied yourself and have done so well in your training, we want to reward you in some way. Since time is short, we felt that the best reward would be some free time to get ready to start private practice. So we want you to have the next two weeks for doing so."

"That's the most wonderful way you could have possibly rewarded me. Thank you, Sister."

"There is one more thing, Doctor."

"Yes, Sister?"

"Here," and she handed me an envelope which I opened immediately. I was flabbergasted. There was a check totaling one month's pay, not just for the remaining two weeks. Tears came to my eyes, and I could barely thank her as I fought back the tears.

She smiled, "That's for the new one to soon enter your lives."

"Thanks, Sister. God bless you." I left, but the tears didn't as they ran down my cheeks.

❖ ❖ ❖

The next two weeks were so hectic that time went by like flashes of light. We first of all had to borrow money to buy a house and furniture since we had neither. We made a flying trip to my parents and arranged a loan from the local bank. With the help of Dad and a brother, we had found a car so we could get around. We found a house, and before I started practice, that was settled. We had to buy furniture to have a place to sleep. How we accomplished all of that in such a short period, I'll never know, but we did! On top of all that, we were expecting our second child later in the month. I guess we felt so lucky that we had such a good possibility for the future, all else was secondary to getting that and just a means to the end.

When we finally settled into our new home and had time to think things over, we came back to reality. We had signed a promissory note for $10,000 and that was a lot of money in 1947. We had obligated ourselves for another $2,000 also. Jessie looked at me in disbelief and asked, "What have we done?"

"I know, honey, but we'll make it one way or the other. I'll just have to work day and night, if necessary." Little did I know that I was a prophet! My words soon came back to haunt me.

Private Practice

July 3, 1947.

"Good morning. I'm Dr. Wilson. Dr. Pearce asked me to come in."

"Good morning, Doctor. We've been expecting you. I'm Mrs. Dunigan and this is Mrs. Pate. We've heard good things about you. We're happy to see you and look forward to your being a part of the office family. Dr. Pearce will see you now."

"Good morning, Dr. Wilson. Come in and have a seat."

"Good morning, Dr. Pearce. How are you?"

"I'm as busy as a one-armed paperhanger with the itch—I'll be glad when you're here to stay."

"I'm looking forward to that day too."

Then Dr. Pearce was all business. "We've talked about everything except salary. Dr. Grobmyer and I feel that we can start you at $350 a month, plus 50 percent of what you book as new patients." That was not as much salary as I had expected, but the incentive was there for me to be aggressive if I hoped to make enough for my family to live on. I hesitated a moment before answering. "That will be agreeable to start. Will I be eligible for a raise at the end of this month?"

"That depends on how well you do and your attitude about work," Dr. Pearce replied.

"You know that I'm willing to work, Dr. Pearce."

"Prove it—then we'll talk about it. Come back on the 5th, and we'll put you to work. There is one other thing we'll need to discuss, and that's hospital rounds. We will want you to make them at each hospital."

Man, they were really testing me. I'll show them that I can do anything they ask. "Ok, I can do that too."

"Very well. We'll see you in two days."

As I left it dawned on me that what I had agreed to do would mean working about 18 hours a day. That was just about what I had been doing for many months anyway. When I got home and told Jessie about the agreement, she thought it was too much to expect of any one man. But when we realized our financial obligations, she agreed that we had little choice but to roll up our sleeves and go to work—and that *we* did. What a wonderful helpmate she would be!

Thursday, July 5, 1947, was my first day in private practice. Office hours were scheduled to start at 1 p.m. Before going to the office, we (Dr. Grobmyer and myself) had done two major surgical procedures and made rounds on all his patients. I had no lunch, but was not hungry; just tense from anticipation of what I was to be doing at the office. I had a pleasant surprise! When I arrived, the nurse told me that I had five patients waiting to see me. "Really. You're kidding me, aren't you?"

"No, I'm serious. I'll show you." She got the list. The very first one was the man I had treated from the train wreck that first Sunday of my internship. What a friend he was! He looked like a million dollars to me. I gave him a big hug, had a visit with him, and checked his blood pressure, looked at his prosthesis, and told him he was as sound as a dollar (in those days), and to come back whenever needed. I saw a total of ten patients that first day and thought I was flying high. At the end of the day Mrs. Pate handed the hospital patient list to me. I saw about thirty patients in three different hospital I was to visit that night. She looked at me and asked: "You think you can handle all that?"

"Sure, no problem." I really thought, *How can I do all this*? That was just the beginning of a continuous daily, *and nightly*, routine. As time passed, my practice grew beyond my wildest dreams. I had registered with the "doctors'-call service." They found that I would accept night calls and pretty soon I was swamped with house calls, sometimes making 10 or 12 in a 24-hour period. My work day usually started at 5 to 6 a.m. and ended about 11 p.m.—but I built a practice.

❖   ❖   ❖

At the end of the first month, my take-home pay was $1,000 ($350 of that was salary; the rest was 50 percent of what I had put on the books from new patients brought to the practice). The major part of that was from house calls at $5 each. An average day went something like this: hospital rounds at 6:30 a.m.; surgery, one to three cases, starting at 8 am.; office hours 1 p.m. until finished, usually around 6 p.m.; emergency surgery after office hours about three nights a week, sometimes lasting three hours; hospital rounds after that. When did we eat? Whenever we had a break. sometimes I would be eating supper at midnight. It was a grueling practice, but I enjoyed it in spite of the long hours, loss of sleep, lack of time with my family, and missed meals. When at times you brought someone "back from the grave" it was well worth all you had been through for all the years.

During all this, my wife, Jessie, went through it with me day and night, taking phone calls, calming anxious patients at the other end of the line, taking care of household chores (washing, ironing, cooking, changing diapers, etc.) and "putting up" with a tired, irritable, and anxious husband. At that time, I didn't realize what a jewel I had. After about two weeks in practice, the obstetrician said that Jessie would be scheduled for a caesarean section on July 26, which was a week from that time. I was so busy that the time came before I realized it was there. It was done under caudal anesthesia by Dr. Hingson, a new procedure started by him, who was known throughout the world. It was a big day for us and the hospital.

The procedure, of course, was reported in medical journals throughout the country. All went well. Our second daughter came into the world a bit prematurely. She weighed only 5 pounds 11 ounces. Her nails were soft, she had no eyebrows, and had to be placed in an incubator for a few days. Grandma came and stayed for two weeks—then Jessie was on her own again. Things got hectic as the baby had feeding problems, vomited a lot, and did not gain weight as she should have. That, coupled with my being gone all the time, the telephone ringing incessantly, and a 3-year-old to take care of, was a wonder Jessie kept her sanity. She was tough, and it showed when everything wasn't going well. As they say, "When the going gets tough, the tough get tougher." She proved it.

One evening I was listening to a football game on the radio while she was in the kitchen preparing dinner. I was thirsty, and not thinking. I said, "Bring me a glass of water, please."

Her reply was, "Get your own damn water. You're not in the Navy now." (Referring to the fact that as the Chief Medical Officer aboard a ship, I had my own cabin boy). That was the last time I tried that for many years.

My practice continued to grow. New patients came to the office every day, and my workload became heavier. At home, it was a merry-go-round with house calls galore at night, a baby that required a lot of attention, 8 to 12 hours in hospital and office practice. We both were chronically tired and irritable. Many times it would be 2 or 3 a.m. before I would get home. A great number of times I would find the house dark and quiet. I would wonder if she had taken the children and headed back to her parents' and a place of sanity. Usually I would find Jessie in a rocking chair with the baby over her shoulder and both sound asleep. Most of these times there would be milk streaming down Mama's back where the baby could not retain it. That went on for another month or so before we finally changed pediatricians (from the young professor-type to the older family-doctor type who used common sense in everyday practice).

The practice became larger and larger. I was building my own patients, and some others also chose to change to me. the surgical part of practice grew, along with the others, and I was happy with that part. Doctors' call service would call me first in most cases that didn't specify a particular specialty, and most did not do so. Because of that I was able to meet many fine people who were new to Memphis, and appreciated my taking care of them. that group would become regular patients and tell their friends about me. within six months, I was seeing 40 to 50 patients daily in the office. By that time I had begun to have problems at night when I could finally get to bed. The patients came back to haunt me. I was having nightmares; people would be screaming, "Help me, doctor!" There would be bloody faces, mangled arms, mothers delivering babies, and others with all types of pain crying for help. that went on for a week or two, and I discussed it with Dr. Pearce. He said, "You're just working too hard and living and dying with your patients. Relax more, take the wife out to dinner, dance a little, weed your house calls, and live a little while you're young. You can help yourself more than anyone else can." I took him seriously, gave myself lectures, and realized that the only way to remedy this problem was not to try putting myself in the patient's place, and accept the fact that I was doing my best—and the rest would have to be left up to the patient, God, and Mother Nature. After that, my nights were still busy, the nightmares did not recur, and I enjoyed a thriving practice in peace with myself.

❖ ❖ ❖

The first few months of practice were hectic because of the things I have related. Then in September, two months after we settled in, my father became ill and was hospitalized in a small hospital near home. A brother called saying Dad was calling for me to come. I talked with his attending physician and found he was planning to schedule him for a prostatectomy in three days. In Memphis, they had been doing a new procedure called "retropubic prostatectomy" for several months. I had assisted in some cases with more than one urologist and decided who was considered the best on our staff. Dad's physician and I discussed all aspects of his case, and I learned he was in serious condition. "Dr. Mac," his doctor, felt that Dad might have some problems with the surgery. We decided that I should fly there and see Dad before doing anything else. I took off that night and found the situation a bit worse than expected.

Dad was weak and pale, his voice weak and hesitant. That was not the man I had seen two months before. At that time he was active, with a firm handshake, a ruddy complexion, and a clear voice. He *was* a sick man.

"How do you feel, Dad?"

"Not so good, Son."

"Do you think you can stand some big surgery?"

"Not right now."

That was enough for me. I had a consultation with Dr. "Mac," and we went over his chart from beginning to end, noting that he still had fever, his blood pressure was below normal, he was anemic, and that a chest x-ray showed a little congestion in the base of both lungs. I thought, *He's not a good surgical risk at all.* Dr. "Mac" said, "Tell me about this new procedure, Wendell."

I outlined the surgery to the best of my ability, comparing to the old, superpubic procedure. He was impressed and said he would like to observe some. The upshot of my visit was that Dad was flown to Memphis the next day.

In the meantime, I had contacted the urologist in Memphis who made arrangements to admit Dad to the hospital immediately upon arrival. Three carloads of Wilsons and some friends left Nashville before the plane and arrived at our home shortly after. Jessie was overwhelmed, but handled everything admirably well. Dad was seen by three of my friends who evaluated him thoroughly, and four days later he had surgery. He was then 70-years-old and had been in good health. He had a good post-operative course and was dismissed in two weeks. My mother had come and was staying with us. She and Jessie enjoyed each other and were able to compare their husband's practices. They were prepared for nursing Dad back to health. That took at least a month before he returned home. Jessie went through hell because she loved my mother like her own. I didn't help the situation by being tense, irritable, and unkind. I was so terrible that my own mother advised Jessie to take the babies and leave. She must have seen some good in me because she stayed.

❖   ❖   ❖

The practice continued unabated. I tried to do it all. Surgical practice and expanded house calls continued, but I became more selective as addicts outwitted me on a few occasions, and the word spread that I was an easy target for them. Two of the last ones I saw I will relate. I got a call about 5 p.m. to see this fellow at an address that was in the down-trodden region of Memphis. He was in such pain with his back that he couldn't move. When I arrived they told me he was on the third floor. "Turn left at the head of the stairs, Doctor." At the head of the stairway, there was a dim light from a small bulb in a high ceiling. I stopped to adjust the light but didn't find a door. Then a muffled voice called out, "In here, Doctor." I went toward the sound and saw a door about 2 x 3 feet that was open to an attic. He called again, "In here." I had to literally crawl through the small door to get into the attic space. When I could see the patient, I realized something was wrong from what I was told. He was lying on a spring and mattress on the attic floor. There was not height enough to stand up.

"What's your problem, Mr. James?"

"My back. I can't move."

On my hands and knees I examined him, finding good mobility, no muscle spasm, and feigned tenderness. "I can't find anything wrong with your back, Mr. James."

"Doc, I've gotta have something for my back. Can't you give me a shot of Morphine or something for this pain?"

"Mr. James, are you addicted?"

"Well, I have a problem, but I have to have something, and I need it now."

He was sweating and shaky. Then I realized he *was* addicted. I gave him a stern lecture and told him he would be reported to the health department, as would his landlord. Then I realized this would be a charity case, and I was not feeling very charitable at that moment.

"Ok, give me ten dollars, and I'll give you a shot." He handed me the money. I gave him a small amount of Codeine and left. On the way out, I saw the landlord and told him of the patient's problems, then added that he had a problem too with the living quarters, and he had better be ready for the health department and the fire marshall to be by the next day.

❖ ❖ ❖

The second case was different. I was taking calls for my friend (and neighbor) who was the house doctor for a large hotel in the city. At about 8 p.m. on a Sunday I received a call from the hotel desk clerk asking me to visit a customer who was in severe pain. He gave me the room number and name. I hurried downtown to help a stricken man, wondering what I might be facing. Entering the hotel I went by the desk and identified myself. An employee took me to the room and left. The "patient" was a well-dressed, 40-year-old man who seemed to be in no paint but couldn't be still.

"Where is your pain, sir?"

"Here"—pointing to his chest.

I proceeded to examine him and found nothing wrong. I said, "I think you're faking your pain, Mister." All this time, I was getting ready to leave.

"I need a shot of Morphine, Doctor."

"I'm not giving you Morphine because you don't need it."

"Yes, I do need it and you're going to give me some!"

I looked up then and was shocked!

He had a pistol pointed at me (it looked as long as a rifle). I was so scared. I would have given him anything he asked for. He saw my fear and added, "I need a grain and a half, Doctor."

"That's a lethal dose, Mr. Jones."

"Not for me," he replied. "I can take two grains."

By then I had regained some composure and knew he would pay any amount for the shot. "Give me twenty dollars, and I'll give you the shot." He put the money in my shaky hand. I gave him the Morphine and was on my way out.

"By the way, Doctor, don't stop by the desk because they won't believe you, and it might cost you a lot of grief." I was so scared and relieved to get out of that room alive that I almost ran to my car. I was still shaking when I got back home 20 minutes later. Every time after that ordeal, whenever I made a call to a hotel, it was a rule that an employee go with me and stay in the room until I left.

❖   ❖   ❖

The last weekend in my Memphis practice I was on duty. I was feeling a little depressed about leaving such a great practice and a wonderful senior associate. I also had realized that my future for success as a General Practitioner was in Old Hickory. After making hospital rounds, I received two calls for home visits. They added to my depression. Both were 18-year-old males with typical signs and symptoms of poliomyelitis. Their examinations also bore that out. What could have been much worse than to tell the parents and patients their fate?

Many other things occurred in our lives during the four years in Memphis, beginning when our senior associate, Dr. Pearce, died rather suddenly from an acute myocardial infarction in the latter part of 1948. That left a void in our lives and the practice. He had treated me like the son he never had. I was very grateful to him and was saddened by is death. Dr.

Grobmyer had been with him for about 10 years and was greatly affected by his death. His passing also meant a much heavier work load for the both of us. We accepted that, along with all their inherent responsibilities. However, we soon had people approaching us to fill the vacancy. This we did within two months, and life went on.

In late May of 1948, we learned that we would have a third child. We had a 4-year-old and a 10-month-old for Jessie to care for, and now this! Thank God she had a wonderful house maid five days a week by then. Except for an unusual amount of pelvic pain and abnormal activity of the baby, things went along normally. In the fourth month of her pregnancy Jessie was called home to be with her mother during and after major surgery. She stayed four weeks before returning in September. At the time, she was scheduled to arrive by plane. I was there (five minutes early) and as the plane was landing I asked to be allowed to go there, but was stopped at the gate (in those days security was still tight). As the passengers were disgorged from the plane, I saw the stewardess carry a baby down the steps and hand her to the mother. I noticed that the mother was obviously pregnant, she was also leading a small child by the hand.

I thought, *Poor woman, I wonder if she has a husband!* Then I recognized her! *That's my wife and children!* I had to wait until they came through a gate before I could help them. What a reunion. While they were away, the house got bigger every day. That's all it was—a house—not a home, without them. It was so quiet at night that I sometimes worried about the cracking, crawling, swishing, and bumping that went on. Boy, was I glad to see all my "women." That same day, the girls and I attended the County Fair a few blocks away and were featured on the front page of the *Commercial Appeal* the next day since the photographer took our picture as I was cleaning tar from Rachel's dress while Mary Beth watched. We all still cherish that picture.

In February, Jessie was scheduled for a third Caesarean section. This occurred at 9 am. on February 19. The spinal didn't take effect for some reason, and she had to be given a general anesthetic. When the baby was delivered, my heart sank. It was limp, gray, and did not cry at all. I thought, *our baby is dead.* It seemed an eternity before she responded to the efforts of Dr. Wilkening (one of my classmates), the house pediatrician. Her cry was weak, her respiration was not full, and she did not move her arms and legs normally. Then I noticed that her head was small. Something was drastically wrong! I thought of a thousand things that could be the problem. When Jessie awoke and asked about the baby, I had a very hard time deciding what to tell her.

Finally I said, "She had a problem when born and will have to be in a special part of the nursery." Then I explained how she was, how she looked, and the response that occurred. Jessie didn't know that I had been to the nursery five or six times already to check on her progress. The baby could not be brought to the mother's room, and Jessie was spared the worst part. When the attending pediatrician explained the situation, Jessie had a difficult time accepting the fact that we did not have a normal baby. Within a few days, the baby did show improvement, was able to go home, and continued to show physical evidence of being normal, if not hyperactive. Before our third child was born we had made the decision to once more try for a son. Even though we realized that our third daughter would probably have a lifetime of problems, we stuck by our decision. That third daughter, Rebecca Susan, is still with us. She keeps us young and is a big help as we grow older.

On September 17, 1950, that fourth child was born. Another girl, Wenda Kaye, came into the world screaming, squirming, and fighting for attention, and is still doing so at age 44.

We quit trying for that son and have never been sorry. Our daughters have enlightened and enriched our lives by their achievements and have blessed us with seven beautiful, intelligent grandchildren.

❖   ❖   ❖

My practice had grown, and we had prospered, but that element of true peace with the practice was lacking. I had been contacted by Dr. E. P. Johnson, the man who delivered our first child, about joining his practice in Old Hickory, Tennessee, on more than one occasion. By the first part of January, 1951, I began to see what was happening to non-board-certified Surgeons in Memphis, Since I had training that was a non-certifying type, I felt it best to look around for a more stable future in general practice and general surgery. The location in Old Hickory would be an ideal place for that type of practice since it was near a large medical center and a medium-sized city also. That way we could rear our children in a small town and also have the advantages of the city. The ever-wily Dr. Johnson invited me to visit him and evaluate the practice. Jessie and I talked it over, and a date was set for me to spend two weeks there and fill in for Dr. Johnson while he was away for medical evaluation in another city. That way I could really get a feel for the practice.

In mid-April, 1951, I arrived in Old Hickory, was introduced to the office staff, and the local hospital management. I presented my credentials and

Doctor From Bugtussle

was duly approved for temporary privileges. The next day I was the "man in charge" for Dr. Johnson's office. Patients came in by the dozens. It was as if he had told all of them to return for follow-ups that week. I was kept *very* busy day and night. The practice was to my liking; a mix of general medicine and surgery, with an active OB practice and a goodly number of house calls. It had a great potential for what I had dreamed of doing. In addition, there was a large, active industrial plant in the heart of the city. A dam was under construction on the Cumberland River that would form a lake, and Dr. Johnson had been asked to take care of the injuries occurring on the construction site. After that two weeks, I made the decision to move to the area as soon as possible. I have never regretted that decision.

Meanwhile, back in Memphis, Jessie had been busy looking for a larger house and had signed a contract to buy one with a contingency clause stating it would be based on my decision to stay or move. When I called to tell her of the decision, she was stunned. Plans were changed. I returned to Memphis and discussed the move with Dr. Grobmyer. He was very gracious and understanding, but thought it best for me to stay in Memphis, and asked that I wait a few days before making a final decision. Each day as I made my way through city traffic to and from hospitals, the office, and making house calls all over the city, I realized even more that our future was brighter in a smaller town. I broke the news to the family first that we would be moving after school was out. The girls reacted with loud "no's," and tears were shed, but we made preparations to move. My mind was made up.

Other things had to be done, such as transferring my membership from Shelby to Davidson County Medical Society, obtaining letters of recommendation to the hospitals, applying for full hospital privileges at the new location, and resigning from the staffs at hospitals where I was in practice. All of that was accomplished quickly, and the patients were notified of the fact that I would be leaving. We bought a house in Old Hickory (sight unseen) and I prepared to depart Memphis, leaving Jessie and the girls there until the house could be sold.

I arrived in the area in the early afternoon on June 22, 1951, and went to work immediately by taking care of an accident victim in the local hospital emergency room as I related in "Where It All Started." Five hours later, I arrived in Old Hickory. Driving up to the "new" house, I went inside and found the power was off. My first thought was, at that instant, I should have stayed in Memphis. I went to the local drugstore for help and explained my plight. Within five minutes two fellows arrived (Mr. Long and Mr. Cunningham), and pretty soon they had bypassed the meter and restored power to the house. At that moment, I knew this was the place the good Lord had chosen for me to live.

The next six weeks I had the experience of being a bachelor. I didn't like that lifestyle one bit. The practice was very active, and I was happy from that standpoint. By the time that six weeks had passed, the practice was experiencing some growth from new patients as word spread that a new doctor was in town. Many patients came from curiosity, some came because they knew my family, and others came to me because they were unable to see Dr. Johnson. So long as they came, I was happy. As busy as I was, my salary was only $650 a month. I had no office expense, a small house note, automobile expense, and notes. Never having had much money, that was no problem. Besides, I was optimistic for the future in this town and in the practice here.

In mid-July, 1951, the family was moved to Old Hickory where we have remained for more than 40 years. In that period we have lived in three different houses, but have stayed in this little, comfortable country town where everybody knows and (I hope) respects the doctor and his family.

I'm sure we created a big stir in this small town with four daughters, nine months to seven years of age. Jessie added further to the gossip when she dressed all four in identical dresses and paraded them through the shopping area. Of course, I was as proud as a peacock of my five "women," as patients would comment favorably about them. Jessie was afraid to say or do anything for fear it might be misunderstood. Pretty soon she felt as if we were living in a fish bowl since we lived in a crowded neighborhood. We soon found a larger house on a 3-acre lot outside of "The Village," as Old Hickory was called. There we lived a more relaxed style of life than before. The girls all grew physically, and all were very bright. We had one problem that haunted all of us—Becky was unable to express herself verbally. She played games without any problems and she made it clear how she felt and what she wanted. Just her lack of speech! Then we began to make an effort to find the cause of her problem. She was evaluated by Neurologists, Speech Pathologists, Audiologists, etc., and we had more than one diagnosis of her problem, and all agreed that she had normal intelligence.

When she was four, we enrolled her in a special school in Racine, Wisconsin, where she spent a year making good progress. We had hoped to establish a definite diagnosis of her problem, but the director of the school died that summer, and that opportunity was lost. After that year she was referred to the speech and hearing center in Nashville, which she attended for several months with some benefits. Her mother took her each day and spent the time reading or taking an extra daily round trip back to take care of business. The second fall, she enrolled at Peabody College, taking courses there and at Vanderbilt. Not only did she pass all subjects, but was an *A* student. The physical and emotional strain was hard on her, but she had the determination and stamina to survive. Becky was then enrolled in special-education classes, going to several different schools over a 5-year period.

Her sisters accepted Becky as she was and treated her as if she had no problems. This, of course, was the best thing that could have been done since it exposed her to many things that she would never have experienced. They were spokesman for her when necessary and helped her to grow socially, as well as to be accepted by their friends. Jessie kept searching for something new that might help us to establish a definite diagnosis and treatment.

During this phase of our life, I was busier than ever with the OB practice growing by leaps and bounds, house calls galore, the number of surgical cases increasing rapidly, the in-hospital patients increasing, and night meetings to attend, I hardly had time to eat or sleep. I was a poor father, but my wife was such a wonderful mother that our girls had plenty of love and attention. Many days I would leave home before they were awake and not be able to get back until they were all in bed asleep. I did find time to be there some, and we had a true family life with occasional picnics, visits to grandparents, and a short vacation each summer. As they got older, the girls accepted the type of lifestyle they had to lead because of my profession.

With my busy practice, I became acquainted with a great many physicians in Nashville, as I needed help in various specialties. Dr. Johnson, my senior partner, was well-known and active in the local medical society, which helped me more in the medical circles. In 1952, I became a member of the Tennessee Academy of General Practice and soon became an active member. In early 1960, somehow I became secretary of the state chapter of that organization. That, of course, led to a greater workload for me (and my wife). The hospital staff members saw fit to elect me to various staff offices over the ensuing years. In the beginning that bolstered my ego, but also increased my responsibility to the organization. The Academy of General Practice had local chapters in which I was also active.

Throughout the 1950s and 1960s, we grew in numbers and activities. I was in the thick of all of this (thanks to my good friend, Irving Hilliard) and subsequently held offices in the organization. Working with both the local and state group, I developed friendships with family physicians throughout the state and had a good rapport with most of them. In 1964, they honored me by electing me to the office of President of the Tennessee Academy of General Practice (later to become the American Academy of Family Physicians). This was the greatest professional honor I had received to that date. During my tenure in office the Academy began to undergo changes and seek more recognition as a specialty group.

To do this meant we had to establish departments of this specialty in medical schools and teaching hospitals. At that time our state chapter started laying the groundwork for meetings with the Dean of U.T. Medical School and various other officials. That was only the beginning, which eventually became a reality through hard work of many colleagues throughout the whole country. The seeds sown by our small organization is now reaping rewards by growing numbers of men and women serving residencies and becoming family physicians nationwide. It pleases me to have played a very small part in our movement in this state. A much larger role by many other members of the academy, along with friends in organized medicine throughout the State of Tennessee, made this a reality. I remained active in general and family practice organizations of the state until 1986. In 1976, I was again honored by the Academy, being named Family Physician of the Year for Tennessee. That was an honor I had never dreamed of achieving. This was the thrill of a lifetime and the highlight of my medical career.

While I was busy with activities in the medical organizations, the practice continued to grown and in 1960, a third man, Dr. Howard Pomeroy, joined the group to help ease the workload, but he was so talented that he attracted patients aplenty. The three of us were seeing 100-plus patients daily in the office, doing ten or more major surgeries weekly, delivering several babies monthly, and making many house calls. We were also taking care of many emergencies at the hospital emergency room day and night. We outgrew our office space, and in 1961 started construction of a new office building to which we moved into in March of 1962. This was a milestone for Old Hickory, as it was the first building constructed solely for M.D.'s in almost 40 years. That was a big feather in our cap! The practice continued to grow, and each of us worked long hours. At that time, I was involved in the state General Practice Organization serving as President, visiting other chapters, organizing a new chapter, and attending various meetings. My associates were good to me, taking care of their patients and mine when I was away. I was fortunate to have such men to be associated with at that time.

Doctor From Bugtussle

Tragedy struck our practice in April of 1964 when our senior partner (and father figure) became ill with a malignant tumor of the pancreas. Surgical procedure were done, but the follow-up treatment was not successful, ad he died four weeks later. It was a devastating loss, not only to our practice, but to the entire area surrounding Nashville. He had been in active practice here for more than 40 years, touching the lives of thousands of people, delivering a few thousand babies, and performing surgery on innumerable patients. he was one of the most devoted physicians I have ever know.

Dr. "E. P." as he was known, was a legend in Old Hickory. He was born in 1897, the fifth of ten children. At the age of nine, he was badly burned and hospitalized. While in the hospital he contracted poliomyelitis which affected the muscles of his right leg. He once told me this was a factor in his becoming a physician. He graduated from Vanderbilt Medical School in 1925, and in 1927 came to Old Hickory where he opened his office. He quickly gained the reputation of being a very dedicated and hard-working practitioner, making house calls, doing home deliveries, performing surgery, and seeing many, many office patients seven days a week. In spite of his physical handicap, he would climb stairways to see patients or deliver babies, walk the hospital corridors, and stay "on the job" 24 hours a day.

In 1944, I became acquainted with Dr. Johnson when he delivered our first child when I was in military service. From the beginning, I admired his attitude, work ethic, judgment, surgical abilities, and patient relationships. He was truly a physician who practiced both the science and art of medicine. His patients had the utmost trust and confidence in him. I saw him briefly a few times when he attended my wife and delivered our first baby by caesarean section. After that our contacts were by mail or telephone until I joined him in practice seven years later. Then I really learned the true intensity of his dedication to the profession. I learned in many ways from Dr. "E. P." Prior to this, I had been associated for four years in private practice with very fine physicians who were excellent in their fields of medicine and surgery, but there was that intangible "something" that Dr. "E. P." possessed which instilled in the patient a desire to overcome an illness or disability.

He taught me the "how" of art in the practice of medicine and surgery. For this, I have always been grateful. Our work days were long and hard, but he never faltered. Surgery was scheduled in the early hours, followed by long office hours, with house calls interspersed, or a run back to the emergency rooms for *true* emergency cases. He always had a cigar in his mouth, sometimes forgetting to take it out before delivering a baby. He would often scrub for surgery while he puffed on that cigar. A nurse would remove the cigar and put his mask in proper position before allowing him in the operating room.

After several months passed, I gradually made most of the house calls, and on many occasions was questioned as to why Dr. Johnson didn't come himself. I had had experience in "playing second fiddle" to older doctors; with my father, Dr. Pearce in Memphis, and now Dr. "E. P." He knew the patients like the back of his hand and would tell me of their idiosyncrasies, which helped in caring for each one. It took some months for patients to trust me completely, especially surgical cases. Although I had five years experience doing major surgery, they still wanted Dr. "E. P." if he had ever cared for them before. One case I recall very well. Dr. "E. P." had not arrived at the office when a lady came in with a classical case of acute appendicitis. I took the history, examined her, did the lab work, gave her the diagnosis, and advised both she and her husband that immediate surgery would have to be done.

The patient spoke up, "Where is Dr. Johnson?"

I knew why she asked. "He's at the hospital. I'll call him right now." After I called him, she went willingly. Then when I showed up in her room with Dr. Johnson she was anxious to know who was to do the surgery. Dr. "E. P." talked to her for a minute to assure her. "We'll both be there!" In the operating room, after the patient was asleep, I was on the assistant's side of the table when Dr. "E. P." came in.

"Move to the other side, Dr. Wilson. This is your case."

Of course, I was pleased that he felt that way, and I performed the surgery. It was an easy case and went smoothly. The next day we made rounds together and both told her how well she did and would soon be home.

She looked at Dr. "E. P.", probing, "Who did my surgery?"

"We both did it," he said.

She wasn't satisfied— "I mean, who made the incision on my stomach."

We looked at each other. Dr. "E. P." came to my rescue. "Dr. Wilson did, and he did a mighty fine job, too."

"Well, I guess it's ok if you were there."

She, luckily, did so well that she counted me as her physician until I retired. Dr. "E. P." used a lot of psychology in practice and taught me its great benefits in general practice. Many patients benefitted more with someone taking time to listen and talk to them, than anything else could have done.

Dr. "E. P." was highly respected by his peers, very ethical in his practice, and expected the same from his associates. Whenever a younger physician would not be as ethical and honest as he should in his work with Dr. "E. P.," a phone call or a private talk with that young man would be held to give him some fatherly advice and recommendations concerning future conduct. More than one good friend has related this to me over the years. He was always honest and forthright with me, and this helped us bond a good relationship during the 13 years we were associated in practice. Taking lessons from him, I didn't hesitate to let him know when I didn't agree with him about a diagnosis or treatment of patients or my stand on a political issue or a community affair. It almost became a "father-son" type of relationship.

In the early years of our practice together each of us had personal, family problems that were burdensome which further strengthened our relationship. Some things had no solution, and we lived with them. Early on in 1952, we had a big problem arise from post-surgical complications in a longtime patient and friend that devastated the both of us. As I was the Principal Surgeon on the case, I felt the greater burden. His advice and counsel helped me through the many years we cared for that patient. In that same period of time, his wife had surgery for a malignant breast tumor, from which she never recovered and expired in 1955.

It was a very touching moment when she died. Only Dr. Johnson, a nurse, and I were at the bedside. He was holding her hand at that moment. As her heart stopped and she ceased breathing, lightning flashed, there was a clap of thunder, and torrents of rain followed. He looked at me with tear-filled eyes. "Even the elements are disturbed at her passing." Not knowing what to say or do, I only nodded. After doing what was necessary, I saw the children briefly and left. Later that night, I visited him and before leaving was assuring him that everything was taken care of with the practice. I was astounded when he told me he would be at the hospital the day following the funeral. I guess it shocked me.

"Dr. Wilson, you and I know everything possible was done for Helen, and she would not want me to grieve over her death. The best thing I can do is to bury myself in work and not sit around worrying."

Of course, he was right, and two days later we were at the hospital doing surgery at 8 a.m. That showed his real strength.

Dr. "E. P." worked like a tiger after that and encouraged me to spend more time with my family. Of course, I didn't listen to him, and the workload was heavier.

Old Hickory Lock and Dam were under construction, and we were the contract physicians for employee injuries, and their families also became patients. DuPont Company was in full production, and we both were busy day and night. He worked a continuous pace and never seemed to tire. His cigar was with him every waking moment—at home, in the office, at the hospital, in the surgical suite, and in OB quarters. He was still delivering a great many babies, doing major surgery, and seeing office patients six days each week and three hours on Sunday. He still found time to attend staff meetings, medical society meetings, and Vanderbilt football games. I felt we could cut down on office hours to a 5-day week. I asked him. "Dr. Johnson, don't you think we should shorten our office hours to a half-day on Saturday?"

"What for? Are you working too hard?"

"No, but I thought it might be better for you to slow down some."

"I'll let you know when I get to that point."

"Ok. If you can dot it, I can too. That ended the discussion, and we kept on working seven days *every* week (we did alternative Sunday office hours).

Dr. "E. P." was still doing tonsillectomies in the office and doing some office deliveries when we became associated. Both continued until he had an accident in 1954 when he fell and fractured his femur. After about two office deliveries, I felt uneasy with the situation. I assumed the entire practice and was working almost 24 hours a day, which was exhausting. I told him that the burden was too great, that most people had insurance which would pay the hospital bill, and that we should stop office deliveries. He didn't think much of the idea, but the office deliveries stopped. I had found that with him I had to stand my ground to get his attention and gain his respect. I also had realized that if something wasn't his idea it would be hard to accept. He was also unable to work for several weeks, and by that time the patients were aware that babies would no longer be delivered in the office.

After more than a year had passed since Helen's death, Dr. "E. P." met a young lady who appealed to him in many ways. Before long he became romantically involved with Marcy, and after a few more months of courtship, they were married. It was the best thing he could have done. She was good to and for him, had a good personality, and was liked by everybody. He seemed to take a new interest in life and to resume doing the things he liked most. She was a bit older than my wife, Jessie, and they became good friends. This also helped to strengthen our professional relationship. Within a year after he and Marcy were married, a son ("Bo") was born. Dr. "E. P." really "strutted his stuff" after that. I had the honor and privilege of being the attending physician of and caring for Mrs. Johnson, and of delivering the baby. I think that was one of the times I felt the greatest pressure and most responsibility of any delivery I had ever performed. Little did I dream when he delivered our first child that someday I would be doing that for him. By another two years they were expecting another child, and you would have thought Dr. "E. P." was 25 instead of nearing 60. This time I bowed out of the responsibility of another delivery. I felt too close to Dr. Johnson to assume that task. The good Lord must have been with me because some problems developed during the pregnancy that were alarming for both mother and the baby. Mary Alice was born near term and without incident.

Dr. Johnson and I continued our busy practice together in the same old building where he had been for more than 30 years. We competed with each other and all of our peers in the surrounding communities. The patient load outgrew the two of us. I felt a third man was needed, and this time we agreed 100 percent. We were fortunate to find the third man, Dr. Howard Pomeroy, who joined us in mid-July of 1960. The place really became crowded then, as he also was soon very busy. I then began the task of finding some land in Old Hickory so we could construct a building large enough to accommodate our practice. Dr. Johnson resisted that idea from every standpoint for about three months. After that I asked for a more formal discussion, at which time there was an impasse. My stubbornness continued and won out. We bought land from the Utility District at the corner of Hadley Avenue and Golf Club Road, and construction fo the building began in October of 1961. In early March of 1962, we moved our offices to that new building where we continued our association until Dr. Johnson's death in May of 1964. He confessed to me, not long after we made the move, that it was a smart thing to have done.

To illustrate his dedication to medicine and his love for obstetrics in particular, at the time of his passing there were 10 or 12 patients he was scheduled to deliver within the next few months. This was just one illustration of his dedication to the profession. Over the years he had cared for thousands of patients, but hundreds of patients were never charged and never paid for services rendered. Many patients have told me of the hours he spent at their bedside or of the number of times he would call or visit them each day during an illness. One man, in particular, who had osteomyelitis at the age of nine, and was critically ill for many weeks, stated he owed his life to Dr. Johnson for his diligent care during those critical times and for years following. His illness occurred in the days before the use of "miracle drugs" such as Penicillin or Mycin drugs or the innumerable ones that are in use today.

At the time I became associated with him, he would send his own car to pick up a patient, bring that patient to the office, examine them, then have an employee take the patient home all for 10 to 12 dollars. Also, if a patient was told to return on a certain day and failed to show up, they would be contacted by phone, and if they had the excuse of having no way to get to the office, he would do the same thing. I'm sure some made this a "racket." He had a remarkable memory and could recite patient's histories from the time he first saw them until that present time. There was one big flaw in this—he didn't always keep records of patient visits. This amazed me, and I chided him about that from time-to-time. That never seemed to bother him until he was asked by a male nurse who was "interning" in our office, if he wasn't concerned about this from a legal standpoint. The nurse was told, in no uncertain terms, to mind his own business. But after that, Dr. "E. P." was more diligent in his record-keeping. I, and his nurse of many years, got a big laugh from that incident.

From the day of my becoming associated with Dr. "E. P." until his death, I had not heard any serious criticism of his methods of practice or of him personally. His presence at the hospital seemed to stimulate nurses and other personnel to be more alert and professional. If patients did not receive proper care, the supervisor, not the floor nurse, would be called in for a conference for not doing her job properly. If there was a problem with the hospital as a whole, then the administration would be paid a visit, and the condition would usually be straightened out in a short time. There was never any doubt as to where Dr. "E. P." stood on any issue. His demeanor and methods of practice were a good example for me to follow.

In early April of 1964, Dr. "E. P." started complaining of "indigestion." This did not seem to be severe, and he continued to work at his usual pace. While I was away attending a medical convention, he was seen by a longtime physician friend. At that time, he was told that he might have a life-threatening problem. I was never made aware of this until just one day before he was scheduled for a "Whipple" procedure for a tumor of the Ampulla-of-Vater (junction of the bile and pancreatic ducts). This was a very major procedure. It was also one that could easily have post-operative complications. Dr. Johnson was one of the unfortunate ones to have that happen. There was a valiant fight to save him from further complications, but—in spite of all efforts—his situation was one of more complications which they were never able to control. Visits to him, while in the hospital, were frequent and each time I left, I cried inside because it was evident that he was losing the battle for his life. Dr. Pomeroy and I visited him at the same time less than a week before his death. "Hi, Dr. Johnson. How are things going?"

"Not good at all."

We surveyed the situation. There was a foul odor from a copious drainage, he was weak, and his eyes were pleading.

"Take me home, boys. You can do more for me than they are doing here."

I was fighting back the tears. "I wish we could, Dr. Johnson, but we have to follow your doctor's orders."

"I'm not going to make it if somebody doesn't come up with something real soon."

"We have had a consultation with your Surgeon, and he will explain everything to you when he makes his rounds in the morning. Maybe he will have good news for you by then."

The nurse came in at that moment. We introduced ourselves, then each held his hand for a moment, saying a silent prayer.

"So long, Doctor. We'll be back as soon as possible." As we left we didn't dare look at each other for fear the tears would start flowing. My last visit was late in the evening, and he had deteriorated so much he barely responded to me then. No one else was there.

"I'm here, Doctor. Is there anything I can get for you?" His eyes barely opened, he shook his head as he barely whispered, "No." I was a coward. "Grown men don't cry," even when you know your best friend is dying, and there's absolutely nothing you can do. I gave his hand a short squeeze and left, going down the stairway so no one could see the tears running down my cheeks. It hurt to know he had suffered so much for that four weeks when he had relieved so many people of their suffering over so many years. It didn't seem fair. "Why him, Lord?" I asked silently.

While Dr. "E. P.'s" body was at the local funeral home, they had the greatest number of visitors on record. Many people would cry openly and unashamedly, not only older ladies, but girls, older men, and boys, as well. Many recalled what he had done for them during his lifetime. Many would say, "I have lost the best friend I have ever had." Our downtown colleagues paid their respects and came to his funeral services at a local church. I thought that was a great tribute to him. Serving as a pallbearer was an honor, but tough to take. Several of the office personnel were weeping as if they had lost a parent. The church was packed, people stood outside, and cars were parked for three blocks as they paid tribute to one of the most beloved men that had ever lived in Old Hickory.

Needless to say I have been most fortunate to have been associated with a high caliber of men in my years of practice. In addition, I have had some wonderful, exciting, scary, unbelievable, sad, happy, and comical experiences during these years. If I could recall a majority of them it would fill a thousand pages. Some I will never forget and will relate to you.

❖ ❖ ❖

In my early years of practice in Memphis, I encountered some things that I have not seen since. I had the misfortune of treating three black-widow-spider bites, one of which was fatal. This case was a 30-year-old dairy route man who lived in the country and had an outdoor toilet. His day started at about 3 a.m. On this day, he was using the toilet just before leaving. While doing so, he had a severe stinging and burning pain on the head of the penis. He then experienced some nausea and, soon thereafter, developed excruciating pain in his abdominal and back muscles. I saw him in the emergency room at 4:30 a.m. in a state of shock, writhing with pain and complaining of being unable to breathe. His pulse was rapid, the blood pressure was low, his color was dusky, and he was deteriorating rapidly. I.V. fluids were started, oxygen was given by mask, a small dose of Morphine given intravenously, and antivenin was requested. After admission, he was given the antivenin and supportive measures continued. We obtained both medical and neurological consultation shortly after his admission, and he was treated vigorously by both. In spite of their heroic efforts, he succumbed to the injury. That was a bitter pill to swallow, but I realized everything possible had been done, and we had to accept it.

The second case had a humorous slant to it and turned out well. A 20-year-old returned home form work, and went to bed, and just before falling asleep experienced a stinging, burning pain in his lower leg. He investigated and found the cause of his pain; a black widow spider! His 9-year-old sister had the spider as a biology project, and it had escaped from the jar and into the patient's bed. The site of the bite, the age of the patient, and early recognition and treatment were successful.

The third case was a 70-year-old man who lived in an older house. He was a gardener and left his work clothes in the closet floor at night. The next day at about 10 a.m., he put his overalls on to garden again but soon took them off because he had a severe pain in his leg behind the knee. I saw him two hours later at home with typical symptoms of back, leg and abdominal pain with cramping which one would see was a black-widow bite. He was immediately hospitalized, treated with appropriate medication, and soon recovered. These demonstrate what can happen to patients with the same problems under very different circumstances.

While in practice in Memphis, I had several unusual cases. One made an indelible impression on me. (I was young and emotional at that time.) A 12-year-old girl contracted chicken pox and had an unusually bad case. She was ill for about three weeks and seemed to be recovering when she developed a fever again and became very ill with nausea, vomiting, and abdominal pain. After hospitalizing her, it was finally determined she had hepatitis as a complication of the chicken pox. She never completely recovered from that illness, and I saw her innumerable times over a 2-year period. During that time, we developed a very close relationship. She was a beautiful redhead with a sparkling personality and loved everything in life. She expressed her love in such a way that it was difficult for me to see her gradually get worse, in spite of everything we could do. When she was in the latter stages of her illness, as she was unable to retain foods of any type and became dehydrated, I had to hospitalize her. As I was leaving, she asked me the one question I had been dreading for a long time. She looked at me with those large, deep-set, hollow eyes that seemed to penetrate ones soul, saying, "Am I going to die, Doctor?" How could I answer that question and be honest with that loveable, innocent child, without her losing faith in my healing power as her physician. Controlling myself, I tried to console her.

"Jennie, all of us have to die sometime. Whenever God has chosen that time He will take us, no matter what we do. If your time is soon, He will call you. We will do everything we can to help keep you from being in pain and make you feel better. Now let's see that big smile again, ok? That's my girl."

"Thank you, Doctor. I love you."

That did it. The tears flowed in spite of all my self-control. A week later "Jennie" died. She went peacefully, a shell of the beautiful, happy, vivacious child who two years earlier had chicken pox that one never dreamed would end in tragedy.

The family wished to have an autopsy performed which revealed the liver to be shrunken to a fourth of normal size and reminded me of a ripe "hedgeapple." It was yellow to orange in color, knotty with fibrous tissue, and very hard. The pathologist remarked, "I don't see how she lived that long with this liver so diseased." I have never seen or heard of a similar case since.

Another rare case we treated in my Memphis practice was a lady who developed a subphrenic, amebic abscess following a clinical case of amebic dysentery. It had been surgically drained but did not heal completely, leaving a sinus tract which we packed every four or five days. This we (I) did for months on end as it finally healed. During all this time, the patient was taking Chloroquine and Emetine medication to prevent further infection by the organism. That was at the time of life in this country when we took care or our own and did not expect a handout from the Federal Government. Nor did we expect to be paid for our professional services because we knew from the beginning that patient had no income and we were obligated to care for her since she had chosen us as her attending physicians.

There were many more interesting cases that I saw but cannot now recall, yet these were so unusual and rare that I could easily and vividly recall them.

❖ ❖ ❖

Some comical ones I recall such as the 300-pound-black logger who came to the office in late afternoon because of a rattlesnake bite. We hustled him into the examining room, expecting to see a patient in severe pain or in shock. To my surprise, he looked comfortable, sitting up, and smiling.

"Hi, John. Did I hear right that you have been bitten by a rattlesnake?"

"Yes, sir, that's right."

"How long has it been?"

"About six hours. It was just a little ole rattler. Didn't hurt."

"Have you been working since then?"

"Yes, sir, 'til about an hour ago."

"Where did he bite you?"

"Right here," pointing at his thigh.

I knew then that he had not injected any venom in the patient. I examined and finally managed to find tiny fang marks that barely scratched the surface. We cleaned him up with soap and alcohol and sent him on his way. I have never seen another rattlesnake bite.

Moving from Memphis altered the type of practice only a little. I still made many house calls, did surgery, and had long office hours. The biggest change was the fact that I began an OB practice which grew rapidly. By 1955, this part of the practice had grown greatly in proportion to the rest of the practice. That meant that I was home even less than I had been before. We had bought a lakeside plot of land, and plans were underway to build a new home. This kept Jessie as busy as bees. Fortunately, she had full-time household help that was very reliable. Minnie had apparently been sent to us by the Divine Master. One day Jessie answered a knock on the door, and there stood a short, stout black lady.

"Does you need somebody to do housework?"

Jessie could hardly believe her ears! "I sure do. Who sent you?"

"The Good Lord, I guess. Nobody else did. I'se jest lookin for work."

"You have come to the right place. Come in." She met the girls and fell in love with the baby and vice-versa. Minnie started the next day and stayed for more than 20 years.

❖ ❖ ❖

In February, 1956, construction was begun on our new home on the lake. This was an exciting time in the lives of the family. We were the talk of the town. Patients would ask about the progress and make comments about how they were building different rooms of the home.

"Thank you, Mrs. Snide. I appreciate that, and I'm sure Mrs. Wilson does also. Come by and see what you're getting for your money."

The house was finished late due to a severe winter, and we moved in October. We have been here ever since. Our girls, at that time, were from 6 to 12 years of age and still call this home. Even though they live from East Tennessee to Pennsylvania and Nevada, have children and careers, this is still home. I consider this a great compliment to their mother, first, and somewhat to me, secondly.

Practice was not altered during this time, except for continued growth from every aspect. This was the period when veterans of World War II were having children and kept us busy. Obstetrics was an interesting part of family practice, and we had an above-average percent for GP's in our practice. From 1955 until 1966, our group averaged 12 to 15 deliveries per month. With all other phases of the practice, that kept us busy day and night. Both Dr. Johnson and I were very fond of that portion, and had many interesting cases. Obstetrical patients, as a whole, were a happy lot. This was something they wanted, far different from an illness that they had to endure.

At least 90 percent had no problems and were overjoyed when *that* baby was born. When complications did occur, it was as sad as the joyful ones were glad. Having to say, "Mr. and Mrs. Jones, there is a problem with your baby, something that is nobody's fault, and everything will be done to correct the problem," or to say, "Your baby has something that cannot be corrected," this devastated families and depressed me when it occurred. Explanations never seemed adequate at those times. This was the times that ministers were called upon to console families and to remind them that there was a Higher Power that controlled our destiny. This group of professionals was a big help to me throughout my career in medicine, at times of family crisis, or deaths. I still owe them a debt of gratitude. Some of the unusual cases I still recall vividly.

Unusual Cases and Unforgettable Families

In early March or April as the waiting room door opened about mid-morning during a busy day in the office, I looked up to see a familiar face enter—someone I had not seen in several months. There was a difference in her appearance this time—she looked scared and anxious. I could see tears in her large, blue eyes. They seemed to be saying, "Help me, Dr. Wilson." My sixth sense told me she had a serious problem. Then I noticed the baby she was so tenderly and carefully carrying in her arms. There was a disproportion of the head and body size; the head was much too large.

"Hello, Ann, I'm glad to see you. Come in and have a seat. How are you, Pappa Clyde?" To the baby I said, "What is your name, young fella?"

"This is Jeff, and I'm afraid he has a problem."

"Yes, I noticed—he does seem to be in trouble. How long have you felt that something was wrong with your baby?"

"For four or five months."

"How old is Jeff now?"

"Six-and-a-half months."

"What have you noticed about him besides the enlarging of his head?"

"He doesn't seem to be as alert or playful as he should be. He's not taking his food as well now either."

"Does he sleep more than your other babies did?"

"Oh, yes."

"Was he ok when he was delivered?"

"So far as I know."

"Have you had him checked regularly?"

"Yes."

"What have you been told?"

"That he'll be fine—just give him more time."

"Do you feel that your baby is ok and that he'll be all right?"

"No! If I had, we wouldn't have driven all the way from West Virginia to see you and Dr. Johnson."

"I realize that, Ann. Furthermore, I can see that your baby has a serious problem. You and Clyde are intelligent people, and I don't have to tell you there is a problem and you know that already. Let me examine Jeff before we do anything else."

"Nurse, would you help Ann undress her baby?"

The examination was soon completed. I noted his lethargy, mild nuchal rigidity, slow response to stimuli. The forehead was bulging, the anterior fontanel (soft spot) was wide and bulging slightly, and the other suture lines of the skull were widening. These were all positive for a progressive increase of fluid pressure within the cranial cavity. This baby needed help now!

"You folks already know that you have a serious problem, but it is one that needs immediate attention. This is a problem for a Neurosurgeon. Let me call one of your choice now and ask them to see your baby as soon as possible."

"We don't know anybody, Doctor. We have heard of some, but will leave it up to you to make the choice."

"I'll choose someone that I would call for my own family. Mrs. Whited, would you please call Dr. Cobb for me?"

On the phone, I explained the problem to the Neurosurgeon, who immediately was anxious to see the infant, feeling that any delay would be taking more risk.

"Could you see him tomorrow, Dr. Cobb?"

"I certainly can," Dr. Cobb answered. "Ask the parents to be here at 9 in the morning."

"Thank you, Dr. Cobb. They'll be there."

As I went back into the room, the parents were both crying their hearts out. "I'm sorry to have upset you, but I couldn't find a better way to tell you of the problem. I want you to be prepared for any unforeseen problems, and there will be some. Let me explain why your baby is in trouble. First of all, don't blame yourselves. It just happens. I don't know why, and I doubt if Dr. Cobb does. I know *what* has caused the head to enlarge. The cerebra-spinal fluid that circulates through the brain and around the spinal cord does so by small canals connecting the entire system. If one of these small, connecting areas becomes blocked, the spinal fluid builds up in certain regions and causes pressure on the brain and skull. This takes time for the symptoms, such as Jeff has, to be noticed by parents or family. If something is not done, there could be irreparable damage to the central nervous system. I'm sure this has not happened in your baby's case, thank God. Now, doctors perform miracles, almost, but not quite. Surgery probably will be necessary, and *soon*, so don't be shocked if you're told that. I hope both of you understand.

"We do, Doctor, and we're ready for something to be done. We appreciate your being so frank and honest with us. I think we can face anything now, if there's a chance it will help our Jeff."

As they left, I was thinking of our own daughter that had as yet an undiagnosed problem from brain damage. I could readily empathize with the parents.

The next day the Neurosurgeon called to say that his workup was not complete, but he felt sure that Jeff would respond favorably to surgery, and he would schedule the procedure when the workup was completed and Jeff had been observed for several weeks.

When Jeff was seven months old, Dr. Cobb performed the surgery for Jeff's hydro-cephalic condition, wherein he inserted a small plastic catheter (long tube) into the area of the brain where the spinal fluid was blocked, then brought it out under the skin, and allowed it to drain into the abdominal cavity. Jeff began to improve soon after his return home and was followed closely by Dr. Cobb, a Pediatrician, and me. He had some rough times during his childhood and adolescent years, but had a normal skeletal growth and body development. By the age of 12, he began to have more problems with irritability, headaches, and visual disturbances.

After further studies were done, it was evident that it would be necessary to replace the tube inserted in early life. This was done without incident, and he began to "blossom out." Although he had some problems, Jeff continued to fight his battles and win. His lifestyle was normal during the teen years, although his social life was somewhat limited and he was not able to participate in sports. He graduated from high school and went on to college. During the first three years of college he had no physical problems, but early in 1984, during his senior year, he again developed signs of increased intracranial pressure and was admitted to Vanderbilt Hospital once again for observation and treatment.

This time he had severe headaches, fever, dizziness, nausea, vomiting, visual disturbances, plus abdominal pain. He once again underwent a thorough workup, including a ventriculogram, which revealed a blockage of cerebra-spinal fluid flow from the third to the fourth ventricle. Because of this, it was necessary again to replace his drainage tube so he would have a normal flow of the spinal fluid. Postoperatively, he continued with fever and abdominal pain, and in addition, he was not alert. Additional x-rays, scans, and laboratory procedures were done to ascertain his problem. It was necessary to surgically explore his abdomen to establish a diagnosis so it could be treated properly.

This was done after Jeff had been treated with antibiotics for several days to protect him against further complications. At surgery, the distal end of the tube in the abdominal cavity was found to be obstructed from adhesions. The tube was replaced, cultures were done, and Jeff once again "made the grade." After a month in the hospital he was released to recover at home. Under the watchful and experienced care of his parents, he progressed steadily, improving more rapidly than expected, and by early spring of 1984, he had recovered well enough to be able to return to college in the fall of that year. He did just that. During the spring and summer, Jeff concentrated on improving his physical health and mental acuity by doing all the right things. He had set a goal for himself and was determined to realize it. In the spring of 1985, Jeff donned his cap and gown and took that walk down the aisle and up to the stage to receive his college diploma. To me, that was a miracle.

Not many victims of hydrocephalus were educable 30 years ago. Those that were could not attain what Jeff had. Most were not supported and encouraged by parents as Jeff was. A great many survivors were not as fortunate as Jeff to have a physician, such as Dr. Cobb, with the God-given ability and foresight to perform the necessary surgeries and give the postoperative care such as Jeff had.

After his graduation from college, Jeff went into social work. Jobs were not easy to find, and he was among the unemployed for some months. He was persistent in searching for the right job, which he found two years ago. Jeff also found the right "girl" and has been happily married since the summer of 1992. Today, he is working regularly in his chosen field of social work with people he loves—mostly the elderly and disabled. He is happily married and head of a household. This young man is surely a miracle wrought by the hand of GOD!

❖ ❖ ❖

"Doctor Wilson, Call 287 STAT!"

I was on duty in the emergency room and when the call came I was just beginning my second meal of the day, and it was now 9 p.m. They paged me again, and I gave up on the plate of beans, macaroni and cheese. Going to the phone, I dialed 287.

Nurse Dalrymple answered immediately. Without waiting she said, "Dr. Wilson, hurry down here. You won't believe what we have for you."

"Ok, I'll be right there. Not waiting for the elevator I ran down two flights, taking two steps at a time. As I burst into the ER, the nurse was waiting and grabbed my arm.

"Wait a minute, Miss Dalrymple, tell me what's going on. What's such a big emergency. I don't see any ambulance, no sirens have been heard, so slow down."

"The patient is in room 3, Doctor. Come on."

As we went into the room I recognized the female as a patient I had seen before. She was pale, anxious, and looked scared.

"Hello, Mrs. Driver. What's the matter?"

"I'm bleeding, Doctor."

"Where are you bleeding from?"

"From my 'privates,' and it hurts too."

"How long have you been bleeding?"

"About an hour. Help me, Doctor."

"I'll do what I can, but first of all I need to know a little about this problem you have."

"Can I talk to you in private, Doctor?"

"Sure. Will you excuse us, Nurse? I'll call when I need you." She gave me a dirty look and left.

"Now, tell me what the problem really is."

"My husband did this to me, Doctor."

"What did he do to make you bleed?"

"He stuck a light bulb 'up me,' 'cause he was mad at me."

"Why was he made at you? Are you and John having trouble again?"

"Yes, and you'll have to ask him about the trouble."

"Ok, I will, but first I'll need to examine you. Nurse, I need you, please. Will you prepare Mrs. Driver for a pelvic exam? We will need plenty of 4 x 4 sponges, a good light, and long forceps. I'll be back in shortly."

"We're ready, Doctor," the nurse called.

"How are her vital signs, Miss Dalrymple."

"All are normal except a pulse rate of 120. I thought it was fright."

"Maybe so, but call the lab to come down for a CBC and do a cross match, just in case. Let's take a look at the patient to see if we can find the cause of this bleeding."

The patient's feet were in stirrups, the knees bent, and her buttocks were on the edge of the table. The light was in focus—the nurse was very efficient—and "antsy."

"We are going to examine you now, Mrs. Driver, so just relax and open your knees. As she did I could see a goodly amount of fresh blood oozing from the vagina, and the underpad was soaked. I inserted the speculum and saw a fresh clot filling the entire vagina. "Sponge forceps, Nurse." Instantly, they were in my hand. As I pulled the clots from the vagina and cleared the field with dry sponges, I was able to see several small lacerations on either side and in the roof, and larger ones were in the floor of the vagina. I also encountered broken pieces of thin glass that were typical of a light bulb. We saved all of these as evidence in case there was a suit from this incident. Some of the larger lacerations would require surgery, and I so informed the patient. Then we packed her vagina with gauze to slow the bleeding until we could repair the lacerations.

"We'll have to take you to surgery, Mrs. Driver. You need to sign a permit for the surgery, ok? I need to talk to your husband also. Miss Dalrymple, can you get the surgery scheduled right away while I talk to Mr. Driver. Also, give her the pre-op one-half hour before surgery is scheduled."

"Yes, Doctor."

Going out into the vestibule I spotted the husband, pacing the floor and smoking a cigarette.

"Mr. Driver, I need to talk to you in private. Come with me, please." In the room, behind closed doors, I confronted him with what the patient had told us.

"Mr. Driver, did you actually push a light bulb into your wife's vagina? If you did, then you must have been very mad or out of your mind."

"Yeah, I did it Doc, and I'll tell you why I did. I was mad enough to kill her at the time. I really just wanted to get even with her for something she did about two weeks ago."

"What happened?"

"I went home, unexpectedly, and she was in bed with another man. You can guess what was going on. I threatened to kill both of them and went for a gun. Of course, he ran out when I left the room. I didn't do anything then, but it had been eating on me all this time. So I decided to do this to her the next time we made love, and tonight it happened. At the right moment I rammed the light bulb in her 'to get even.'"

"I can't believe you could do such a thing, Mr. Driver."

"When somebody hurts you so much and you get mad enough, Doc, I think a person might do anything. They might just go off the deep end and kill the one they love most."

"You're probably right. How did your wife react to your attack?"

"Aw, she screamed and hollered 'You bastard, you've ruint me, I'm bleeding to death. Call a doctor.' I let her wait a few minutes, then brought her here so you could help her. Now I'm real sorry I did it, Doctor."

"You should be. She really is not badly injured, but she has several 'cuts' in her vagina, and some of them will have to be sutured."

"What do you mean sutured, Doctor?"

"We'll have to put some stitches in the larger ones. To do it right, we will have to take her to surgery where we will have the proper light and instruments to work with."

"Ok, whatever you say, Doc. I trust you, and I'll pay you too."

The surgery went well, requiring several sutures. The procedure lasted about an hour, and during this time the husband had time to think everything through and decided he was not entirely blameless in the incident, confessing to me that maybe he had "sinned" a time or two also, but didn't get caught. Before Mrs. Driver was dismissed, the couple had reconciled, and they went away happy. Her follow-up visits showed her to be well-healed in three weeks, and they were anxious to resume their "love life." Mrs. Driver was dismissed from our care, and I presumed that all was well with the marriage.

❖ ❖ ❖

"Dr. Wilson, you have an urgent call from Madison Hospital. This way to the phone." We were in a meeting 30 miles from the hospital, and I was the presiding officer.

"Hello, this is Dr. Wilson. What's the problem?"

"This is Mrs. Youngblood in OB, and we have an emergency that needs something done as soon as possible."

"Who is the patient?"

"Your 16-year-old primipara, Mrs. Eaves, that's due in two weeks. She is bleeding and has some abdominal pain. Looks like a premature separation of the placenta (afterbirth). Blood pressure is going down, and pulse is going up."

"Yes, I agree. Start an IV, type and cross match for four units of blood. Call surgery and anesthesia. Also, see if you can find Dr. Pittman and ask her to be there when surgery is ready. Dr. Johnson and I will be there as soon as we can drive from Springfield."

I asked the vice-chairman to take over, collected my wife with Dr. and Mrs. Johnson, and we were on our way. Fortunately, there was not much traffic and no Highway Patrol. Time was of the essence, and I drove at break-neck speed, sometimes nearing 100 m.p.h. In about 20 minutes we arrived at the hospital. Dr. Johnson broke the silence for the first time since we left Springfield. "Dr. Wilson, you're a good driver, but I'll never ride with you again on an emergency call." I looked at Jessie, and she was staring straight ahead with a scared look on her face and still clutching the door.

"Are you ok, honey?"

"Y-yes, I guess so."

"Well, we made it. You drive Marcy (Mrs. Johnson) home, and I'll call when we are finished."

"Ok." She never looked at me.

I ran to the OB floor as the nurses were pushing the gurney up a curved incline toward the operating room. As I looked, a strap holding the patient gave way. The nurse saw the patient falling off the stretcher and caught her to prevent a catastrophe.

She yelled, "Stop! Somebody help me!"

By that time, we were all there, got the patient back on the gurney, to OR, and onto the operating table.

"Are you ok, Mrs. Youngblood?"

"No, I think I have ruptured a disc."

"We'll check that in the operating room. Let's get her to OR rapidly."

Within five minutes we had changed into scrub suits, and the surgery crew was prepping the patient. The Pediatrician was there, IV fluids were going, and the patient was stabilized.

The nurse said, "The fetal heart is still ok, doctor."

"How is the bleeding and her blood pressure?"

"Blood pressure 110/60. Pulse 100. Bleeding has decreased."

"Good. Go ahead and drape the patient. We'll be ready in two more minutes." It took me about two minutes to put on the gown and gloves, and

I was ready. Dr. Johnson said, "Go ahead, Dr. Wilson, I'll be with you by the time you make the incision."

Everybody was poised and ready. "How is the patient, Mr. Bowen?"

"She's doing fine. You can go ahead." (I always waited for the anesthetist to say ok.)

"I'm making the incision, a long one, from the pubis to the umbilicus in this case since we have to deliver the baby very rapidly. Everything is fine. Is she all right now, Mr. B?"

"She's fine. How are you doing?"

"A-ok. The uterus is exposed and looks good. We'll open the uterus now." I glanced at Dr. Pittman. She nodded and smiled.

"We are opening the uterus now." I was making the incision through the thick muscle of the uterus as my assistant clamped bleeders. "Suction, Miss Jacobs!" The blood and amniotic fluid was flowing out and over the drapes. Dr. Johnson was rapidly extracting the baby as I began to suction the infant's mouth and nose while the nurse was wiping the face with a "lap" sponge. I was clamping the cutting the cord as Dr. Johnson gave the baby a sharp slap on the buttocks. The baby was crying lustily and was handed to the Pediatrician. Everybody breathed a sigh of relief as we turned our attention, once again, to the patient.

"Look at this placenta, Dr. Johnson. It's a good thing we got here in a hurry."

"Yes, it is, but I'd rather not hurry so fast next time" (referring to my driving).

"Is the patient ok now, Mr. Bowen?"

"She's fine doctor."

Now I was separating the spongy-like tissue of the placenta from the wall of the uterus. As I did so we could easily see that it had separated about 25 percent of its surface from the uterine wall. This would have extended and endangered the life of both mother and baby.

The mother was given Pitocin to contract the uterine muscle, and some was also injected into the uterus. "We are now ready to close the uterus and abdominal wall."

"Saline, Miss Jacobs." She was pouring the solution into the cavities as we suctioned out the bloody collections of amniotic and peritoneal fluids.

With a large, curved needle and heavy catgut suture, I was closing the uterus with several interrupted sutures that would withstand any pressure on the walls. I next closed the abdomen with four layers of sutures. Now we covered this with a heavy gauze dressing and taped it onto the skin.

"How is the baby now, Dr. Pittman?"

"He's fine. I'll take him to the nursery and let the family see him."

"Thank you for coming to help us, Doctor," I added.

"Mrs. Eaves, you have a healthy baby boy."

Hardly awake, she whispered, "Thank you, Doctor."

"Everything is fine. Why don't you sleep a while, then I'll talk to you more."

She had an uneventful recovery from the surgery and later had another child, which was delivered uneventfully. She was under my care for the next 30 years until the time of my retirement.

❖ ❖ ❖

Another complicated OB patient was a primipara at the other end of the age group. A 40-year-old with Addison's Disease came to us for prenatal care and delivery. Because of her illness she was referred to the nearby University Medical Center where she could be monitored closely for her endocrine problem. All was apparently well for the next six weeks. Then one day as I check the appointments, I noted her name listed for the last one of that day. When she came in, her husband was with her. Hmn—something is wrong, or Harry wouldn't be here.

"Hello, Mrs. Hosey, come in. And how are you, Harry? Have a seat."

"We're fine."

"I'm glad to hear that. How are things going with your pregnancy?"

"That's what we came to see you about," said Harry.

"I want you and Dr. Johnson to take care of Alice and deliver our baby."

I was stunned! "Alice, you have a big problem, and you really need to stay under the care of the University obstetricians. They are certainly more capable of handling any complications that may arise."

"That is the problem. I don't feel comfortable with them. To them, I am just patient number 1001, not an individual that needs personal attention. They don't seem to care as you folks do."

Deep inside I knew she was right. After all is said and done, *caring* is what our profession is all about.

"Alice, give me a day or two to consult with Dr. Johnson, and we'll call you. I do appreciate the confidence you have in me. Take care of yourself. I'll call as soon as we can work things out."

The next day I presented the problem to Dr. Johnson for his sage advice.

"Well, doctor, I tell you, we can probably care for her as well as they can if she feels that way about the situation."

In his slow drawl, puffing on his ever-present cigar between words, he suggested, "Why don't you take care of her and I'll be your consultant." That was really what I wanted to hear him say.

"I'm ready to accept the challenge with your help. I'll call Alice and let her know of our decision."

At the end of that day, I called her from the office to let her know that we could accept her as a patient on condition that she would inform the OB department at the University that this was their (she and Harry's) decision. After we obtained her clinic records, she was seen regularly and often so we could monitor her progress and watch for any possible complications. Near the calculated time of delivery, pelvic measurements were done, as in all OB patients. I could not believe the readings. There was no way she could deliver a baby through that small pelvic outlet.

I must have had a look of doom on my face after reading the measurements.

"Is the baby all right, Doctor?"

"Oh, yes, the baby is perfectly normal, but we'll have to take some x-rays of your pelvis. The measurements show that you're too small to deliver a baby in a normal way. Let's take the x-ray and have the radiologist read them and be our consultant."

"Whatever you say, Doctor."

We sent her to the nearby hospital with a request for pelvic outlet measurements. They called back almost immediately.

"Dr. Wilson, this is Dr. Gilbert. I've seen your patient's x-rays, and I agree that she'll have to be delivered by caesarean section due to an unusually small pelvis."

"Thank you, doctor. I'll await your report."

"Mrs. Smith, call Mrs. Hosey, please."

"Dr. Wilson, Mrs. Hosey is on line two."

"Hello, Alice. How are you today? I'm calling about your x-ray reports. As we told you, the baby is fine, and your x-rays do confirm our findings of a small pelvis. I need to schedule you for the surgery. Can you and your husband come in tomorrow?"

The next day Harry and Alice came as frightened as two younger people because the baby would come into the world by a method other than what God had intended. "There is really no problem concerning the baby, Mrs. Hosey. On the other hand, we have to recognize the fact that you have been on steroids, and that trauma of any type can effect your problem. For this reason, you'll need to increase your dosage by 50 percent for two days before the surgery. We will also be giving the medication by IV route, immediately before and after surgery, to further protect you. Are there any questions?"

"When do you plan to do the surgery?"

"Let's see. This is April 30. How about a week from today?"

"That's fine with me. Ok with you, Harry?"

"Fine, whenever Doc," said Harry.

On May 6, 1956, we performed a caesarean section on Mrs. Hosey under spinal anesthesia, delivering a normal, healthy male infant who cried lustily, was pink and flailing both arms and legs. Everything went well with the procedure, and the patient made an uneventful recovery. I visited her twice daily for a week and monitored her dose of steroids around the clock. By then she was stable and ready to be discharged.

"How do you feel, Alice? Are you ready to go home?"

"I feel fine and I'm ready to go home now!"

"Can you manage your steroid injections at home, or do you want the nurse to come by for a few days?"

"I can take care of that all right."

"Good. Don't forget to keep your salt intake high at all times. Remember what we have discussed about that need when you have to control your problem of Addison's Disease."

"I will. I promise." She held her arms out and we embraced as she said a tearful "Thank you, Doctor. You did a wonderful job." At that moment, I felt proud, humbled, and thankful that this woman had been able to conceive, carry a fetus to term, then have a seemingly healthy, normal baby. Here she was with a life-threatening illness, she had lost one ovary and part of the other one, and was 40 years of age. It was almost a miracle. God was surely watching over this woman (and her doctor).

❖   ❖   ❖

A third unusual OB case I recalled happened shortly after the last one. Again, the good Lord must have been looking over my shoulder.

Mrs. Ballou was a 32-year primipara that was in her eighth week of pregnancy when I first saw her. She was a large woman, not obese, just with a large body. Her initial examination showed nothing abnormal except a "borderline" blood pressure. The initial pelvic measurements were adequate, the fetal size was normal, and I felt she would have no problems with delivering babies. The prenatal course was uneventful, with little weight gain, and the blood pressure stayed controlled. Near the EDC we repeated her pelvic measurements, and they were great. In about 10 days I got a call at 6 a.m.

"Doc, this is Avery Ballou. I think my wife is ready to go to the hospital."

"How often are her pains, Mr. Ballou?"

"About every five minutes. She's hurtin' bad, Doc."

"Take her to the hospital. I'll be there by that time. On the way, I kept reviewing her case. Everything should be all right with her, unless her blood pressure could go up.

As I walked into the OB department they were paging, "Dr. Wilson, call 3458." I entered the nurses station and was greeted with, "Boy! I'm glad to see you."

"Do you have a problem?"

"Could be. I think the patient is scared and needs something for her pain. Her blood pressure is up a bit—150/90. I haven't had time to check her as yet.

"Let me take a look, so we can see what's going on."

As we walked into the room the patient was groaning, tossing about, and had a wild look on her face.

"Hi, Mrs. Ballou. Are you ok?"

"I'm having hard pains, Doctor. Can't you give me something right now?"

"Let me check you first. We want to be sure your baby is all right before we give you something that might hurt him.

As I check the baby's heart, a contraction started. It was a good, strong one, but it did not affect the fetal heart sounds. That was a good sign. Her blood pressure was still 150/90. Her heart sounded very strong, regular, and normal.

"Everything seems to be fine with you and the baby. Here, let me examine you further." I slipped on a pair of sterile gloves and examined the birth canal. The fetal head was down to a 1+ station. The cervix was beginning to thin out and was dilated about 2 cm. All of this was normal for her hours of labor and a first pregnancy. "You're doing great, Mrs. Ballou, and the baby is ok also. We'll give you a shot to ease the pain some so you can relax between contractions. The nurse will be here all the time and will check you both. She'll take good care of you. Try to relax between pains so you can rest some. I'll be back in an hour or two, just as soon as we finish in surgery."

"Mrs. Goodnite, give this patient 50 mg. of Meperidine IM now, and I'll leave more orders on her chart."

I made an admission note, observing her appearance and all of the physical findings that were pertinent, underscoring the blood pressure level. Left orders for more pain medication when indicated. Then I talked with the husband, explaining what we found on examining her, and that it was all normal. I reassured him that I felt everything would be all right and that she would be closely watched by capable and experienced nurses. Then I added that I would be back to check her before I left for the office. I saw four or five patients on the floors, did a case of surgery and went back to OB. I presumed everything was progressing normally.

"How is our patient, Mrs. Goodnite?"

"She's doing well. I have checked her once, and she had made a little progress."

That had been about two hours since I examined her. Let me have a sterile glove, please."

The patient was drowsy. "Mrs. Ballou, I need to examine you again so we can tell if you're progressing." I examined her; she didn't resist. The cervix had thinned, but very little since the first exam—the station was now 1.5+, and dilation was 2.5 cm. Progress would be slow. I checked the fetal heart. It was 118/min., regular and strong.

"You're ok now, Mrs. Ballou. Push a little with your pains, and that will help." I saw the husband again, gave him a report and left for the office. The OB nurse checked with me every two hours, and things began to pick up about 5 p.m. After I finished office hours and checked with OB, all was still quiet. I went home for a quick meal (the first food since 6 am.). Just as I was finishing, the phone rang.

"Dr. Wilson, this is Goodnite in OB. I think you had best come, no big rush, but Mrs. Ballou is progressing pretty fast now."

"Ok, I'll be there in 15 minutes."

Traffic was a little slow, and I was delayed some. When I arrive they had Mrs. Ballou on the delivery table. I greeted the family, changed to a scrub suit quickly, and was in the delivery room in three minutes. Examination of the patient revealed that she was fully dilated, but the station was only +3. The fetal heart was still 120, strong and regular. I had a premonition that we might have a problem if we should give her a general anesthetic.

"Mrs. Ballou, we need to give you something that will keep you from having any pain when the baby's born."

By then the patient was awake. She protested, "I don't want a needle in my back doctor."

"It would really be the best for you and the baby if we could give you a spinal anesthetic, Mrs. Ballou."

"No, I don't want a spinal. I won't take one."

"Ok, if that's how you feel. Mrs. Goodnite, have her husband come to the door so we can explain it to him." He felt the same as his wife and signed papers to that effect. By now, she was straining and pushing with each contraction, but making little, if any, progress.

"Nurse, check the fetal heart now and with the next contraction."

After check she reported, "It's 126 now, regular and strong. Here comes a contraction." She kept listening.

"Is it ok now?"

"No, its only 50. The patient is now asleep."

"How is the patient, Mr. B?"

"Her blood pressure has dropped some, but she's all right."

"If the fetal heart is still low with the next contraction, I'll have to do an emergency C-section," I said.

"Check it right now, Nurse!" I looked at her as she was shaking her head as she listened and timed the beat. It was still the same.

"Call surgery, stat!"

"The supervisor has called. They're doing a case now and can't be ready for another hour."

"We can't wait 15 minutes, or we'll lose this baby and could lose the mother too," I shouted. "Get the emergency tray. Intubate her, Mr. Bowen. Prep her abdomen, and I'll need two more people to assist. Ask lab to type and cross match for two units of blood STAT. Have the husband sign a permit for surgery. Now let's get going before it's too late."

Within five minutes all of those things had been done, and we were ready to do the section. I looked at Mr. B. He nodded for us to go ahead.

"Scalpel, Mrs. Goodnite. We have to do this one real quickly. I'm making the long incision as I talk. Clamp those bleeders!" I was now opening the fascia (the glistening, white, tough membrane protecting the muscle and supporting the abdominal wall).

"How is she, Mr. B?"

"Everything is under control."

"Retractors, please." The assistant pulled the skin and fatty layers to each side. Now I was opening the peritoneum (the last layer before getting inside the abdominal cavity). The assistant and I each picked up a small bit of tissue with a hemostat. I made a nick in the thin tissue and fluid came flowing out. We then opened this layer the entire length of the incision, inserted a Balfour retractor, and I suctioned fluid as we exposed the uterus.

"Let's get this baby out! Everybody ready?"

"Scalpel!" I made the incision. "Heavy scissors, Nurse." I was enlarging the incision in the uterus while the assistants clamped bleeders, and the scrub nurse was suctioning blood and fluids from the incision.

I was working as fast as possible, frantically extracting the baby. He was a big baby. The umbilical cord was wrapped around his neck twice. That was the problem. I clamped and cut the cord while the nurse was suctioning the amniotic fluid and blood from his nose and mouth. A slap to his buttocks, and he cried. (What beautiful music.) The supervisor, who had a sterile blanket, took the baby to the nursery. Now I had time to survey the situation. We had worked so fast that instruments were thrown instead of handled and had to be retrieved. The blood and fluids had soaked the drapes, and they were changed. Then we all became calm.

"How is the mother, Mr. B?"

"She's still doing fine."

"Thank you. I didn't have time to think about her. I knew she was in good hands!"

"Thank you, Doctor. You did a good, fast one this time."

"I *had to*. How long did it take?"

"About 12 minutes from the skin until the baby was out."

"It felt like an eternity to me. Let's close her abdomen."

The uterus was closed with large catgut sutures, then reinforced with a second layer of fine sutures. Now I was ready to close the abdominal layers.

"Scissors!" The didn't appear in my hand. Again, I yelled, "Scissors!"

"I can't find them, Doctor."

My heart sank. "Where are they?" Then I thought of how we had slung instruments in our hurry to delivery the baby. *Please, Lord, let them be in her tummy.* I groped and searched in the abdomen and pelvic region. I touched something that felt like metal! A second feel, and there was the pair of missing scissors. "Thank God we found them." I had to calm myself for a minute to continue.

"Saline, Mrs. Goodnite."

She poured two quarts in the abdominal cavity as we suctioned and sponged it dry.

"All instruments are now accounted for, Doctor."

That broke the ice, and I closed the abdomen as we rehashed what had transpired during that frantic half-hour. By the time we finished the surgery the mother was beginning to react; her BP was normal, and she was sent to recovery.

I saw the new father, explained in detail what had happened, what we did and why, also that mother and baby were well off. They continued to do well and were dismissed one week later.

As a sequel to this, two years later that lady was back with her second pregnancy. All went well, and I followed the adage, "Once a C-section, always a C-section." We scheduled her for a time just before the EDC. Somehow it happened that was the same time as our vacation some 300 miles away. The patient was very insistent that I take care of her and do the surgery. Since we would be at my mother-in-laws, I assured her that I would be back and do the C-section. After four days, Jessie and I drove back home and left the children with "Maw-Maw." I did the surgery, visited the patient twice, and left her in the care of my partner. We had a 2-day "honeymoon" at a Kentucky state park, then returned to Indiana, and everybody was happy.

❖ ❖ ❖

During the 15-year period that I delivered babies (roughly 1,000), I saw several born into the world with congenital deformities, some that were ill when born, and delivered a few stillborns. In this part of practice one can be praised to high heaven or damned to the depths of purgatory. Most of the time there was a happy ending for the families, and one was praised much more than damned. I thoroughly enjoyed the years when I was doing obstetrics.

One of the most unusual cases I had in my OB practice was a surprise and a shocker. A 19-year-old with her second pregnancy had an uneventful antepartum course, went into labor at her expected date of delivery, and delivered after eight hours of labor. The baby was normal in all respects, and everything seemed to be fine. As I cared for the newborn I noted some unusual bleeding.

"Massage the fundus, Nurse."

That didn't seem to help much, and I massaged the fundus myself. It is very firm, which was normal, and yet the bleeding continued. I kept massaging as I pulled on the umbilical cord. There was no "give" to the pressure and pulling. That bothered me more than a little. *That placenta (after birth) should be separating by this time,* I thought.

"How is her blood pressure, Nurse?"

"Ok, 110/70. Pulse 100."

"What was her Hemoglobin and RBC count on admission?"

"RBC 4 million, Hgb 13—all else normal."

"Call lab for a repeat of both STAT. Also ask them to type and cross match for three units of packed RBC."

We kept trying to deliver the placenta with usual methods. Nothing happened. By this time I was getting anxious and pulled much harder on the cord. It was as if I were pulling on an immovable object. "Is Dr. Cothren in the building?"

"Yes. He happens to be on the OB floor."

"Ask him if he can come in. I need his opinion on how to treat this case."

By this time, the lab report was back.

"Here's her lab report, Doctor. She reads: RBC 3 M, Hgb. 10.5." That shook me. Something had to be done soon! An hour or two had passed, and the placenta was not separating, and the bleeding continued. I knew we had to open her abdomen and look at the uterus. This was an unusual problem.

"What is your problem, Dr. Wilson?"

"I'm not sure. We may have a placenta accretia." Then I recited everything that happened and what we had done—with negative results.

"Would you check her and give an opinion, please."

"Sure, I'll be glad to."

He examined her very carefully, pulled on the cord, and nothing happened. Another hard pull, and there was a gush of blood. He looked at me, shaking his head. "I think you're right. I suggest you get her to surgery right now before she bleeds out. You will have to do a hysterectomy to save this girl. I'll write a consult for you."

"Thank you, Dr. Cothren, I appreciate your help and advice."

"You're welcome. Let me know what you find." He left to take care of his own patients.

"Call surgery, Ms. Youngblood, and ask them to hurry. I'll need an assistant. I also want you to be there, if possible."

"Ask Mr. Woods to come to the dressing room."

"How is my wife, Dr. Wilson?"

"She's ok, but we have an unusual problem that needs attention immediately.

In layman terms, I explained what the problem was and what had to be done to be sure his wife would be all right. As I was talking he began to tremble and I saw small beads of sweat on his lip and forehead.

"Sit down, James. How are you? Nurse! Ask this man's mother to come here."

"Amanda, we have a problem with Nora. We will have to take her to surgery right now. You need to help James through this. I'll explain more later. Come up to the surgical waiting room."

Within a half-hour we were in OR and ready to do a hysterectomy. I didn't like to think of doing a hysterectomy on a 19-year-old, but knew that was the only route to take to salvage her. But I was still hesitant.

"Let's start a unit of blood, Mrs. Sweet. Is she ready to be prepped?"

"Yes, Doctor. The catheter is in place, and everything is ready for you to start."

"May I start the surgery, Mr. B.?" He nodded "Yes."

The abdomen was draped. My hand was trembling slightly as I made the incision in her lower abdomen. We were proceeding swiftly with the procedure, and all was going well.

"Let me sponge your forehead, Doctor." I wasn't aware I was sweating so profusely.

Mr. Bowen said, "Just relax, Doctor. Everything is fine."

What a friend. "I'm fine now, thanks."

Now we were through the last layer of the abdominal wall and could see the uterus. It was firm, purplish in color, firm to touch, and a bit lumpy. As I was feeling it there seemed to be a mass that I could outline. This had to be the placenta. I was massaging it, but nothing was happening."

"Let's go ahead with the procedure. Retractors in place, we pulled the uterus up for better exposure and proceeded with the surgery."

"Large Kellys, please." Swiftly, surely, and firmly they appeared in my hand. I was clamping the fallopian tubes and dividing them at the edge of the uterus. The supporting ligaments were treated in the same way. Then I incised some tissue and pushed the urinary bladder away from the uterus. As I was clamping and dividing the arteries (blood supply) to the uterus, I had a twinge of guilt at having to do this to a 19-year-old, but knew it was the only answer to the problem. As we removed the enlarged, purplish organ, with the umbilical cord protruding form the mouth dangling 18 inches away, I was thinking of what had happened to this young woman during the last 10 hours. The urge to open the uterus overwhelmed me, but I remembered the words of our pathology professor: "Leave all surgical specimens intact." I placed it in the specimen basin and proceeded to close the incision, swiftly and in silence. Although I knew we had done everything we could to prevent the surgery, I still had that twinge of guilt.

Arriving back at the hospital the next morning, my first stop was the pathology lab. Nobody was in. It was *7:00. They should be here*! The time dragged by as I made rounds. AT 8:30, I dialed pathology. "Dr. Stegall, have you had a chance to look at the uterus I had to remove last night?"

"No, but I was just about to start. Come on down and give me a history as we open."

I took the stairs—the elevator was too slow. I knocked on the door. As I went in, Dr. Stegall was ready to open the "specimen."

"This is unusual. Tell me about the case," Dr. Stegall asked. I outlined the entire night, starting with the delivery, my diagnosis, the consult, and finally the procedure.

"Sounds like you had no choice. Let's see what we can find." He proceeded to open the uterus with an incision from the fundus (top) and through the entire length, being careful to avoid the still intact placenta and cord.

"You were right, Doctor. This placenta could not have been removed. It was growing into the walls of the uterus. This looks like placenta accretia all right. After I do the microscopic then we'll know."

Back up to Minerva's room I went to give them the news that her problem was rare, and that the surgery was the only route we could have taken.

"Good morning, Minerva. How do you feel?"

"I feel fine. I'm a little sore and have some pain."

"Have you seen your baby?"

"Yes, he's beautiful." She named him Antonio.

"That is a beautiful name. Sounds romantic. I want to tell you about your problem and what we had to do. After the baby was born, the afterbirth wouldn't let go. You began to bleed some, and we had to transfuse you and operate because we were afraid of losing you. We had to remove your womb in order to save your life. The afterbirth had grown into the wall of your womb so deeply that it was impossible to remove it without risking the chance of your hemorrhaging to death. That is so rare that I have never before seen such a case, and neither has Dr. Johnson who has been delivering babies for 30 years. Your tubes and ovaries are fine, and you can lead a normal life, but you won't be able to have more children."

"That's all right, Doctor. Two is enough anyway. Thank you for what you did."

"You do understand the problem?"

"Yes, I do."

The next day the pathology report was back. The pathologist had described his findings in detail—of how the placenta had grown into the wall of the uterus, that there was partial loss of the decidua basalis and spongiosum layers to the point that the placenta was a part of the wall of the uterus with no chance of separating the two. This relieved me completely of any guilt feelings I had when doing the surgery. The word spread, and each doctor that delivered babies would go by pathology lab to see the gross specimen and take a look at the microscopic too.

❖ ❖ ❖

During my years of practice, I was fortunate enough to treat many families, some of whom were patients of five generations, such as the McMahons, the Meadors, and the Slates. The latter two I had known as a child, since they were patients of my father. They moved to this area and had children. After I came into their neighborhood to practice, they became patients of mine and remained loyal to me until they died or I retired. All families made an impression on me of some type; some much more than others. None left as deep an impression as a special one—the Hosey family.

My first visit to the Hoseys was about 7 a.m. in the latter part of 1951. About 6:30 a.m. the phone rang. When I answered, a friendly voice identified himself as Harry Hosey.

"Yes, Mr. Hosey, what can I do for you?"

"I need you to stop by the house to see my sick children."

"I'll stop by in half an hour."

"Thanks, Doc. Oh, bring your penicillin. I think they all need a shot."

"We'll take care of that. See you in half an hour."

When I arrived there were ten children seated at the long table preparing to eat breakfast. "Come in, Doc. Join us as we say grace." Pointing to a 6-year-old, he said, "Harry, it's your turn—now let's join hands." As we bowed our heads, he said a beautiful prayer. Each child and the father crossed themselves, and all prepared to eat.

"Just a minute. Doc needs to examine you sick ones." He called out five names: Johnny, Harry, Wanda, Charlie, and Mike. "Come over here and meet Doc Wilson." Each child offered their hand as they lined up for the examinations. Then a vivacious, blue-eyed brunette appeared from somewhere. As she came into the room the childrens' faces lit up, and someone said, "That's *Alice!*" The voice was one of adoration.

"Good morning, Doctor. I'm Alice Brittian, a friend of the family."

"Good morning, Miss Brittian, I'm glad to meet you."

"Come on, kids, line up so Doc can look at you," said Harry.

As I went down the line looking at throats and ears, listening to their hearts and lungs, feeling of the neck glands, I would tease each one to help them relax. All had fiery red throats and tonsils that were swollen and covered with white exudate in some. Neck glands (lymph nodes) were enlarged and tender. They all had a strep infection which should respond quickly to penicillin.

"They have strep throat and tonsillitis, Harry. All of them need a shot of penicillin, then more by mouth for three or four days. They should be ok by then."

"Good. Here, kids, pull your pants down. Dr. Wilson is going to give you a shot in the butt to make you well. Who wants to go first? here, Mike, you're the oldest—bend over."

I had the alcohol swabs and penicillin all ready. As I went down the line and gave each an injection, nobody made an objection, nobody cried out, and no tears were shed. I thought I had never seen such self-disciplined children. I was really impressed! When I left, they all said, "Thank you, Doctor."

Driving away from the home, I was thinking of what they had experienced the year before when their mother had died unexpectedly, immediately after giving birth to her twelfth child. They were remarkable children. I was so impressed by them, I called my wife to relate the experience at the Hosey home.

Not long after my visit to the Hoseys, Miss Alice Brittian became Mrs. Harry Hosey, Sr. Within a year, she became ill, had a downhill course, and almost lost her life. She was diagnosed as having Addison's disease caused by the loss of function of the adrenal gland. She was treated at Mayo Clinic and returned there periodically for several months before being released by the Clinic.

After she was released from Mayo Clinic and returned home, we received her medical records from them, along with a letter outlining her treatment, underscoring the necessity of close observation and laboratory follow-ups. She was on large daily doses of cortisone and Flourinef by injection. She was also on a high-sodium (salt) diet and enforced periods of bed rest each day. After several months, she was completely under our care, as well-controlled, and made steady rapid improvement. By the end of 1954, she was her same vivacious self again. In late October or early November, 1955, Mrs. Hosey came to the office because she had missed two menstrual periods and had symptoms of early pregnancy. Our examination was compatible with her history, and she was so informed.

"Are you sure, Doctor?"

"Well, I have done hundreds of pelvic examinations during the last ten years, and I would stake my last dollar that you are pregnant."

"But I've been told that I had very little chance of ever conceiving. You do know that I have lost one ovary and half of the other one?"

"Yes, I know that, but you have been on steroids for two years. *And* you have been 'exposed' to a very potent male during this time. *You are pregnant, Alice Hosey*!"

"But I'm almost 42-years-old, Doctor. Do you think I can carry a baby?"

"We'll have to wait and see. Is your husband with you?"

"No, he's out of town and won't be back for three days."

"We'll need to talk to the both of you about your prenatal care. You do know that you are a high-risk patient because of the Addison's disease and the necessary medication? There could be complications. I feel you should be under the care of an Endocrinologist and an Obstetrician who are well-trained and have dealt with similar problems, preferably at Vanderbilt, which is nearby. Come back in a few days when your husband can come with you."

"We'll do that, Doctor."

"Everything is fine right now. Don't change your lifestyle and be sure to take your shots each day and keep on the diet. See you next week."

The pair returned. I persuaded them to go to the University for her prenatal care, and all was well, I thought. Six weeks later, they showed up in the office for a conference because they were not happy with her care and wanted us to care for her. After a long discussion, and our stipulating certain requirements, we did take her back. Everything went well, and a normal male infant was delivered by caesarean section in May of 1956. A year later, Mrs. Hosey conceived again. In her third month, she hemorrhaged and lost the fetus, but continued to bleed for several hours. Then she called.

"I'm in trouble, Doctor. I think I'm miscarrying. Can you stop by?"

"Sure. I'm leaving for home, and it's on my way. See you in 15 minutes."

I had been at the hospital in surgery for about two hours. During this time there had been a thunderstorm with strong winds and some hail. Outside I realized it was worse than I thought. Limbs were down, power was out in some places, and twigs, leaves, and debris were strewn all along the streets. As I came nearer to the Hosey's home, it was even worse, but power was on. As I drove up, someone came to the door and quickly led me to the patient. Alice was pale, anxious, and sweating.

"Hi, Alice, looks like you're in trouble. Tell me what happened."

"Like I said on the phone, I'm cramping and bleeding. Just before you came I passed some large clots. I feel better now, but I'm still bleeding. We saved the clots for you to see. They're in the bathroom."

Someone showed me the specimen. I examined it, and there was no doubt what the problem was. "Can we find a jar to put this in? I want a pathologist to check it to be sure of what we have."

After checking further, finding the blood pressure down, the pulse up, and the patient still bleeding, I asked them to take her to the hospital immediately.

"We will, but before you leave take a look at Wanda. She's had a stomachache for about six hours, and it's worse than it was earlier. She's in here."

"Hello, Wanda. I hear you have a tummy ache."

"Yes, sir, I do. I've had it since 4 o'clock."

"Are you sick to your stomach?"

"A little, but I haven't vomited."

"Where's your pain now?"

"Around my navel and in my right side."

"Let me take a look at you, Wanda." Feeling of her abdomen it was a bit tight. As I check her peri-umbilical region, there was mild tenderness. When I touched the right, lower abdomen (McBurney's Point) she pushed my hand away, and the abdomen became rigid. There was no doubt of her diagnosis—she had an acutely inflamed appendix (appendicitis). "Looks like you'll have two patients to go to the emergency room, Bill. This young lady has appendicitis and needs surgery immediately. May I use your phone? Emergency room? I have two surgical patients coming in by car. One is for D & C and the other, for an appendectomy. Get the lab work started as soon as they arrive. Get in touch with surgery to schedule the D & C and follow with the appendix. We'll need to type and cross match for two units of packed cells for the D & C. I'll see you in 45 minutes."

"Everything all set to go, fellows?"

"Yes, sir."

"Mrs. Hosey, you'll have to sign the operative permit for both you and Wanda before we give you any pain medication. I'll see you at the hospital."

When I arrived at the emergency room, the nurse greeted me with, "You just left here. Don't you ever stay home?" (Surprisingly, I didn't feel tired at that moment.)

"Oh, I've been home for supper."

Surgery personnel arrived in the emergency room almost immediately, and we went to the operating room.

"We'll be ready for you in 10 minutes, Doctor."

As I dressed, my thoughts were of the family and all their problems and how they faced them so matter-of-factly. I was confident the surgeries would go well, and they did.

Some five months later, I saw one of the young, teenage boys with acute appendicitis. This was near the end of office hours, and we scheduled the surgery to start around 6 p.m. This was late summer, the time of year when thunderstorms came quickly and severely, usually accompanied by a lot of lightning.

About the time we began, the thunder started. Lights would blink as the lightning flashed, and then thunder came crashing down, shaking the hospital at times. In spite of the storm, the surgery went well. We found the "hot" appendix and freed it up enough to visualize the base and the artery to the appendix. Just as we applied the hemostat to the artery, a bolt of lightning struck nearby, the lights went out, and we were in near-total darkness. At the same time, a loud roar of thunder shook the entire building, the auxiliary flashed momentarily, and we were in total darkness for sure. We were to the point of no return and had to remove that appendix. Ever resourceful, the operating room supervisor came up with two or three flashlights, and we finished the operation by that light source. This type of thing could happen only to the Hosey family. All went well. The patient had a good postoperative course, and went home in five days.

During that same year I delivered a baby for one of the older married girls. Also during that calendar year, Mrs. Hosey conceived for the third time, and all went along normally until within three weeks of the expected date of confinement. It was early on Sunday afternoon when I got the call from Alice! "Doctor, I'm bleeding. What shall I do?"

"Get to the hospital as fast as you can. I'll meet you there." I arrived first, as anxious as if I were the father expecting the firstborn. Soon, Alice arrived pale, weak, feeling faint, and sweating freely. Examination revealed blood pressure was low, pulse rapid (110). Fetal heart tones normal. There was a moderate amount of vaginal bleeding.

"Mrs. Vest, call the laboratory for stat counts, then type, and cross match for four units of packed red cells."

"They've been called and are on their way."

"Let's get surgery here, STAT. We will have to section her as soon as possible. Call Dr. Pittman, too, please, and let me talk to her. Have the patient sign an operative permit now."

Within a 30-minute period, Mrs. Hosey was in the operating room, a spinal anesthetic had been given, and we were doing the "C section." All went well in spite of the fact she had a 40 percent separation of the placenta (after birth). Thank God that was her last pregnancy. I might not have made it through a fourth one!

❖ ❖ ❖

Several years went by without any unusual happenings in that family. Alice stayed under control with her steroids, the children grew up, married, and had children of their own. They had a family business that grew successfully, and opened a second business that kept all of them busy. Grandchildren came in great numbers, until it reached near 50. But tragedy struck again in 1982, when one of the sons-in-law lost his life from a malignancy. His illness was dramatic and sudden in onset. He lived about one year after the onset.

In the summer of 1984, Mr. Hosey had an accident—bumping his head on the door frame of the car when getting in, striking the left temple region. I saw him about two weeks later because of his headaches, slurred speech, and unsteady gait. This symptom complex, along with his history, was typical of a subdural hematoma (a blood clot on the brain) caused by the blow to his head. He was immediately referred to a Neurosurgeon, had surgery the next day, recovered nicely, regaining all of his faculties. Now (1993) well past the age of 80 years, he makes regular trips to Haiti where he has been building schools and medical clinics for the natives.

It is almost unbelievable that I have been so fortunate to have so many interesting experiences while taking care of many wonderful families. If I were able to recall even 10 percent of the dramatic events with families during the 40 years of practice, it would fill a thousand pages.

House Calls and Emergencies

The practice of medicine is a fascinating life. To me, doing general practice had to be the most interesting phase of all medicine. You touched the lives of all ages, from conception to the grave. In my years of practice, doctors and patients had good relationships. There was a bonding effect between us like no other type. Doctors knew the innermost secrets of their patients, those things that so affected their lives that it unburdened them to talk to someone about it. Who was better than the family physician?

It also helped me personally when I went into a home to see the lifestyle they led, the filth or cleanliness of the home, the memorabilia they kept or discussed. It gave me an insight into the life of that person, their loves, their dislikes, and how they related to spouses and children. Proper treatment of many "illnesses" depended on that knowledge that could not be gained in a 20-minute office visit. House calls were frequent and varied in my early practice. Of course, some were unforgettable, and a few I will recall.

Being reared by a country-doctor father where 90 percent of his practice was in patient's homes, I assumed that house calls were to be expected, day or night. In addition, I had four years of private practice, in which house calls were an integral part of practice, and I knew they were often abused. Many were the times I would go with my father to a home 8 to 10 miles away to see someone with a very minor problem or a simple tension headache, or a woman distraught over a family quarrel. In those days, I learned that when a patient called, the doctor was supposed to go to their aid, regardless of the hour or the reason.

❖   ❖   ❖

My first house call in Old Hickory came at 2 a.m. It was at the time I was here to "evaluate" the practice while Dr. Johnson was out of town for medical reasons. They telephone jangled, and I was wide awake.

"Hello, this is Dr. Wilson."

"Doc, this is Watson. Can you come to my wife?"

"What's the problem, Mr. Watson?"

"She's not feeling good, Doc. She's got a terrible headache."

"Ok, I'll come. Where do you live?"

"At 908 Birdsall Street."

"Where is Birdsall Street?" (I was staying with a brother at 1208 Birdsall).

He snickered, "Why, Doc, hit's jist three block from where you are right now."

"Oh, that's right. I'll be right there." Five minutes later I was knocking on his door.

He was smiling. "I see you found me all right. Come in, Doctor." I didn't bother to introduce myself at 2 a.m. I had already "smelled a rat."

"Mama is right puny. She's upstairs." He was leading the way. "The doctor is here, hon. He'll take care of you."

"Good morning, Mrs. Watson. I'm Dr. Wilson. Do you have a problem?" I sure stuck my neck out.

"I sure do, or I wouldn't have called you. I have a terrible headache, and I haven't slept all night."

"Where's this headache, Mrs. Watson?"

"All over. It starts in my forehead, then spreads over the rest of my head."

"Is it throbbing?"

"Sometimes it does."

I was examining the back of her head and neck. The muscles were tight, but not tender. As I gently massaged the muscles, they were relaxing.

"How is your headache now?"

"A little better. What you did helped."

"Let me take your blood pressure"—BP 134/78. I checked her pulse (longer than usual)—P 88, regular. I then listened to the carotid arteries (in her neck), then her heart, then her reflexes. Everything was normal, and Mrs. Watson was smiling.

"Are you on any medicines at present?"

"Oh, yes. I have to take medicine all of the time."

"May I see them?" Mr. Watson handed me two bottles. I check the labels: Empirin with Codeine, 1/2 grain; Phenobarbital, 1 grain—take one 3 times daily for nerves.

"Mrs. Watson, I can't find anything wrong at this moment. I think we can give you a little shot that will relieve this headache." As I prepared an injection of Codeine, I asked, "Did you have a son in college at MTSU? I knew a Fount Watson in my class there."

"Oh, yes, that's our boy."

"I thought maybe he was. He favors you with the same black eyes and hair. Let's give you this little shot. You should feel a lot better in another ten minutes. If your headache continues, come by the office tomorrow afternoon so we can check you better. Good-bye."

When Mr. Watson was letting me out, I remarked that the call was not an emergency.

"Doc, when you put yourself up for a target, somebody is gonna shoot at you. So anytime Mama says she needs a doctor, I'll call one, day or night."

He taught me a lesson! Do your job and keep your mouth shut.

As I made house calls, I remembered what Mr. Watson said to me that night, and I got "shot at" many times over for 20 years.

❖   ❖   ❖

As I rushed from the hospital to my office one day, just as I came into Old Hickory, a man appeared on the corner waving his arms wildly. Then he stepped off the curb, and I was forced to stop. Then I recognized the "wild one." "Mac, what in the world's wrong? Do you have an emergency?"

"I have a very sick child, Doc. Too sick to come to that office and wait two hours."

"What's wrong?"

"She has a high fever and a sore throat. She needs a shot of penicillin." He always knew what to do because he lived with his doctor uncle 30 years ago.

"Ok, come on. Let's go." Old Hickory was a small town, two minutes from end to end by car. We arrived, and I saw Mrs. "Mac," looking harried and worried as she welcomed us.

"Thank you for coming, Doctor. Pam is in here. She has a real high fever and can hardly swallow."

"She still has her tonsils, doesn't she?"

"Yes, she does, and I think that's her problem."

"Have you taken her temperature?"

"We don't have a thermometer."

Mac said, "We don't need a thermometer. I can tell by feeling of her forehead."

"Okay, Mac, tell me what her temperature is now." He placed his hand on her forehead."

"It's 101."

"Let me see what the thermometer says." While I took her temp, I checked her pulse and it was 110/min. The thermometer read 103.5!

"How do you feel, Pam?"

She frowned and spoke in a hoarse whisper, "I feel bad, and my throat hurts too."

"Let me look at you, honey." I check the lymph nodes in her neck; they were three times normal size and 4+ tender. The neck was not stiff, the ears were not red.

"Open your mouth and stick out your tongue. Let me see your tonsils." They were 4+ in size and badly inflamed. The surface was covered with a purulent exudate (pus).

"Let me check your lungs. Breathe deeply, Pam." Heart and lungs were clear.

"Pam, you have a real bad case of tonsillitis. You need a shot of penicillin now because you are real sick."

"I don't want a shot, Doctor. Can't you just give me some medicine?" She was so hoarse that I could barely hear her.

"Honey, you really need a shot. Your throat is bad. It'll hurt some, but it'll make you well a lot faster. If we don't give you this shot, we might have to go to the hospital." That did it!

"Let daddy hold you when I give the shot—then it won't hurt so much." I gave the shot, wrote a prescription, gave instructions, and then looked at the mother. Wow! She looked beat!

"What else is wrong, Mrs. Mac?"

"I was up all night with Pam and my dog started having puppies about five hours ago and is really in trouble. Why don't you help me deliver the puppies so I won't have to take her to the vet?"

"Ok, let's see what we can do." I took off my coat, rolled up my sleeves, put on a pair of surgical gloves, and lubricated them with KY jelly. "Don't let her bite me. I'm allergic to dog bites, not the dog." I examined her and found the head and one foot trying to come through the birth canal together. Pushing both back a few inches, I rotated and delivered the head—then the entire puppy came out easily. Mama dog did the rest. I asked, "Are you ok, now, Mama?" The dog actually seemed to smile at me.

I knew Mac had the reputation of being "tight-fisted." "Ok, Mac, I'll send you a bill for a house call and for delivering a puppy."

"Now, wait a minute, Doctor. I didn't ask you to deliver that puppy. You volunteered for that."

Mac still likes to tell that story. We have had a good relationship for a span of more than 40 years.

❖ ❖ ❖

It was a slow day, and I was waiting for some activity. A call came with, "I need you to come see my sick children."

"Where do you live?"

"Here in Madison. It's just a little ways from your office."

"Ok, I'll be there soon." We went prepared for minor emergencies, always carrying a good supply of penicillin for injections and something for pain and anxiety.

This should have been a quick, easy call with no problems. As I arrived on the porch, I could hear grumbling from inside.

"Come in, Doctor. These boys have a high fever and sore throats. It may be their tonsils."

That was the usual situation, often with a strep infection.

"Hi, fellows, what's wrong?" Sullen faces stared back at me. No answer.

"Who wants to be first? Come on Billy Joe, you're the oldest. Let's look at your tonsils. Open your mouth and say ah. Uh huh. That's the problem. Ok. Now let me check your ears and chest. Now it's your time Paul." He resisted more, and Mama came into play.

"Open that mouth, boy! Let the doctor look at you, and be still!" Evidently Mama carried some weight. He complied. His findings were similar to big brother.

"They both have tonsillitis and strep throat. The ears are fair. They need a penicillin injection to protect them from strep."

"I was hoping you would say that. It does them more good than anything," Mama said.

I began rummaging in the bag and brought out the syringe filled with penicillin and a needle attached. As I did so, one of them (Paul) catapulted from the bed and out the back door with his mother chasing him, at the same time yelling, "Young man, you're going to get it now." About 60 feet from the house she caught him. I watched as she turned him across her knee and gave him a hard spanking. I thought, *That's a good mother that will be respected by her children for life.* With sullen faces, each took his shot in silence. Over the years as I continued to care for the family, the story was recalled many times.

❖ ❖ ❖

The house calls I dreaded most were the ones that came at the end of the work day, usually when the supper had been eaten. There were many men that had heart attacks doing chores or playing sports just after a heavy meal. I would usually rush to these homes when called because I soon learned most of them were dire emergencies. It was not uncommon to find a man of fifty to sixty years of age lying dead beside a lawn mower or on the floor near a work bench. I have been called to find them sitting slumped over dead at the steering wheel of a tractor.

I have crawled under houses to find them dead with plumbing tools still in their hands. Probably the most dramatic ones were the patients that were dying in agony. The scenario was usually of a distraught, shocked family, crying uncontrollably with neighbors rushing in to help.

"Hurry, Doctor, do something for Daddy! Hurry up here." I have sprinted up many stairways to get there in time to do something. In the cases I mentioned, it was usually too late. The patient would be writhing, very cyanotic, struggling desperately to breathe, or in a convulsive state. If he showed any signs of life, such as a pulse, heart sounds, or breath sounds, I would pump his chest and give him Morphine to relax him and hope to relieve his pain. At least 98 percent of these patients were beyond help. In those days, we had not yet developed the modern-day CPR. The only ambulance service available were local funeral homes who did not have lifesaving equipment. Old Hickory was fortunate to have a well-equipped fire hall in the center of the city that had resuscitative equipment and oxygen. We called on them frequently, and those men saved lives with the knowledge and training they had. I am sure that if we had been more knowledgeable in emergency medicine, and had equipment as they have today, some of the patients I saw in those years could have been saved. We didn't, and patients died as a result.

❖ ❖ ❖

House calls in general were a pleasure, and I made many, many of them. Some were unforgettable. Some were near tragedies, some were comical, some were needless, and sometimes they waited too long for anyone to help. Early in my career in Memphis, I made a call at 2 a.m. As I made my way through the house I had to watch closely to keep from stepping on sleeping bodies. As we went out the back door, a sleepy girl spoke up, "Mama, don't let the dogs bite the doctor." By the time she got the words out, I was being attacked by two small dogs biting at my pants legs. My hair stood on end. I started kicking them, and slinging my bag around to ward them off, and made it to the door of a garage apartment without more than a bad scare. That made me cautious from that time on, even to the point that I would ask if they had a dog if I had not been there before, when someone requested that I make a house call.

❖ ❖ ❖

Here are some other things I experienced on house calls. A lady called for me to come see her about 6 p.m. I asked if anyone was with her, and she replied, "Yes, my sister is here."

"Okay, I'll see you in about 30 minutes." I drive about 15 miles, arrived at the house, and knocked on the door.

A melodious voice answered, "Come on in, Doctor." I smelled trouble! The living room was semi-dark and as I went through she called again, "Come on back, Doctor. I'm in here." I stopped at her bedroom door—the picture was like a scene in a movie where the alluring female is dressed in a pink negligee, and she had too much perfume and makeup for a sick woman.

"Where is your sister, Mrs. 'Allure'?"

"She had to go home to see about her kids. It's ok, I won't bite."

I wasn't too sure and wasn't about to take a chance of being accused of attacking an 'innocent' ill female who was alone and helpless. I got close enough to take her pulse and blood pressure. As I was finishing she made an implicit request that angered and frightened me.

"Mrs. Allure, I came here to see you because you said you were ill. Now I find that you have been dishonest and have behaved disgustingly. I am a professional and try to act as one. I think it is best that you find yourself another doctor." I left before I might have said too much.

❖ ❖ ❖

There was the lady who was having an acute asthma attack when I arrived at her home. She was alone. I gave her the then-standard treatment, IV Aminophylline, very slowly. Just as I wa giving her the last bit, she turned pale and did not respond to my questions. My heart sank, but I reacted to what I had been taught. I gave her Adrenalin IV and then "pumped" her chest. She responded immediately, and was soon ok, but I wasn't. My adrenalin kept me shaking all the way back to the office.

❖ ❖ ❖

There was the lady whose daughter called me, panic-stricken, asking that I come to her mother immediately. I left the hospital expecting to see a patient in shock. I found a distraught "old-maid" daughter who had a domineering mother. She demanded that I do something for her right that minute. After a brief history and exam, I found she had a fecal impaction. I called Dr. Price, and he asked if I could remove the impaction.

"Yes, I can." I went to work. Explaining what I was going to do to relieve her, she was screaming like a banshee, while her dutiful daughter held a large pan in one hand and her mother's hand in the other. I proceeded to manually remove about two pounds of hard feces from the elderly woman's rectum and lower colon. When I finally finished the task and prepared to leave, she smiled and thanked me, saying, "If I have any more trouble, I know who to call." I must have smelled pretty bad that day, as my nurse avoided me all afternoon.

❖ ❖ ❖

Another case was the man with heart disease who was told to take his medication on a regular basis. My neighbor and I had been seeing him on alternate visits, and both noted his prescriptions never seemed to need refilling. Also, the patient was not improving.

"Mr. Burns, are you taking you medicine like you're supposed to?"

"Doc, I'm afraid to take that stuff."

"If you don't take it you will never get any better. In fact, you will have heart failure and die." Three days later I had an emergency call to the home. When I arrived, a son was waiting at the door.

"I think you're too late, Doctor. He's gone."

He was right. There were no heart sounds, no pulse, and no pupillary reaction. I looked for his medication and found that he had never taken any. The cotton was still inside the bottle, and not a pill was missing.

❖ ❖ ❖

A dramatic case I saw immediately after office hours one day: "This one sounds like trouble," my nurse said as I left. She was right again. When I stopped at the curb, I could hear him screaming in pain. I literally ran to him.

"He's in awful pain, doctor." I saw a 60-year-old man writhing in pain, holding his leg, which was snow-white from his toes to mid-thigh.

"Give me something quick, Doctor, this is killing me!"

I felt his leg—no pulse—the nails were white, and the skin was cool. I gave him Morphine immediately while his wife called an ambulance. I told them this was a dire emergency and to hurry. They were there in five minutes.

"Mr. Bates, you have a blood clot in your artery that is cutting off the blood supply and oxygen to that leg and foot. You will have to have immediate emergency surgery to save the leg and foot." By this time the Morphine was taking effect and I examined him further. The upper thigh was warm and pink. The femoral pulse was strong in the triangle, but the leg and foot were still white and cold. I called Dr. Grayson, who was at the hospital, and gave him the details, saying, "I'm pretty sure he has an embolus blocking the femoral artery."

"I'll get the operating room set up right away. Thanks. I'm on my way to assist." Fifteen minutes later we were prepared to operate. At surgery we found a pencil-size clot blocking the artery almost exactly where the leg had lost its color. As Dr. Grayson was suctioning the clot out, he remarked, "The quick house call and early recognition of the problem saved this man's leg." I point this out as an example of how timing, and the proper action, are so important in emergency cases.

❖ ❖ ❖

Here are a couple of more cases I must recite as examples of what we had to take care of as we made house calls.

The call came at about 11 a.m. on a Saturday morning. "This is Jim Sinnett. Can you come to see Betty right away? I think she may have had a stroke."

"Yes, I'll be right there."

On the way I wondered what I would find. He didn't sound too upset, but he was apparently an unemotional man. He and his whole family were disciplined and rigid. They were also all highly intelligent individuals. Well, I would soon find out.

As I hurried up the steps, he met me and I knew by the look on his face it was a serious problem. "Betty" was sitting upright on the couch with a tearful daughter on either side. Her head was bent forward, chin on chest, tongue lolled out and drooling. Her face and neck were cyanotic, and she was unresponsive. I lifted her chin, and her color improved immediately as we improved her airway.

"Let's lay her down. Get a pillow, Jim." I supported her head as we laid her down. Then as I was lifting her chin she took a deep breath, and her skin "pinked up."

"Call an ambulance right now, Jim." I examined her. BP was elevated 165/105, pulse 110, respiration 16, heart regular with grade 3 systolic murmur. Breath sounds came through ok. Reflexes 000.

"How bad is it, Doctor?"

"Very bad. This is a life-threatening stroke. I'm afraid she may have suffered a great deal of brain damage. Let's get her to the hospital immediately."

The ambulance arrived quickly, and with oxygen being given, she seemed to improve. We had no intensive-care units in those days and had to admit her to a regular private room. She remained unconscious for two days, and things looked bleak. In the meantime, she had been seen by consultants in cardiology and neurology. They both gave a poor prognosis. Her EEG showed brain activity, but severe damage. It was likely she would never be functional again. Long-term care in a nursing home was suggested by both consultants.

We continued her supportive care for another two weeks with little change. By this time, arrangements had been made to transfer Betty to a nursing home. Then tragedy struck! One night as her husband was visiting, he stood, leaned over her bed to move her foot, and fell dead across the bed! The door to her room was open, a passing nurse saw him, and reported the incident to us. That was a shock to everybody concerned.

❖   ❖   ❖

Suicides were always a dreadful situation for me. I never felt comfortable with families at those times. Maybe it was because I always felt that somehow it was my fault if the patient had been under my care. I saw a few during my 40 years of practice. They varied from purposeful overdosing, drinking insecticide, hanging, slitting the throat, to shooting themselves. The last one I recall was a patient I had known since childhood. He had not lived peacefully for many years after developing several allergies that were manifest by skin diseases. He became severely depressed, and late one Sunday afternoon made the decision to end his life. His method was to put a loaded shotgun under his chin and pull the trigger. I got the call immediately afterward. "Come quickly. 'Joe Cash' has shot himself." Within 10 minutes I was at the home. It was a grisly scene. He did this standing at an open, sliding closet door as he faced the room. It was a sickening, gruesome sight. He literally "blew his brains out."

That particular case really bothered me, probably because I recalled some instances in his youth, such as the time I had witnessed someone slash him across the face with a knife as they stood talking inside a church. I recalled how my brother and I reacted by chasing after the attacker, not thinking that we might suffer the same fate. Following the attack, we assisted our Dad as he sutured the laceration. 'Joe's' life had not been filled with pleasure.

❖ ❖ ❖

House calls were an education within themselves. The variety of illnesses equaled what we saw in office practice. The number of cases almost equaled the variety. A "banner" number made in one day was 15. This was a day when I was the only doctor available in Old Hickory. There was flu epidemic, and the other four doctors were sick with the flu. That day I began by delivering a baby at 5 a.m., did an emergency appendectomy, made hospital rounds, then two or three house calls, followed by seeing 30 to 40 office patients, and then finished the day by making more house calls, finally getting home about 2 a.m. I really felt I had "earned my keep" that day.

In the late 1960s, the profession began to make a change in policy in making home visits. We were so busy in the office practice that it was next to impossible, timewise, to continue making house calls during office hours. They had to be limited to dire emergencies to conserve time in order to care for the office patients. There were exceptions, such as the elderly and totally disabled patients. After a few years, hospital emergency rooms hired full-time doctors, and patients began to use them for emergencies. That was the era in which the insurance companies began to pay for these visits, and most patients were covered by the companies where they were employed. In present-day practice, house calls are a rarity. This change has caused a rift in doctor-patient relationship that I feel are bonded by the personal visits in the home. To me that was the one place a physician really learned about family habits, relationships, attitudes, and beliefs. After 20+

years of making house calls, I really missed the closeness to families after we phased out that part of practice.

❖   ❖   ❖

Although hospital emergency rooms had full-time M.D.s, we still made many calls to the emergency rooms to see problem cases. One evening I received a call to see one such patient. As I arrived and walked into the ER, they were paging: "Dr. Wilson, emergency STAT!" As I opened the door, a nurse grabbed my arm to hurry me inside.

"We need some help in here." I saw the Pediatrician working frantically with an adult patient who was bleeding profusely from the mouth. I recognized the patient as one of the student nurses.

"Dr. Wilson, I need you to help me. Thelma has post-op bleeding from the nasopharynx where she had a repair of her cleft palate two days ago. I have done what I know to do, but can't stop the bleeding."

"I'll be glad to see what I can do. May I have a mask and some sterile gloves, Ms. Adams?" I suctioned the site and could see the general area, but not the one bleeder that was the culprit.

"I need six 2" x 2" sponges, Miss Adams. Also a #10, red-rubber catheter, and someone to suction and keep the light in focus."

"Thelma, can you hear me?" She nodded *yes*. "I'll have to insert this small catheter into your nostril, ok?" She nodded *yes*. I lubricated the catheter and slowly pushed it into the nostril as the nurse was suctioning blood from the nasopharynx.

"Miss Adams, I need umbilical tape and the 2" x 2"s. I tied two 12-inch lengths of umbilical tape to the rolled-up gauze 2" x 2"s, tied one end to the catheter, then slowly withdrew the catheter from the nostril. As the gauze pad neared the soft palate, it was guided beneath to enter the nasopharynx up under the soft palate. I pulled it snugly and watched for bleeding. It soon stopped. The loose string of umbilical tape was then brought out and secured to her face with tape, along with the end that was tied to the catheter, holding the pack firmly against the bleeding site. The bleeding stopped in two minutes and I felt relieved when it did.

The patient was returned to the Plastic Surgeon the next day. I received a call from him thanking me for what we did and asking me to follow her with him. As it happened so often, I was in the right place at the right time.

Thelma went on to graduate and became a nursing supervisor. She also remained a faithful and loyal patient as long as I continued to practice.

Doctor From Bugtussle

During her career, she married and became a mother. I was honored to be her Obstetrician and to deliver her baby by caesarian section.

❖   ❖   ❖

"Dr. Wilson, call 4587 STAT!" That meant an emergency. I was in the midst of an operation as the supervisor came with a message. "You have a patient on the way to ER that has been injured in an automobile accident. She has a head injury, but is conscious. What shall I tell ER?"

"We will be finished in 15 minutes and will be down by the time she arrives. Ask them to page me when she gets here."

Before we closed the skin, the page came, and I rushed to the ER.

"Your patient is a mess, but I don't think there is anything critically wrong."

As I walked in I recognized the patient as a nurse's aid that worked at Baptist Hospital in downtown Nashville. She was bloody from head to mid-chest.

"What happened, Mrs. Hull?"

"Is that you, Dr. Wilson? I don't remember. My head hurts."

"Yes, I'm here." I was looking at a bleeding scalp and face. I check her pupils as the nurse took the BP and P. I did a brief neurological check. Then I checked the heart, lungs, and extremities. Everything was ok here.

"Do you have a suture tray ready, Miss Adams?"

"Yes, sir. It's all ready with 000 catgut, 00 and 000 silk, 7-1/2 gloves, and 2 percent carbocaine."

"You're on the ball. Thank you! Let's go to work and stop the bleeding. We need to shave a larger area so we can see better."

As I was talking, the nurse was shaving and prepping the area. I could see a small scalp artery pumping away and quickly clamped it. I injected the carbocaine around an inch-long, jagged laceration of the posterior scalp, then irrigated it with normal saline, smoothed the ragged edges with tissue scissors, then closed the laceration in two layers with catgut and then silk. I then turned my attention to the facial laceration, caring for it in the same manner.

By the time we finished repairing the lacerations, Mrs. Hull was awake but somewhat disoriented. We got head, neck, and chest x-rays, and admitted her to the surgical floor. By this time, I had spent 1-1/2 hours in the emergency room, and it was time for office hours. The patient was later seen by the neurology department, and there was no deficit. She recovered well and had no residual problems.

❖ ❖ ❖

Other cases came more frequently than expected. They were mostly the usual things one would expect to see—acute appendicitis, pneumonia, high blood pressure, minor lacerations, etc. These I tended not to remember. The unusual and dramatic ones I do recall, such as the man with the lateral side of his left hand torn away when it was caught in a pulley as he held onto a cable, not aware that his hand was endangered until it was too late. He jerked his hand back, but lost the outer half, along with the ring and little fingers. It was a clean tear; the tendons to the other fingers were not torn, and he had a hand that was still usable.

❖ ❖ ❖

Then there was the man working in construction of the Old Hickory Dam who had a "bucket" of concrete dumped on him as he worked inside forms while the footings were being poured. He was buried up to his armpits before being rescued. He lived, but has been totally disabled since the accident.

❖ ❖ ❖

Of course, there were many automobile accident victims with a few fatalities. While making rounds at Memorial Hospital there was a call to ER. "Dr. Wilson, you have two accident victims here. Can you come?" I went immediately.

"They're in here, Doctor." I recognized both victims as regular patients. The first did not show any signs of trauma except a large bruise on the forehead. He was DOA. The second was groaning with pain, holding his chest and having difficulty breathing. His exam showed severe bruising of the chest and shoulder girdle with small lacerations in the same area. There was a large bruise of the lower abdomen also. Extremities were not injured. X-rays revealed four fractured ribs, but the spine was not fractured. He was treated and make an uneventful recovery.

❖ ❖ ❖

I was not at the hospital when the most dramatic and depressing accident victim was admitted to the ER.

A 15-year-old female was brought in by ambulance with injuries to the anterior neck. She was a passenger in a Volkswagen "bug," sitting in the right front seat, halfway off and facing the driver. As they were driving along, a second car, going in the same direction, pulled into their car, throwing the patient into the dashboard. Her anterior neck struck the edge of the dash just above the instrument panel, injuring the cartilage in the neck. A former associate saw the patient almost immediately, called me from ER, and described the injury. We both knew that this was a case for the ENT department to care for. She was seen in minutes and rushed to surgery for repair of the fractured cartilage. Her airway became obstructed before they could do the planned surgery, and by the time a tracheotomy could be completed, there was oxygen depletion to the brain with damage that was irreversible. That beautiful, intelligent, blonde, 15-year-old became a spastic, brain-damaged, wholly dependent individual, unable to verbally express herself, not able to feed herself, or care for her bodily functions. Thank God there were very few tragedies of this magnitude.

❖   ❖   ❖

Surgical practice was the most exciting and dramatic part of general practice outside of OB. I was busy in the operating room almost from the day I came to Old Hickory. Dr. Johnson had a tremendous patient load, many of whom I naturally cared for, and many of them were surgical problems. Since having four years' experience in surgery in my Memphis practice, it helped a lot. Dr. Johnson being my sponsor helped even more. We did an average to ten elective cases per week within a year from the time we became associated. In addition, we had emergencies very frequently, oftentimes at night or in early-morning hours. The emergency cases were mostly acute appendicitis or "C" sections, strangulated hernias, intestinal obstructions, fractures, and other trauma cases. Our track record in surgery was good, and patients referred other patients.

❖   ❖   ❖

House calls were often a good source of surgical cases. I recall seeing a variety of acutely-ill patients at home that proved to need emergency surgery. As in other phases of practice, only a small number can be easily recalled. I do remember these cases. The first was a 75-year-old man with an acute abdomen that proved to be a mesenteric thrombosis. Although he was operated on within an hour from the time I saw him at home, at least 50 percent of the intestines were gangrenous. There was too much bowel damage and shock for him to survive.

❖   ❖   ❖

Another case was a 1-year-old baby that had cried and vomited for 12 hours before the mother called. I saw him within half an hour.

"Has he been able to keep any food down today?"

"No, he's vomited a lot too."

"Does he have fever?"

"He feels hot, but we don't have a thermometer."

"Can you tell if he hurts at any particular part of his body?"

"No, but I noticed his stomach seems to be swollen."

"Let's see what we find." If it was an adult there would be little doubt of the diagnosis: appendicitis. Then I recalled what our revered pediatric professor told us: pediatric patients have many of the same things as adults, so when you have an acutely ill infant or small child, think as if you would be seeing an adult. Findings on baby John were temperature of 101, pulse 110, respiration 30, chest clear, and heart normal. Ear, nose, and throat normal. Abdomen mildly distended with absent bowel sounds. Peri-umbilical tenderness 1+. Four+ tender right lower quadrant with marked rebound tenderness. This was noted as I checked his tummy. He screamed, his abdomen became rigid, and he tried to escape my hand.

"Mrs. Brake, I think your baby has acute appendicitis and needs immediate surgery."

"I never heard of babies having appendicitis. He's too little to be operated on, isn't he, Doctor?"

"No. He can tolerate the surgery as well as you or I."

"Are you sure, Doctor?"

"Yes, I'm sure. I'll be glad to get another opinion if you want one."

"No. If you're sure of the problem, I believe you. If I hadn't, I would have had some other doctor."

We did surgery an hour later and found an acutely inflamed appendix with a small area of gangrene near the tip. Being blessed by having penicillin and intravenous fluids to give baby John, he made an uneventful recovery. I also add that he was treated by me for his ills during the next 30 years.

❖ ❖ ❖

The next case I recall was a remarkable one in that the patient was so grateful then and for many years afterwards. The home telephone rang at 7 at night. "This is Mr. Whitehouse. My wife is sick and needs a doctor. Can you come?"

"Yes, I'll be glad to see her. Where do you live?"

"406 Neely's Bend Road in Madison."

"I'll be there in half an hour," and I was.

"Mr. Whitehouse, I'm Dr. Wilson."

"Come in, Doctor. This is my wife Marjorie. She's right sick."

We shook hands. "Glad to meet you, Mrs. Whitehouse."

"Hello, Dr. Wilson. Thank you for coming." She had a decided British accent.

"What is your problem, Mrs. Whitehouse?"

"I have this pain in my stomach. It's been here all day. Now I'm sick to my stomach."

"Where did the pain start?"

"Around my navel at first. Now it's in my right side. It's so bad now that I can't walk."

"Ever had a pain like this before?"

"No, sir, I have not."

"Let me examine you. First we'll take your temperature and blood pressure." Temperature was 100, blood pressure was 110/70. "Let me see your tummy." I examined her abdomen which was flat without scars or masses. She was slightly tender under the umbilicus. When I touched her right lower quadrant, she jumped and grabbed my hand. "That spot is really tender, huh?"

"Yes, it is."

"Mrs. Whitehouse, you have acute appendicitis. We need to get you to the hospital for some lab work to further help make a diagnosis. Regardless of what the blood count is, you need surgery tonight."

Mr. Whitehouse said, "How soon does she need to go?"

"Right now, as soon as you can." Within 45 minutes the patient was admitted, the lab work was done, and surgery had been scheduled. At 9 p.m. surgery was started. As I made the incision the nurse remarked, "This had better be a hot one. I was looking forward to a good night's sleep after our all-night stand last night."

"Here it is, Ms. Marcum, see for yourself." The appendix was swollen, badly inflamed, and covered with stringy pus. It was ready to become gangrenous or rupture. Time was on Mrs. Whitehouse's side this time.

The patient was one of the most grateful I encountered throughout practice. As a result of that call, I gained several new patients who were friends and family members.

❖ ❖ ❖

Surgery, with all its glamor and glory, had its downside and complications. Whenever we found unexpected things, such as a malignancy or spread of a known malignancy to other areas, it was heartbreaking. To have a patient have a cardiac arrest during surgery was one of the worse complications I have experienced. When such things happen, some hurt so deeply that you never forget. Here are two or three of the unforgettable ones.

❖ ❖ ❖

"Dr. Wilson, can you see my husband before you go home?"

"What's wrong, Ruby?"

"Jake has an awful pain in his right side. He's had it all night, but he wouldn't let me call you."

"Yes, I'll see him. Bring him on."

"This was in 1965 at 1 p.m. on a Saturday, the end of a long, busy week (some of the nights with two hours of sleep). I was ready to relax and not too happy about waiting for a patient coming from 20 miles away. But I waited.

"Mr. West is here, Doctor."

"Put him in Room 4."

"Hello, Jake. I hear you have a belly ache."

"Yeah, I have, Doctor, and it's getting worse. Now I'm sick to my stummick. Hit hurt me about all nite, and I thought it wuz jist a 'green-apple' bellyache, but dogs if I don't thank I got sumpin' bad a-goin' on."

"Miss Smith, get a WBC and Hgb on Mr. West."

I examined him with typical findings of appendicitis. The WBC was typical also.

"Jake, you have appendicitis. From your history, it started last night, and from our examination, it could be at a bad stage. You had best go to the hospital from here. We will call to get a room, and I'll be over within an hour or so. We will schedule surgery at 2:30. Take these orders with you so they can get started with everything to prepare you for the operation."

This man had been a patient for five or six years and had never had a life-threatening illness. He had had normal chest x-rays and EKGs. To me he was a good surgical risk, and he certainly had all indications for emergency surgery. The surgery crew was called in. I talked to anesthesia, got the lab reports, and started the procedure at about 2:45 p.m. About 15 minutes into the surgery, just as the appendix was being exposed, the anesthetist yelled out: "Dr. Wilson, there are no heart sounds."

"Has his heart stopped?"

"Yes!"

"See if Dr. Evans is in the house." We instinctively went into action as in any emergency. The abdomen was abandoned, drapes were stripped off, and I started pounding on the chest. The anesthetist continued the endotracheal oxygen, then Dr. Evans came rushing in dressed for action.

"Open his chest, Dr. Wilson. I did so instantly, and somehow we were able to stimulate his heart, and it quickly picked up a normal rhythm. His blood pressure rose to normal, and the shocked crew started breathing normally once more. By this time a Cardiologist came in to help. He checked the EKG, which I had interpreted as being normal, and he assured me it was.

"Thank you, Dr. Grant. Would you mind following him with us until he stabilizes?"

"I'll be happy to."

"Thank you, Doctor. Now let's close the incisions."

The man kept his appendix as we all feared any further surgical activity and deep anesthesia might result in a second arrest. With the help of good medical friends, constant nursing care, antibiotics, and a lot of prayer, Mr. West recovered and lived another five or six years.

❖   ❖   ❖

I had patients to become "shocky" during a surgical procedure, but never had one to arrest. It is hard to describe the shock one feels as this type of thing happens. First, there is disbelief, then realization. As this occurs, a cold chill engulfs your body—then you feel hot over the entire body, and as this happens, the heart and pulse race as you go into action (the fight or flight syndrome). After the action is over and everything is under control, an uncontrollable weakness overtakes the entire body to the point I personally wondered if the body could withstand the insults over again.

❖ ❖ ❖

Other cases that occurred took their toll on both me and the patients.

One of the first gallbladder operations I did after coming to Old Hickory was a near disaster. The patient had a congenital anomaly of her common bile duct that was not recognized, resulting in an injury to the duct, which necessitated many surgical procedures later on. Only by the help of an excellent minister and a strong belief in a Higher Being, were the patient, family, and I able to withstand that ordeal. That was when I really began to appreciate ministers.

❖ ❖ ❖

A 34-year-old, obese white male came to the emergency room with abdominal pain he had had for two days. He asked for me. I was called and subsequently saw the man, made a diagnosis of acute appendicitis, and did the surgery. At the time of surgery, he had a gangrenous appendix that had a foul, fecal odor. Cultures were done on the peritoneal fluids and from the appendix. Appropriate surgical measures were taken to prevent complications. Cultures came back positive for E-Coli and Pseudomonas organisms. At that time (1960), we did not have antibiotics to kill certain organisms such as pseudomonas, and we had to rely on what we had to fight infection. After medical consultation, we gave him the whole gamut of antibiotics to ward off further infection. By the seventh post-op day, his temperature was 103 degrees, and I knew the battle was lost. He died on the tenth post-op day. It was depressing and frustrating to me and my colleagues to lose a battle for life under such circumstances. Families are devastated, and often bitter, by such happenings, even if they knew everybody did their best for the patient.

❖ ❖ ❖

She was 52-years-old, the mother of five children, and in apparent good health. Then she started having abdominal pain, then a heavy feeling in her abdomen, then she began to menstruate again. This continued to occur, and after a month or so she came to me with her problem.

"Why didn't you come sooner, Mrs. Borden?"

"Oh, I just thought it would stop. And I was scared of what you might tell me."

"Afraid you might have cancer, Mrs. Borden?"

"Yes," she said in a tearful voice. Then a flood of tears followed.

"Let's look at the practical side of this, Mrs. Borden. First, less than 30 percent of this type of problem are caused by malignancy. If they are malignant, 95 percent can be cured by early diagnosis and treatment. Secondly, if we see you early on, for any problem, it is much easier to solve than if you keep waiting. You haven't had your complaints a very long time, so I think we can help you."

"Whatever you think is best, Doctor. I just know that I can't keep on doing as I am."

"I'll need to examine you first. Miss Slate, prepare Mrs. Borden for an abdominal and pelvic exam."

On examination, I found an abdominal mass that was felt to be of the uterus. The mass was irregular and firm, compatible with a benign tumor. The pelvic examination did show the uterus to contain a tumor about the size of an orange. The cervix appeared to be healthy, and there was no enlargement of either tubes or ovaries.

"Mrs. Borden, you have a fairly large tumor in your womb, which is most likely the cause for your abnormal bleeding. I see no signs of cancer, but we did a pap smear to be safe. Your tubes and ovaries are normal for your age. I recommend we hospitalize you, get a second opinion, and if they agree, we need to do a hysterectomy to cure the bleeding."

The patient was hospitalized the next day, and consultation was given to the effect that the surgery was indicated, and he agreed with our diagnosis. Two days later, my associate, Dr. Rivas, and I did an abdominal hysterectomy, removing the tubes, ovaries, and appendix at the same time. The surgery was uneventful, and the patient did well until the fourth hospital day when she complained of more than the usual amount of pain, became restless, and within an hour was in a state of shock. She was intubated almost immediately, placed on the Ambu bag for oxygen exchange, and rushed to intensive care where she was placed on a respirator and a cardiac monitor. The heart monitor showed a normal pattern, which ruled out a heart attack. A chest x-ray was done also. We found the problem. She had thrown an embolus to the right lung. It was a huge one. A medical consult was given, and we treated her vigorously and appropriately from that minute. There was too much involvement, and the shock was too great. All efforts were in vain, and she died within a few hours from time of the embolus occurring. That was another shocker. There was a tragic sequel to her death. About two years after her death, a daughter gave birth in another hospital and lost her life on the second post-partum day, also from a pulmonary embolism.

❖ ❖ ❖

During the 15 years I had delivered babies, I was honored to deliver more than 1,000; 95 percent of these were normal. Parents were happy and celebrated. This was a culmination of marriage and continuing their bloodline. The other five percent were sad to tragic endings to the union of man and wife. I have had the burden of telling mothers before labor began that there was no sign of life in the baby—no movement and no heart sounds. Delivering a stillborn gave me a guilt complex. It was depressing to deliver any type of congenital deformity or an infant that was obviously ill. I was fortunate to have delivered babies with club feet, polydactylism (extra toes and fingers), cleft palate, hare lip, palm-sized, polk-berry-stained moles of the body (some with heavy hair growing in the mole), and one encephalic (born without a skull, but with a small brain). These were the heartbreakers for me and soul-rending for parents. Delivering premature infants was always a dread. We did not have the facilities to care for high risk, immature babies anywhere in this area at that time. Consequently, we lost a high percentage of them. I went through the ordeal a few times also.

In 1966, it was suggested by my physician that I give up obstetrics due to the fact I began to have chest pains after long hours (16 to 20) of work, which involved many night deliveries. It was difficult to do, but I followed his advice, and made the last delivery in early 1967. That was a sad landmark in my practice.

The Doctor As A Patient

In early summer of 1984, I had begun to have chest pain on exertion, when upset or after having worked for long hours. I would go home dog tired to have Jessie say, "You look gray again. Why don't you lie down while I finish supper?" The couch just swallowed my tired body. After a few months, I told her of my chest pain. She chided me, saying, "If you don't slow down you'll have a heart attack." I didn't slow down much and kept having exertional angina. I am a definite type A Personality, one that is in constant motion, wanting everything done the moment it is mentioned—also the high-risk-heart-attack type.

By December, 1985, I myself had undergone three surgeries. The last of these, I was lucky to escape the grim reaper. The first two were minor in comparison. The first was a minute retinal separation in my right eye. The second one was a ureteral calculus (kidney stone) which was removed from below. That made me sit up and take notice. The movement of that stone down the ureter caused an unforgettable pain. Up until that time I had never experienced pain that severe. It would first hurt, then ache, then kick me in the kidney, then I would vomit, and following the vomiting a "fainty" feeling would overcome me. This was all accompanied with a cold sweat and extreme weakness that would last for several minutes. After three days of this I was ready for anything that spelled R-E-L-I-E-F.

The third surgery was the big one. On December 2, 1985, I underwent quadruple, coronary-artery bypass surgery. For some reason I was not bothered as much then as I was when the minor procedure was done on the eye. I was depressed, ashamed, and felt as if I was letting my family down by taking a brush with death. I survived and have been in apparent good health since. During that time and through the three months of recovery at home, Dr. Rivas carried on the practice with the help of a wonderful friend of mine. I have been forever grateful to him for accepting the responsibility and keeping the practice going during that time. I did very few surgeries in 1986 as I suffered a minor myocardial infarction in May of that year. Dr. Rivas remained in practice with me until I made a decision to retire from the practice. This decision was made in July of 1987, and made known to my patients in early September of that year. I saw 29 patients on December 31, 1987, walked out, and have not actively practiced since.

❖   ❖   ❖

November of that year (1984) was when I had been served papers notifying me that I was being sued for malpractice. This came as quite a shock. When the papers were served I had more than the usual amount of chest pain, which soon left, and then the pains gradually worsened. Within six months I had to quit rushing, climbing stairs, or undergoing known stressful situations. When I did any of these I experienced substernal pain and momentary shortness of breath.

By November, 1985, I knew the problem was serious. At about that time my annual physical examination was due, and I presented the symptom complex to my physician and friend, Dr. George B. Hagan. We had a long discussion of the problem, discussing all phases and their pros and cons.

"Are you under much stress, Dr. Wilson?"

"Yes, more than usual." Then I told him of the impending lawsuit.

"You may be in trouble. Let's take a look at everything first, and then we'll do a stress test."

My physical showed a mild rise in the resting blood pressure, a pre-existing heart murmur was more distinct, and all else was normal. The resting EKG was normal, and all reports normal. Then the stress test was done! By the time I walked one minute I felt pressure in my chest, my head began to throb, then to pain, and my vision blurred a bit.

"Are you all right, Dr. Wilson?"

"I think we had better stop. I have a terrific headache and some chest pain."

"Ok. Lie down and let me take your blood pressure." As she did the mercury level rose to more than 200. I was momentarily dizzy, had a pressure feeling in my chest, and was thinking, *I may be having an infarction or a stroke.* "Lord, please don't let it happen here," I prayed.

"Put this under your tongue, Doctor!" It was the nurse bringing me back to reality. Then a buzzer sounded, and Dr. Hagan came bounding in to the room.

"What's wrong, Ms. Ruby?"

"His blood pressure went up to 210/120. He had some chest pain and shortness of breath. Take a look at this EKG too!"

As he looked, his head was shaking. "How do you feel now, Wendell?"

"Better, but I still have a headache."

"Your EKG shows that you have a real problem. You need to have an arteriogram real soon." Then he showed me the changes in the EKG, and that frightened me a lot more. "Who do you want to do this?"

"The Cardiology Group at Baptist Hospital."

"I'll call right now and make an appointment one week from today."

That would be Friday, November 29, the day after Thanksgiving. That was fine with me since all of the married daughters would be home for that day (Thanksgiving). We had a great visit, and the appointment was barely mentioned. When I was alone, that feeling of weight on my chest would come back, and I thought it was anxiety and not really true angina. *This couldn't happen to me now*! Boy, was I ever wrong!

It was Friday, November 22, 1985, when Dr. Hagan told me of my serious problem. I was not surprised or shocked about the diagnosis. I was hesitant to tell Jessie. The girls and families were to visit us on Thanksgiving day, and I had an appointment with the Cardiologist, Dr. Charles Mayes, on Friday, November 29, the day after. Our youngest daughter went with us to Baptist Hospital where I was scheduled to have a coronary arteriogram. As we turned into the parking area I made the statement: "You know, I'm not having any bypass surgery done." After being seen by the Cardiologist, who ran and interpreted an EKG, I was admitted for the coronary arteriogram.

Following that, I was told that it showed seven different areas of the coronary arteries that were blocked. They also informed me that it would be risky to leave the hospital, that I should be on constant cardiac monitoring, and they recommended that I have bypass surgery as soon as they could get me on the schedule. That sobered me, and I had second thoughts about having surgery. The Cardiologist and Vascular Surgeon said without surgery I would be at great risk, from hour to hour, of having a myocardial infarction. I was really in a quandary. Jessie actually helped me make the decision by saying, in effect, "The risk you will take by not having the surgery is greater than the surgical risk will be. Why would you not choose the route of the lesser risk?" That did it!

The decision was made to have the surgery which was scheduled for December 2 at 8 a.m. I remained in Baptist Hospital over the weekend, on the monitor and medication, preparing for the surgery. Tranquilizers kept my anxiety under control until just an hour or two from the scheduled time, when I finally realized what the possibilities were. Then I became just another patient and not a sane, sober, practical-thinking doctor I had always been. I became a frightened, blubbering child and shed tears of anguish—anguish because I felt I was deserting my family and all the people depending on me. I had no real fear of the surgery itself, but fear of what it would do to the ones I care for most of all.

Then that merciful injection, the kind I had ordered so many hundreds of times, was given, and I soon had no fear of anything. Neither did I have any realization as to what was happening.

The next thing I recall is being in a dream world with voices that spoke to me from a great distance, so far away that I could barely hear. When I opened my eyes there seemed to be a mist covering the whole room with vague shadows of people moving slowly about as if they were floating. There was a large endotracheal tube protruding from the corner of my mouth, and I felt as though it was slowly choking me. Then I felt my chest expanding and realized the respirator was my salvation—I wouldn't choke to death. Visitors came to hover over me and talk in far-off voices, "How are you doing Dr. Wilson?" It was Camille, one of my ex-nurses with her new boss "big John" (Dr. John Hollifield). They both wore glasses that seemed to be a foot in diameter, dwarfing their faces.

I had very little pain as I began to react and become conscious of what was going on. Some 18 hours later they removed the endotracheal tube, and I knew I would live again. Another 24 hours and I was moved to the post-op cardiac care ward, where most of the patients were recovering from bypass surgery. The following day I sat and dangled my legs. The next day I sat in a chair for 15 minutes every eight hours. After three more days of increasing activity I was moved to a private room where I remained for another ten days before leaving the hospital. During all this time Jessie or a daughter was with me day and night. At this time I realized what a caring family I had. It had been said that doctors were the world's worst patients, and I was determined to change this belief. I cooperated 100 percent so the nurses and family wouldn't say, "Whew, I'm glad he's going home, we couldn't take much more of him." My recovery was smooth, except for a minor infection of the incision of a leg.

At home, things improved from hour to hour as I received the tender, loving care of my wife, the most wonderful nurse and person I have ever known. By mid-March I was back in the office seeing patients; first for four hours a day the first week, but before long the hours gradually became longer, and by the third week I was spending eight hours there for four days a week. By May 15, I was making hospital rounds as before, which meant longer hours and much greater pressure. Soon I began to tire more than I should have, but I kept the pace. Not long after that Jessie remarked: "You're looking tired and gray again. You had better slow down, or you'll be back in the hospital as a patient." Little did she know how soon that would be. At about 2 a.m. on May 18, 1986, I awoke with pain in my chest, with mild shortness of breath. I knew immediately what was happening and awoke Jessie. She called Baptist Emergency Room with the history, gave them the doctor's name, and was advised to call 911 to get me there as soon as possible. I heard the conversation and shook my head "No!"

"Don't wait for an ambulance. I'm not critical and we can be there before an emergency vehicle can get here from four miles away." I saw the fear in her eyes. "I promise not to die on you, honey."

I walked the ten steps to the car and we were on our way!

Another nitroglycerin under my tongue gave me some relief, but within five or six minutes the pain came back. I used another one. By now I was beginning to feel a little apprehensive and looked at the speedometer. She was going 65 m.p.h. I was thinking, *She needs to "step on the gas."*

"Honey, floorboard this thing."

"The patrol might stop us."

"Let him do that, and then we'll have an escort to the emergency room." She "floorboarded it." I saw 85 m.p.h. appear on the speedometer, then 90 m.p.h., and in another ten minutes we arrived at the emergency room.

As we wheeled in a nurse and orderly were waiting with a stretcher. Boy, was that a welcome sight. Then I saw Dr. Potanin, Dr. Mayes' associate, appear by their side. He wasn't Jesus, but he was my savior at that moment. An I.V. was in my arm by the time the stretcher stopped. Then a small dose of morphine was given through the I.V. tubing, and I was relieved of pain. As this was being done, they were doing an EKG and examining me. Dr. Potanin was reading the EKG as it spilled out of the machine with all of the electrical impulses of each beat of my heart, revealing the T wave, P waves, R waves, ST segments, and QRS complexes, showing what was happening to the muscle fiber of the organ.

"Wendell, you have some changes compatible with a minor acute myocardial infarction."

"What area is it in?"

"Left posterior. Looks like a small branch is effected."

"Thanks, Dr. Potanin."

The area and the minor branch meant the danger of a major attack was not likely. I breathed a sigh of relief with the news I had just gotten. That oxygen mask I was wearing didn't bother me one bit. In the room on the cardiac ward, I was back in familiar surroundings, which made me less apprehensive. All went well for the next two days with very little to no pain. My EKG had stabilized, I was allowed bathroom privileges, and I felt good. The fourth day I was showering and about the time I finished toweling off, I experienced a sharp pain in my chest, and felt lightheaded and dizzy. Managing to get back to bed, I called the nurse. She immediately called for oxygen and paged the Cardiologist. Both appeared within minutes. Dr. Wray assessed the situation and gave me SL Nitroglycerin, which relieved the pain quickly. I went back on monitoring for another 24 hours with no new changes. EKGs were unchanged. The next day I got a good lecture from the Cardiologist, reminding me that I was 68 years of age, working long hours, and under stress, and that I also had recent bypass surgery, all of which made me more susceptible to a heart attack. Then he recommended that I immediately retire from practice. This I could not readily accept.

"I'll have to think about your recommendation, Dr. Mayes."

"I think you should seriously consider the whole picture, then we'll talk about this again."

"I will, Doctor. Thank you."

Three more days and I was up walking the halls with no pain or discomfort. After a total stay of two weeks, I was dismissed on a strict rehabilitation program, plus a change of medication. They also forbade me to practice for another three months, and saw me on a monthly basis for that period. I returned to work in August and continued, with limitations, until I retired.

❖ ❖ ❖

We had a third doctor with us from September 1, 1986 until October 1, 1987. This relieved some of the workload and made it possible to continue the practice during that period.

A very unusual and noble thing happened to me when I underwent bypass surgery. A good friend, who had retired a few months prior, came to the hospital to see me shortly after and informed me that he wanted to help by taking care of part of the office practice. I was elated! It was almost beyond belief that that could happen. That man, Dr. Lee Kramer, had a heart as big as all outdoors. He stayed with the office, helping Dr. Rivas carry the practice, until I returned in May. What a friend! I will be forever grateful to Dr. Kramer. Wherever he is I know that he will bring joy and sunshine into any life he might touch.

Not too many months after I returned to practice, I decided to stop doing any major surgery for two reasons. First, my capabilities were not as they were before I had bypass surgery, and second, Dr. Rivas was very capable and qualified to do all of the surgery that might be done in our practice. It was a tough decision but proved far better for both the patients and me. It was well-accepted by most of the patients, and we had no problems to arise. With the three of us we were able to stagger office hours so that someone would be in the office at all times from 9 a.m. to 5 p.m. This took care of the patient load and allowed us to relax a bit more.

By mid-1987, I realized the physical and emotional strain was becoming too great for me to continue in practice. Besides the workload being great, I still had the threat of the malpractice suit haunting me day and night with dreams and nightmares. It did more to destroy my practice than the heart attack ever could. It was not a visible something, but it ate at me all the time, making me feel like a criminal, although I knew I had done nothing wrong. In August, the office personnel were told of my decision to retire. By September 1, a letter was sent to all patients telling them that I would retire as of January 1, 1988.

A Forty-Year Career

During my 40 years in practice, I performed innumerable surgical procedures. At one time, we did some reviews of certain types of cases to find the numbers we had done. That was in 1966. By that date, I had done over 1,000 hysterectomies, almost that many cholecystectomies, innumerable appendectomies, plus a few hundred tonsillectomies, not to mention other procedures. Some of those numbers were most likely doubled, as I continued to do surgery until 1986. Anyone doing the number of cases my associates and I did were bound to have complications along the way. You would expect to have a few post-operative deaths also. We were very fortunate in that I can recall fewer than 15 during the years. The small percentage of the total number of cases done hurt deeply each time and always made on cognizant that every case could result in death or tragedy if not handled properly. All things considered, I feel that my years in surgery were successful—and, I hope, helpful to all, plus lifesaving to many.

Surgery and obstetrics were certainly not the only phases of practice. Those and the emergency part were the more dramatic and exciting ones. The other patients were just as important, challenging, and interesting as the dramatic ones. Many patients had chronic medical ills that changed their lives for them and their families. The diseases which, I feel, affected most were diabetes, kidney disease, heart ailments, high blood pressure, and psychiatric problems. Lifestyles had to be changed, sudden deaths occurred, social lives became non-existent, and small children had to accept adult responsibilities. Many of these patients were helped most by having someone to listen to their problems. My adage was to lend a big ear and a broad shoulder to the patient, which would improve their ills more than a thousand pills. Taking time to do this was often difficult, and I'm sure many were neglected from that standpoint. I did my best to listen to the ones that needed this time and treat the medical problems diligently and to the best of my ability.

For the first 20 years of practice, I made house calls to the chronically-ill patients and emergencies. I, in turn, was happy to be chose as their doctor. They referred so many patients to me to the point that I was almost

Doctor From Bugtussle

overburdened. It was at this time in 1960 that the third man, Dr. Pomeroy, joined our group. He was welcomed with open arms. He was a very intelligent young man, and soon, he too, was very busy. Since he did not do major surgery, Dr. Johnson and I each had an increase in the number of surgical cases we did. This continued for the next four years as the three of us worked day and night. Dr. Pomeroy and I made house calls mostly at night, except in emergencies. The chronically-ill patients were sometimes scheduled between hospital rounds and office hours. If you promised an elderly patient to be there at a certain hour, and did not arrive near the time, they would put a call in to find out why the doctor wasn't there.

Sometimes we made house calls on post-op patients as a follow-up on their progress. This I called their "luxury item" in medical care. One such case was one on whom I had performed a hemorrhoidectomy. I visited him on a weekly basis for about six weeks. Before he left the hospital I explained what he would have to do: take warm sitz baths twice daily, take mineral oil once daily, eat oatmeal or bran flakes each day, and I would dilate him weekly to prevent stricture from forming (the latter was very painful). Each time I did the dilation he would scream, curse, and threaten me. Then afterwards he would always apologize. I realize this was almost barbarous treatment, but he had good results and referred several friends to me for the same problem.

This type of care had to be discontinued for the simple fact that I was so busy and there was not enough time to justify offering the service. And it also meant sacrificing office and hospital practice. By 1964, we had lost Dr. E. P. Johnson and were "swamped" with patients. Although we mourned his loss, we had to take care of our obligations to the patients. Again, good fortune came our way. Dr. Robert Pilkinton joined the practice shortly after Dr. Johnson's death. He was also a fine young man, a pharmacist turned physician, with a good personality who had a good grasp of general medicine and an interest in surgery. He, of course, was soon busy also, seeing new patients, taking overflow ones, assisting me in surgery, making emergency calls, and delivering babies. After three years, he decided to leave to establish his own practice. Naturally, he took a number of patients with him, but we seemed to be as busy as ever following his departure.

Dr. Pomeroy and I continued on together for a total of 10 years. The practice was extremely busy and hectic, as we both carried a heavy load of office patients. We were each seeing 40 to 50 patients daily, plus having nearly that number (combined) in two hospitals. The workload took its toll on both of us. Then we tried a third man, but his work ethic was not compatible with ours. He soon became a liability to the practice and "relieved" of his association with us. He, at that time, was able to start a residency in urology. There was no letup in practice at Old Hickory Clinic at that time, as the patients continued to be seen in great numbers at the office, the hospital, and in the emergency rooms.

During all the changes they remained loyal and supportive. By 1966, Madison Hospital was employing full-time resident physicians to assist in surgery and to handle the emergency rooms. Most all of them had two to three years surgical training, and this was a tremendous help to our practice as it relieved Dr. Pomeroy from assisting in many cases, as well as giving him more freedom in office hours. The surgical practice continued to grow as we did as many as ten scheduled cases per week, plus emergency cases as well. I recall returning from vacation on Sunday, and the following day did two scheduled cases, and by late that afternoon we had scheduled three emergency appendectomies beginning at 6 p.m. That was a bit unusual, but not uncommon. We kept up the pace pretty well until 1970 when he decided to leave the practice and establish his own.

As Dr. Pomeroy prepared to leave, I contacted Dr. Agbunag, one of the fellows who had been with Madison Hospital for two or three years. He was an excellent surgeon who had had three years of formal training in General Surgery and was Board-qualified. He joined the practice in mid-1970 and remained for five years. Then I began to feel I had more freedom to be away from the practice as he wa doing many of the major cases. After he came, our surgical practice took on a different phase, as he did colon resections and other cases I was not doing. His surgical skills were appreciated by me and soon made known to our patients. He was a great asset to the practice and was soon also very busy. The practice seemed to grow more and more, and by 1974, a third man. Dr. Sator, joined us. He too had three years of surgical training, and all three of us were doing surgery. In spite of the fact I had less training, the number of cases I did was still the greatest of all. This was simply caused by my being in active practice many more years and with patients being more comfortable with my caring for them.

Again, I went through losing yet another associate. Dr. Agbunag decided the time had come for him to establish his own private practice. He departed in July, 1975, began his own practice and has continued to grow and become a well-known surgeon in the suburbs of Nashville. Some patients were lost to my practice, but that was to be expected. Any physician as capable as Dr. Agbunag would be busy, build a good practice, and be successful by his known capabilities. I would like to think that his association with me was helpful in being successful with his practice. I was grateful to him for the years he spent with me and for the boost he gave to the practice. I learned from him in the surgical field, and I hope he learned other things from me that have helped in his practice.

Dr. Sator was my associate until January, 1980. He, too, started his own practice in Old Hickory. He was also a big help to me. We had a good relationship, did many surgical cases together, kept busy in the office and emergency rooms, and cared for the hospitalized medical patients. Again, I felt more like taking some time away from practice, knowing he would be able to take care of any surgical emergency that might occur. He was a quiet, unassuming young man, and a very capable surgeon who did not receive as much credit as he should have for his surgical skills.

When Dr. Sator left my office, a third well-trained, Board-qualified General Surgeon joined me in practice in January, 1980. We had never met. He was highly recommended by a mutual friend and proved to be everything this friend said he would be; a fine Surgeon, a hard worker dedicated to his profession, dependable, and conscientious. He did an appendectomy the day he arrived before he had been to the office and had been fully approved for staff privileges. His surgical skills were very evident when we did the procedure, and as time went by, he proved his abilities many, many times.

Fortunately, my surgical practice was still on the upswing, so we were busy beyond his hopes. The first few months of our association, I had a record number of cholecystectomies to perform, and that really pleased him since he had done research on gall bladder surgery during his residency training. He proved to be even more helpful since he had a year of practice in rural Mexico as part of his training in medical school. He also had two years of private practice in Illinois. During the next eight years he proved to be a loyal associate and friend as I had to face another enemy: a malpractice suit. This proved to be a very disturbing problem for me. Even though I knew there was no gross malpractice, of which I was accused, it haunted me day and night. Many nights were sleepless or nightmarish from the accusation. During the daytime I was usually too busy to think of anything more than patients currently being cared for. The case never came to trial as the patient's attorney could not find a Gynecologist or General Surgeon to testify in court that I was guilty of any malpractice. Therefore I was absolved of any wrongdoing.

Dr. Rivas supported me in every way, giving depositions on my behalf, taking care of the practice while I was away, and many other necessary, daily problems that arose.

He came at a time that was mutually beneficial. he had decided to return to the Nashville area where he had trained for four years and had not found a suitable practice to associate with. I was searching for someone with surgical training and skills such as he had. I was able to afford the right place for him to practice, and he had the skills needed for the practice. The association worked well for both.

The eight years we spent together were mostly amiable, very productive, and rewarding for both. We had many interesting surgical cases. Since he did the cases that were complicated or had malignancies, there was a larger number of complications than usual in the practice. Some cases were unusual, such as the elderly lady with a malignant breast tumor that she had known she had for two or three years, but by the time she came to us, the tumor had eroded to be an open sore. Because of Dr. Rivas' skills, it was surgically removed. The incision healed well, and she lived a pain-free life for two years, at which time she fell and fractured a hip. After the fall she had a downhill course and died from complications of pneumonia and heart disease.

Another elderly lady of 82-years came after having a complete prolapse of the uterus for several months, to the point an erosion of its surface caused bleeding, and she became frightened. Gynecological consultation was sought, a vaginal hysterectomy and repair were performed, and she made an uneventful recovery.

Once when we had done a breast biopsy that was positive for malignancy, as we were preparing to do a modified radical mastectomy, the Anesthesiologist noted a sudden, radical change in her blood pressure, and the EKG monitor showed changes in both T waves and P waves compatible with an infarction (heart attack). Surgery was stopped, a Cardiologist was called to the operating room to assess the situation, and she was moved to the coronary care unit. Those were scary moments, not knowing what might happen any second, as we watched and waited. This patient had no signs or symptoms of heart disease, and had had more than one EKG that was interpreted as normal. The lady made a good recovery from the heart attack. The pathology report was encouraging, not showing any spread of the malignancy which was a low-grade type. Today she is leading a normal life.

One more case stands out in my memory as Dr. Rivas and I worked together. A very obese, 65-year-old man came to me with typical gall bladder disease history and physical findings. Gall bladder x-rays and ultrasound were positive for gallstones. We did no scans of the abdomen as we saw no indication for that expensive procedure.

Surgery was scheduled. His admission lab work and electrocardiogram were normal. We felt good about his status and were confident of our diagnosis.

As I made the abdominal incision, someone said, "He sure is a fat one." I replied, "We can handle that ok. We'll just have to pull a little harder to expose everything."

As we opened the peritoneum and began to explore with our hands, we both felt a mass that was below and medial to the gall bladder. There was a startled look on Dr. Rivas' face, and I felt foolish and a bit shocked as we both realized we had not found the baseball-sized tumor either on physical examination or by x-rays. This changed our plans. We had to do two procedures instead of one. The mesenteric mass was a low-grade malignancy. It had to be removed first and was done by Dr. Rivas who did an excellent job in record time. Then we did a cholecystectomy after that. By the time we had finished we had been operating 3-1/2 hours, not the anticipated one hour procedure we had planned on. I was worn out, physically, and somewhat depressed over the new problem.

There were many acute surgical emergencies during the eight years we were associated. Most all of them came out well, but not 100 percent. There were times that a patient was not salvageable, or had an unforeseen complication, such as a stroke or had such severe accidental injuries that they were beyond help.

❖ ❖ ❖

A great task now faced me: how could I attract someone to buy, or take, the practice? Dr. Rivas would not stay, nor did he want to buy. Again, luck was with me. Two young family physicians contacted me concerning the practice. We met on two or three occasions discussing all facets of the practice, and within a few days had agreed on terms of a sale. It was what I had hoped for. I knew both from our professional association. They had been in practice together for about ten years, and were successful in the practice. In addition, they were leaders in their field of family practice, with each being chief of that section at the two local hospitals. The community would be in good hands. I was relieved from a professional standpoint, as well as from a personal one. Now I could retire with a clear conscience.

Retirement came too soon! Drs. Moore and Seeley asked me to stay with them for two or three months on a part-time basis to make the transition more gradual. I chose to not do that. I left the office on December 31, 1987. Little did I realize how that decision would affect me!

After 40 years of active general practice which came to a sudden halt, I soon began to wish I had something to do. I felt useless and within a few months became depressed. After that, I soon reached the point that I had rather not see anyone or go anywhere for fear I would have to talk with people. The feeling of uselessness continued for several weeks before I realized it was creating problems. I had a personality change from an extrovert to an introvert. Realizing it was caused from the depression, I tried to find an answer to the problem.

At that time, a friend came to see me to ask that I become involved with the Senior Outreach program in our communities. It was the best thing that could have happened for me. Being with my age group and becoming involved in their activities woke me up to reality. *I was not useless.* With the involvement, I was soon asked to do various things that helped other people, and pretty soon I wanted to be involved again. After more than two years I became overloaded with the work and felt it best to pursue other things. As we had started a walking group and I was active in community theater, these two kept me involved enough to relax and become interested in being with people again. Now I look forward to seeing people even more and am enjoying retirement to the fullest.

❖   ❖   ❖

On two occasions I have been honored by the communities of Old Hickory, Lakewood, and surrounding communities. In 1976, after I was named "Tennessee Family Physician of the Year," a congratulatory party was held at Lakewood City Hall, sponsored by the Community Club. That event was attended by some one hundred and fifty guests of family, friends, and colleagues, and members of Nashville Metropolitan Government as well. On that occasion, one of the Metro representatives presented me with a key to the city as I was interviewed by a local television station. That was a wonderful gesture by that group, one that I have always remembered as being among the highest honors of my life. I have never felt that I adequately expressed my appreciation to the group that honored me then.

The second occasion was in April, 1988, shortly after my retirement. On this date both Dr. E.B. Rhea and I were honored, he for fifty years and I for thirty-six years of practice in the area. The party was held at Old Hickory

Country Club and hosted by local community organizations along with two area hospitals, Nashville Memorial and Tennessee Christian Medical Center. Both were very generous in their involvement, furnishing all the food and trolley/bus transportation from distant parking lots to the club. The president of each institution came to pay tribute and present plaques to each of us. It humbled me as I'm sure it did Dr. Rhea.

There were local (Metro) and state representatives present to make short speeches and present certificates for our community services. Local ministers also presented community service plaques to each of us, which I greatly appreciated.

Old friends from college years and some from earlier years came to congratulate us, as did colleagues of the area, and one came from Alabama to honor Dr. Rhea. Most importantly to me, family members came to show their love and pride for us. By my side was Jessie, my wife of (then) forty-five years, along with our four daughters from Pennsylvania, Nevada, and East Tennessee as well as one from home. With each of our married daughters came husbands and seven grandchildren (our pride and joy). Scattered through the five to six hundred people attending was another twenty family members who had come to see their kin honored on this occasion.

Ex-office staff members came to boost my morale by telling me what a great boss I had been and how much they enjoyed working at the clinic. I'll have to admit it became a little emotional with the reminiscing. The most appreciated visitor of all, outside the family, was a colleague of many years who was not able to come inside, as he was a victim of Parkinson's Disease. I didn't know about this until after the fact, and have always regretted not seeing him.

After all the celebration it was Dr. Rhea's turn and mine to express our thanks and gratitude to the many people, which was not an easy task. Somehow we got through it all, and we were left with fond memories of a wonderful day made by so many, many wonderful people.

Looking back over the years makes me realize what a wonderfully full life I have had. Much good luck came my way throughout life. There were not many disappointments for me during my lifetime. We had intelligent, hard-working parents that taught good life values, good morals, the value of honesty and hard work, how to be self-sufficient, and above all, the love of God and country. Our mother taught us always to be honest and truthful, to set a high goal in life, and to work toward that goal. I never forgot those teachings. Now that I am approaching that 78th year of life, I can see the value of my early teachings more clearly than ever before.

What more can a man ask for than what I have had? God-fearing parents, the love of a wonderful wife and helpmate, four beautiful children, who are successful in their lives and have blessed us with seven beautiful, handsome, and highly intelligent grandchildren. The support and praise of both Jessie's and my families. The support and assistance of friends in college and medical school. The trust and support of colleagues that helped me be successful throughout my career. The honors bestowed on me by those same friends and colleagues. No man could be successful in life without the love and help of family and friends.

The period of life in which I was born, grew up, and lived, was one of the most devastating, yet enlightening, thrilling, and exciting times ever to have lived. We lived in a time of great discoveries, a time when history was made. In my chosen profession, we were able to see the development of sulfa drugs, the discovery of penicillin, and the mycin drugs. The discovery of polio vaccine, followed by the development of mumps, measles, flu, and pneumonia vaccines.

In my childhood years, there had been the development of vaccines for diphtheria, tetanus, typhoid, and whooping cough. Each of the discoveries has saved millions of lives worldwide. In the latter years of medical school, the great scientific minds of this universe were working feverishly to find a way to split the atom so they could harness its energy. It was done because of a war that threatened to destroy a great percentage of the world's population. To me it was the deterrent to that world destruction. Following the discovery, an atomic bomb was developed by coordinating the scientific minds of several geniuses. Now atomic energy is used in so many different ways that it is inconceivable to most human beings. Because of that discovery, we have been able to put people in space, develop ways and means for them to live there, produce many foods and clothing that we use every day, and develop new surgical techniques that save millions of lives each year. Not only that, it saves people from pain and suffering by decreasing the great majority of invasive surgeries that people required in the past centuries. Other medical and surgical advances have also resulted from this. The laser beam was discovered to be a wonderful method in which to perform many types of surgery such as deep within the body and deep in the brain. Many eye surgeries are done with laser beam, and I am sure there are many, many more in addition to these.

Today, drugs have been developed to treat a specific disease or a specific type of malignancy. Some of the most dreaded types of cancer I recall (such as malignant melanoma) today can possibly be wiped out with a new vaccine. Think of how much pain, mental anguish, family destruction, and family financial burdens this one instance will save. People have come to expect this to happen whenever they have any type of illness, injury, or malignancy. They expect miracles! I blame our profession in some respects because we try to ease a patient and family of anguish or anxiety by minimizing an illness or surgical procedure. All of us fail to appreciate the many advantages we have that much of the world's population does not have.

It is hard for me to realize and appreciate the multitude of discoveries and developments in our world today. Yet, when I recall what my father had with which to treat the sick, diseased, and injured people, I marvel that he was so successful in his practice. Then as I compare what my generation had to utilize in the way of drugs, diagnostic tools, and surgical procedures to today's sophisticated varieties of each, I sometimes wonder *how* we did as well as *we* did. Medicine progressed in great strides during World War II. We all learned to make do with what we had. Again, "necessity was the mother of invention." Surgical procedures were done on the battlefield and as the battles progressed, all patients had to move on.

Surgeons noted how much more quickly post-operative patients recovered by being more physically active and began the short time in bed following surgery. They also developed new procedures to accommodate the military life. These practices carried over into routines in civilian life. Our Army and Navy learned from our allies and enemy medical and surgical teams as they cared for each country's wounded and ill. Like religion, medicine was a common ground for everybody, be he friend or foe. That was progress, and today the whole world is reaping the rewards from that era of learning. Since my retirement of seven years, I marvel at what great strides have been made in medicine during this time and realize that they will continue to do so.

As the attrition rate of our generation mounts from retirement, disabilities, and death, the next generation, with their brilliant minds and desire for further knowledge, will discover more and better ways to relieve the pains and suffering of humanity. And I'm sure they will discover preventions or cures for many dread conditions and diseases such as AIDS, Alzheimer's, Parkinson's, and many malignancies, etc. They will be the guardians of life and health for the entire world.

How fortunate I have been to live and enjoy the wonderful years during my lifetime. No one could have been more rewarded than I have to experience the many things along the way, and especially to be blessed with the God-given abilities to care for and treat the ills of my fellow man. Above all this, I have the honor of being married to a wonderful woman and helpmate for 52 years, Jessie Elizabeth Bess Wilson. What more could any man ask for? It has been a wonderfully rich life.

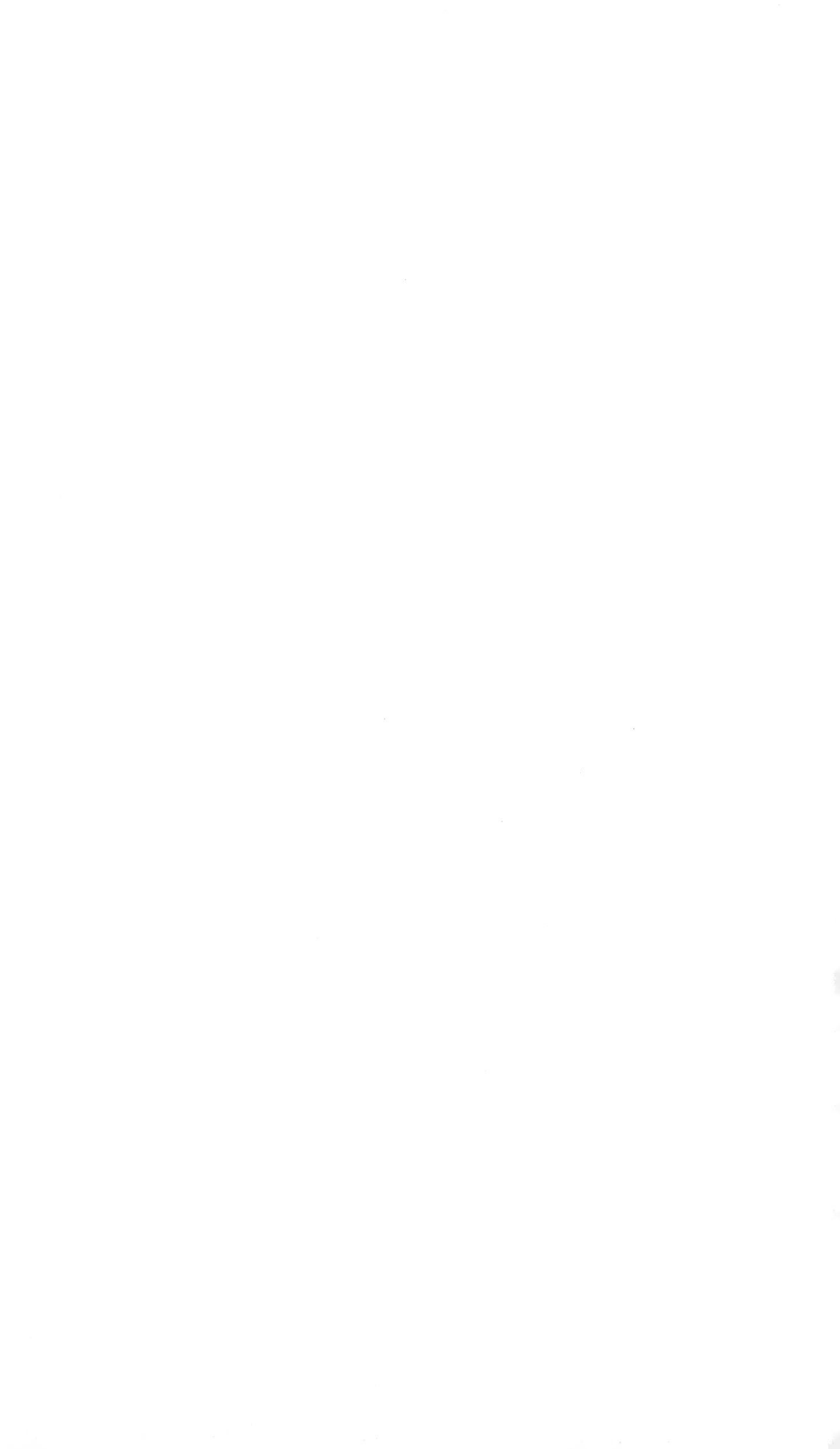

About the Author

After graduating from Middle Tennessee State University, Wendell W. Wilson attended the University of Tennessee School of Medicine, receiving his M.D. degree in 1943. He served an Internship at St. Joseph's Hospital in Memphis during that year, and was called to active duty in the Navy Medical Corp for 30 months, with the last 19 months being on sea duty. Upon release from active duty, he served a one-year General Practice/Surgery residency at St. Joseph's Hospital followed by a four-year Surgery/Family Practice Preceptorship in Memphis. In 1951 he left his practice in Memphis and settled in Old Hickory, Tennessee, where he remained until retirement in January, 1988.

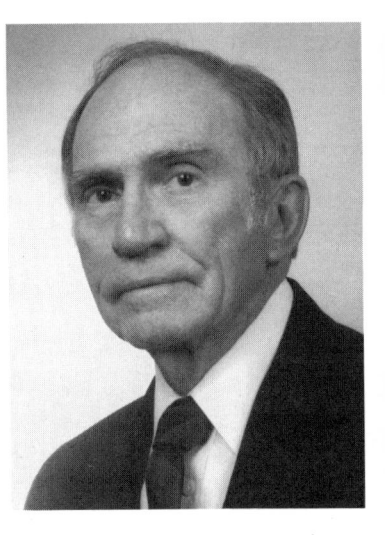

Dr. Wilson is a member of the American Medical Association, member and Fellow of the American Academy of Family Physicians, Southern Medical Association, Tennessee Medical Association, Tennessee Academy of Family Physicians and Nashville Academy of Medicine.

Dr. Wilson's long and distinguished career includes being named Tennessee Family Physician of the Year in 1976. He was President of Tennessee Academy of Family Physicians in 1964-65 and was Board Chairman of that academy in 1965-66. He served on the Board of Managers of Tennessee Christian Medical Center and was one of the Founding Fathers of Nashville Memorial Hospital where he served on the initial Board of Directors.

Since his retirement, Dr. Wilson has been active in community theater, where he serves as Chairman of the Board of Lakewood Theater Company. He is a member and an elder of Old Hickory First Presbyterian Church.